The New York Times
GUIDE TO
Alternative
HEALTH

The New York Times
GUIDE TO
Alternative
HEALTH
A CONSUMER REFERENCE

by Jane E. Brody, Denise Grady

and Reporters of *The New York Times*

Edited by Denise Grady

Times Books

Henry Holt and Company / New York

Times Books
Henry Holt and Company, LLC
Publishers since 1866
115 West 18th Street
New York, New York 10011

Henry Holt® is a registered trademark of
Henry Holt and Company, LLC.

Library of Congress Cataloging-in-Publication Data

The New York Times guide to alternative health : a consumer reference / by
Jane E. Brody, Denise Grady and reporters of the New York Times.
    p. cm.
  Includes index.
  ISBN 0-8050-6743-4 (pbk.)
  1. Alternative medicine—Popular works.   2. Consumer education.
  I. Title: Guide to alternative health.   II. Brody, Jane E.   III. Grady, Denise.
  IV. New York times.

R733 .N49 2001
615.5—dc21   2001017160

Henry Holt books are available for special
promotions and premiums. For details contact:
Director, Special Markets.

First Edition 2001

Designed by Paula Russell Szafranski

Printed in the United States of America

1   3   5   7   9   10   8   6   4   2

CONTENTS

Contents

Contents

Contents

Contents

INTRODUCTION

It may come as a shock to many practicing physicians to learn that the most popular form of medical care in America falls outside the realm of conventional medicine. It includes such practices as acupuncture, aromatherapy, massage, t'ai chi, magnet therapy, chiropractic, soy foods, herbal remedies and a long list of other so-called dietary supplements, including vitamins and "natural" hormones as well as many supplements that, though purported to be nutrients, have no established role in human nutrition.

It may also surprise some doctors to learn that many of their colleagues, along with a dozen or so of the nation's leading medical centers, are studying and using such alternative—or, as they are now often called, complementary—forms of care along with more conventional remedies and preventives. Some experts make this distinction between the two terms: they reserve "alternative" for treatments used in place of conventional medicine, and "complementary" for treatments used along with the conventional ones. Indeed, some complementary techniques, such as dietary changes and regular exercise, are now standard practice for treating such health problems as heart disease, hypertension, diabetes and osteoporosis. However, complementary medicine is now making even more extensive inroads into traditional care.

For example, Memorial Sloan-Kettering Cancer Center in New York, long regarded as a bastion of conventional therapies, now has a full department of "integrative medicine" to help patients better withstand their diagnosis of cancer and its treatment, and thereby increase both their quality of life and, possibly, their chances of survival. At ten other leading medical centers, complementary medicine is being studied and applied under grants from the National Institutes of Health, which now has a division devoted to the field thanks to funding authorized by Congress. And acupuncture, long dismissed by conventional medicine as a mystical placebo from the Orient, has become an integral part of modern medical care in treating stubborn pain syndromes. Magnet therapy, even more mysterious, has begun to make inroads in treating chronic and acute pain.

Why the sudden growth in alternatives to conventional care? After all, many of these techniques have been around for hundreds, even thousands, of years. But following the birth of scientifically based medicine they were usually spurned by those licensed to practice medicine and abandoned by patients in favor of potent prescription drugs and other remedies established as effective through well-designed scientific research.

Explanations for the public's interest in alternative methods start with the changes that have occurred in the practice of medicine in recent years. Medical care has become increasingly impersonal and fragmented. Gone is the family doctor who is both friend and physician, who has cared for several generations of family members and knows not only what may go wrong in their bodies but also what happens in their lives that can affect their physical and mental well-being. Gone, too, is the opportunity for physicians to spend thirty to sixty minutes with a patient during a routine medical visit, time that is needed to unearth reasons for health problems that do not show up in a laboratory test, time that is needed to provide assurance, comfort and caring that cannot be dispensed through a prescription pad.

Dr. David Spiegel, professor of psychiatry and behavioral medicine at Stanford University, says: "Patients want to be treated as a whole person, not just a disease. They want to be active participants in treatment, they want better communication with the practitioner and they want treatments that are not worse than their disease."

Another major reason for the attraction to alternatives is that conventional medicine does not have all the answers patients need. Half to two-thirds of patients who visit a primary care provider for a health problem are suffering mainly from the wages of psychological stress manifested as a physical complaint, like backaches, headaches, gastrointestinal disturbances, excessive fatigue and eating disorders. The prescriptions of physical remedies offered by doctors may provide temporary relief, but unless the contributing cause—the stress—is also addressed, the problem is likely to recur. Few doctors are schooled in recognizing and managing stress-related health problems, which takes more time than the typical ten-minute office visit now mandated by managed care.

Whether they acknowledge it or not, practitioners of complementary medicine often treat the mind as well as the body. Many of their techniques, like massage, aromatherapy, t'ai chi, meditation, etc., are profoundly relaxing and can help patients cope better and feel better. In addition, patients are naturally attracted to practitioners who see them as whole people, not just a diagnosis or collection of body parts. When no physical reason can be found for a symptom, the practitioner of alternative medicine does not tell the patient "There's nothing wrong with you," when clearly something is wrong, even though it may not show up on an X ray or blood test.

Finally, too many conventional physicians adopt a paternalistic approach, with the doctor as the authority and the patient as the supplicant. But patients who feel in control of their fate, who participate in decisions related to their health, become "empowered," and this power in itself can minimize their discomfort, if not speed their recovery.

The appeal of alternative medicine notwithstanding, an ill-informed foray into that world can be counterproductive and even dangerous. Not a few patients have abandoned scientifically proved treatments, say, for cancer, in favor of remedies like coffee enemas, laetrile and dietary supplements, which have no basis in science or physiology. And, of course, they all die, when at least some might have had their lives prolonged or even been cured had they stuck with established treatments.

Furthermore, the vast and still-growing array of herbal remedies and other so-called dietary supplements is totally unregulated. No government agency assures that these products are safe, effective or even contain what the labels claim. Consumers are at the mercy of manufacturers, some of whom are unscrupulous. The fox is watching the henhouse. Manufacturers are forbidden to make direct medical claims about these products, and they are also not required to list possible side effects, precautions or adverse interactions with drugs or foods.

There have been numerous instances of adverse consequences associated with herbal remedies and other dietary supplements, and the potential for disaster exists. For example, a toxicologist at the University of California, Berkeley, has pointed out that while flavonoids found in low doses in foods like soybeans may be beneficial, the very large doses contained in commercial supplements can be carcinogenic. Flavonoids at high doses can also change the activity of certain enzymes and interfere with the metabolism of estrogen and thyroid hormone. "Some Americans could be poisoning themselves with these supplements," the toxicologist, Martyn Smith, said. "The idea that natural is safe is completely wrong." After all, botulism toxin and hemlock are perfectly natural; they are also deadly. The name of the game is caveat emptor.

A responsible approach to alternative medicine requires that patients steer clear of alternative practitioners who tell them to abandon conventional care, claiming that medically prescribed remedies can "interfere" with the workings of the alternative treatment. Patients who use unconventional therapies should also be sure to tell their doctors what they are doing or taking, in case the alternative method could aggravate an underlying medical problem or interact badly with what the doctor has prescribed. Or perhaps some medical monitoring, say, of blood pressure or liver enzymes or the clotting ability of blood, is needed to assure that the alternative method is not causing harm.

At the same time, as you will see throughout this book, people may stand to gain from any number of reasonably well-studied alternative medicine techniques, among them acupuncture, massage therapy and some vitamins and herbal remedies like Saint-John's-wort. And as researchers explore others using scientific research methods, there is the promise of more effective alternative techniques to come. But remember, in most cases, the idea is to integrate these alternative methods with more traditional preventives and treatments so that you don't end up throwing the baby out with the bathwater.

—Jane E. Brody,
Personal Health columnist for the New York Times

The New York Times

GUIDE TO

Alternative
HEALTH

[1]

Patients Seek Kinder, Gentler Cures

Alternative Medicine as a Social Trend

Consider the case of a woman in her late seventies, battling colon cancer that had spread to her liver. She had a graduate-level education, as did her husband, who was a science professor at a university. And she had a will to live: children and grandchildren who loved and delighted her, endless lists of books to read and places to see with her husband. One of her children, a physician, helped her navigate the complicated paths of clinical trials and experimental chemotherapy once the standard treatments failed.

But along with the established therapies, her doctor daughter and scientist husband also encouraged her to try complementary approaches: a vegetarian diet, shark cartilage, green tea. Gamely, she took up the regimen, figuring it couldn't hurt and might help. It seemed to boost her spirits to think she was doing all she could to help herself. The cancer specialists treating her did not object.

Ultimately, she lost the fight. She survived for about two years, and until the last few months, her quality of life was decent.

Did the complementary treatments make a difference either way? There is no way of knowing; one person does not a study make. But neither she nor her family were sorry they had tried.

1

Some readers will think, good for her, she had nothing to lose. Maybe the stuff helped, maybe not, but at the least it might have given her some peace of mind. Others will think she and her family should have known better than to throw common sense out the window and waste their money on quackery in a desperate and deluded attempt to fight the inevitable.

Whatever your perspective, the fact is that millions of people are trying alternative or complementary medicine in one form or another. There is no profile of the average user: there is no average user. Consumers range from people who try a few herbs or vitamins now and then when they catch a cold to those who faithfully swallow handfuls of pills every day as insurance against old age and illness. Some make use of health food stores along with conventional medicine, but others prefer to take their chances, doctor themselves and shun the health care establishment. Many turn to alternative treatments for minor problems like small burns or cold sores that aren't worth a trip to the doctor, or when conventional treatments do not help ailments like arthritis or chronic pain. In big cities, many immigrants rely on herbal medicine, because it is what they knew in their own countries, because it is all they can afford or perhaps because they fear that the mainstream health care system will ultimately land them in legal trouble over their immigration status.

Echinacea, magnets and Saint-John's-wort may have few fans among doctors, but even some of the skeptics have begun to say alternative medicine deserves attention, if only because it has become so popular, and doctors need to know what their patients are taking, and why. Some herbal remedies can interact badly with prescription medicines and some can be toxic, but some may actually make the patient feel better.

ALTERNATIVE MEDICINE: PROMISES AND PROBLEMS

Alternative medicine is clearly the largest growth industry in health care today. In 1997, 42 percent of American adults used some type of alternative care—herbal therapy, chiropractic, acupuncture, massage therapy or any of a number of other methods not taught in medical school, according to a nationwide telephone survey conducted for

Landmark Healthcare Inc., a managed alternative care company in Sacramento, California.

Of the 1,500 adults interviewed in November 1997, 44 percent said they would use an alternative method if traditional medical care was not producing the desired results, and 71 percent predicted that consumer demand for alternative, or complementary, care would be moderate to strong in the future.

While most doctors shun such care and question its merits and reliability, Americans are voting with their feet and pocketbooks. Studies have shown that patients make more visits each year to alternative care practitioners than to primary care physicians, and most of them pay out of their own pockets for the care they receive.

Now, however, in response to the growing demand and in hopes of reducing health care costs, more and more health plans are including options for alternative methods, and a number of hospitals across the country have complementary care clinics.

Promises . . .

At a meeting on complementary medicine sponsored by the Northern California Cancer Center and held at Stanford University, Dr. David Spiegel, a professor of psychiatry and behavioral science at Stanford, said patients who availed themselves of alternative care were seeking "caring attention, something they are getting less and less of from physicians under managed care."

Alternative care practitioners, including acupuncturists, chiropractors, herbalists and massage therapists, spend more time with patients— thirty minutes on average, or four times more than physicians now devote to each patient, Dr. Spiegel said.

He said: "Patients want to be treated as a whole person, not just a disease. They want to be active participants in treatment, they want better communication with the practitioner and they want treatments that are not worse than their disease."

According to a 1993 study by the Kaiser-Permanente health care system, 56 percent of those who seek alternative care suffer chronic pain and 22 percent cite stress or a mental health problem as their chief complaint. Among the most common problems are back pain, anxiety, allergies, arthritis, depression and insomnia. Evidence is mounting that alternative techniques like acupuncture, hypnosis and some herbal remedies can help relieve such conditions.

Decades ago, physicians made an arbitrary separation between mind and body, and modern medicine is only now beginning to reintegrate them and more fully appreciate how they affect each other. Alternative care practitioners never forgot that people can get sick and can heal as much through their heads as through their bodies.

Perhaps the most powerful testament to the healing power of the mind

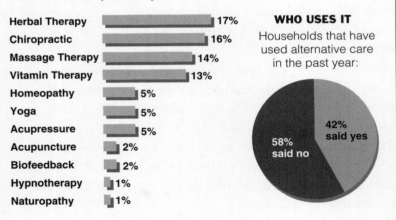

Public Perceptions Of Alternative Care

Many Americans are turning to alternative health care, from massage therapy to acupuncture to hypnosis. But many others remain cautious and skeptical of various techniques. Shown are findings of a nationwide random survey of 1,500 people, conducted by a marketing-research firm for Landmark Healthcare Inc. The margin of error is 2.5 percent. Findings were released this year.

WHERE AMERICANS TURN

Shown are the therapies that respondents have used in the previous year:

Therapy	Percent
Herbal Therapy	17%
Chiropractic	16%
Massage Therapy	14%
Vitamin Therapy	13%
Homeopathy	5%
Yoga	5%
Acupressure	5%
Acupuncture	2%
Biofeedback	2%
Hypnotherapy	1%
Naturopathy	1%

WHO USES IT

Households that have used alternative care in the past year:

42% said yes
58% said no

Source: "The Landmark Report on Public Perceptions of Alternative Care," 1998; survey conducted by InterActive Solutions of Grand Rapids, Mich.

The New York Times

is the placebo, a look-alike but inactive remedy that, on average, benefits about one-third of those who receive it when active treatments are tested in clinical trials. Dr. Spiegel asked, "Even if an alternative remedy is just a placebo, if patients get better and there are no side effects, what's the harm in trying it?" (In some cases, of course, people will recover from an illness whether they take a drug, a placebo or nothing.)

. . . and Problems

Disastrous consequences, however, can come from an uneducated and careless foray into alternative medicine. Here are some important issues to keep in mind:

- Be sure you have received a correct diagnosis from a conventional doctor before seeking alternative care. Medical literature is filled with stories of patients receiving months of useless alternative remedies as an undiagnosed cancer grew unimpeded.
- Tell your medical doctor about any alternative methods, including dietary supplements, you are using or thinking of using. Discuss the risks and benefits and possible interactions with other treatments you are receiving.
- No matter what you may be told by a friend, neighbor or alternative care practitioner, never stop an existing treatment without first consulting the doctor who prescribed it.
- Don't be fooled by the word *natural*. Natural is not synonymous with safe. Arsenic, pennyroyal, botulinum toxin and urushiol (the rash-inducing substance in poison ivy) are perfectly natural—and highly poisonous.
- Beware of phony practitioners. Everyone who hangs out a shingle is not necessarily schooled or licensed. Anyone, including you and me, can take on the title "nutritionist" or "herbologist" because there are no such professions, and anyone can

impress the uninitiated with phony credentials and certificates.

- Don't assume that products labeled "dietary supplement"—herbs, vitamins and minerals and other potions—are safe and contain what they say they do. Some are hormones, and others are stimulants or sedatives that can have serious adverse effects.

These products are virtually unregulated. No one outside the company that produces them monitors them for quality control: the types and amounts of active ingredients, presence of contaminants or honest labeling. Independent studies have shown that some of these products contain little or none of the ingredient they are supposed to have, especially if that ingredient is a costly one.

Furthermore, companies are not required to warn consumers of possible side effects or interactions. There are no guidelines for who should and should not use the product. To make matters worse, the Food and Drug Administration, which cannot require premarket clearance based on tests of safety and effectiveness for any dietary supplement, can act against a product only after a disaster.

Jane E. Brody, April 1998

LET THE SCIENTIFIC GAMES BEGIN

In the year he has suffered from osteoarthritis, Harold Katcoff has followed his doctors' advice, to no avail: aspirin, steroids, the latest anti-inflammatory drugs. The pills, he says, offer little relief from the stabbing pain in the back of his knees. So Mr. Katcoff, an eighty-year-old retired pharmacist, is trying Chinese medicine instead. Or at least, he thinks he is.

Every Tuesday and Thursday since late November 1999, Mr. Katcoff has come here, to Kernan Hospital in Baltimore, to see an acupuncturist who pokes him with twenty needles, nine in each leg and two in the belly, and then hooks the probes to a mild electrical current. The patient is convinced that the therapy works. "It's fantastic," Mr. Katcoff says. But in the same breath, he admits that he cannot be certain if the effect is real, or imagined.

That is because Mr. Katcoff may be receiving sham acupuncture—needle sticks in places where, according to the theories of traditional Chinese medicine, they should not do any good. He is a volunteer in a $2.5 million federally financed study, run by a rheumatology professor and a family-practice doctor at the University of Maryland. The study represents a new wave in academic medicine: the application of rigorous, Western scientific methods—including the gold standard of medical research, the placebo, or fake therapy, as a control—to test alternative therapies, from ginkgo biloba to shark cartilage to a mystical Chinese healing art known as qigong.

Just five years ago, many academics would not have gone near such studies, for fear they would become a laughingstock. And while alternative therapies remain hugely controversial in the staid world of science—"quackupuncture" is how one vocal critic, Dr. Victor Herbert of the Mount Sinai School of Medicine, summed up the University of Maryland's work—large, multimillion-dollar clinical trials are getting under way this year at some of the nation's most prestigious university hospitals.

"The scientific games have begun," declared Dr. David Eisenberg, director of the Center for Alternative Medicine Research and Education at Beth Israel Deaconess Medical Center in Boston. Or, as Dr. Barrie Cassileth, chief of integrative medicine at Memorial Sloan-Kettering Cancer Center in Manhattan, said: "The research is just coming into its maturity. It's bar mitzvah time."

The boom is being driven by the National Institutes of Health, which, under pressure from Congress, has sharply increased its budget for studies of alternative medicine. In 1992, much to the chagrin of the institutes' leadership, Congress required the institutes to establish an Office of Alternative Medicine, a tiny operation with a budget to match, just $2 million.

"It was," said Dr. Dan Molerman, a medical anthropologist at the University of Michigan, "like setting up an office of deviltry within the Catholic Church."

But the office is gaining acceptance at the institutes and is setting the tone for scientists around the country. In 1999, Congress upgraded the office, making it the National Center for Complementary and Alternative Medicine, which means it now has grant-making authority. Its yearly budget has grown to $68 million. In October 1999, a new director came on board, Dr. Stephen E. Straus, a virologist and longtime NIH insider whom Dr. Harold Varmus, the former director of the institutes and once one of the program's biggest detractors, describes as "a really distinguished scientist."

At the same time, hospitals and medical schools are bowing to economic reality: alternative medicine is big business. According to the *Nutrition Business Journal,* an industry trade publication, Americans spent $27.2 billion in 1998 on providers of alternative health care, including those in chiropractic, traditional Chinese medicine, homeopathy, naturopathy and massage therapy. Sales of herbs are also growing, to $4.4 billion last year, from nearly $2.5 billion in 1995, the journal said.

And a survey of more than two thousand adults, conducted by Dr. Eisenberg and published in November 1998 in the *Journal of the American Medical Association,* estimated that 46 percent of the American population had visited a practitioner of alternative health care in 1997, up from 36 percent in 1990. Patients like Mr. Katcoff, who had never before tried alternative therapies, are increasingly doing so.

"Consumers are saying, I want some type of care and I will pay for it out of pocket if I need to," said Dr. Brian Berman, the principal investigator in the Maryland acupuncture study.

But applying Western methods to Eastern traditions may be easier said than done, as Dr. Berman well knows. For one thing, how do you do placebo acupuncture? Dr. Berman and a Chinese colleague, Dr. Lixing Lao, ran several experiments just to figure out a technique that, they say, can reliably fool patients. And medical concepts do not easily translate. The diagnosis "osteoarthritis of the knee" does not exist in traditional Chinese medicine. The closest translation, Dr. Lao said, was "the knee area is energy blocked."

Cultural clashes aside, the work proceeds: a study at Duke University comparing Saint-John's-wort to the antidepressant Zoloft; a study at the

M.D. Anderson Cancer Center to test shark cartilage as a treatment for lung cancer; and at the University of Michigan, Dr. Steven F. Bolling, a heart transplant surgeon who describes himself as "the high priest of techno-medicine," is surprised to find himself examining whether practitioners of the Chinese art of qigong can help his cardiac surgery patients recover faster. One-third of the patients in the clinical trial will be visited by a qigong master, who performs slow-motion exercises that are said to release a healing energy. One-third will be visited by an impostor and one-third will not have visits.

"If it's proven, it works and it helps my patients," Dr. Bolling said, "so be it."

The trend is affecting the training of young doctors as well. Two-thirds of the nation's medical schools now have courses on alternative medicine, many of them to teach doctors how to handle questions from patients. Harvard Medical School is about to begin a fellowship program to train internists in how to conduct research on alternative therapies.

"We need a small army of clinician researchers who will do this work now," said Dr. Eisenberg, the codirector, "and for the next generation."

The story of how alternative medicine has worked its way into the mainstream of research begins not with scientists, but politicians.

In the late 1980s, Senator Tom Harkin, Democrat of Iowa, became chairman of the subcommittee that holds the purse strings to NIH. At about that time, Mr. Harkin said, a friend, Representative Berkley Bedell of Iowa, became ill with Lyme disease and prostate cancer, and resigned from Congress. "A couple of years after that, Berkley came to see me and he looked like a new man," Mr. Harkin said. "He told me about a strange cure he had taken, an alternative approach. I was just amazed."

Mr. Harkin has since become an aficionado of alternative medicine himself: he takes bee pollen for his allergies, a practice that critics find silly. But Mr. Harkin may have had the last laugh. In 1991, he inserted a provision into the NIH appropriations bill requiring the institutes to create an Office of Alternative Medicine, with a $2 million budget.

"They fought it and fought it and fought it," he said in an interview. "You'd think I was single-handedly destroying NIH by spending $2 million on alternative therapies."

The amount was indeed a drop in the bucket for the institutes, an agency that now has a $15 billion annual budget. The tiny office on alternative care was set up in a remote outpost, nowhere near the institutes' main campus in Bethesda, Maryland. Its mission was complicated. Alternative medicine is such a vast conglomeration of practices, ranging from the use of vitamins and herbs to meditation, massage, movement therapy and acupuncture, that even its practitioners cannot agree on what to call it. (The terms *complementary, integrative* and *alternative* are used interchangeably.)

The office began by offering small grants of $30,000 each. Soon, it was drawing fierce criticism for spending taxpayers' money on projects of dubious scientific merit. "The quality was incredibly low," said Dr. Varmus, who is now executive director of Memorial Sloan-Kettering. "The investigators who were applying didn't really know much about science."

In 1994, Congress took a step that would have a major effect on patients' access to alternative therapies. It passed a law that permits manufacturers to make claims about health benefits for herbal medicines whose safety and effectiveness have not been proved by the usual standards applied to prescription drugs. "Now," said Dr. Cassileth, of Memorial Sloan-Kettering, "everybody can play doctor and buy anything they want over the counter and treat themselves." Good research became even more necessary, she said.

But the battles at NIH continued. The alternative medicine office ran through a string of directors. The man who took the job in 1995, Dr. Wayne B. Jonas, drew criticism because he practiced homeopathy, a two-hundred-year-old system of medicine in which illnesses are often treated with diluted solutions of plant extracts. Most mainstream scientists, including Dr. Varmus, take a dim view of homeopathy. As a result, said Dr. Jonas, who left the institutes at the end of 1998, he had a difficult time getting approval of proposals to finance research.

But as Congress continued to appropriate more money for the office and public interest grew, Dr. Varmus said, "I came to feel that there was a real public health concern that NIH had a responsibility to address."

By 1996, the alternative medicine office had moved onto the main institutes' campus, and Dr. Varmus had formed an advisory group of government scientists to set priorities. The alternative medicine literature contains thousands of studies, but the majority are scientifically flawed. Dr. Varmus wants scientists to test the most promising and most widely used therapies.

But the critics remain. Dr. Herbert, the Mount Sinai professor, calls the center on alternative medicine "a worthless waste of money" that was "set up to promote fraud."

Dr. Marcia Angell, the editor of the *New England Journal of Medicine*, said the center had so far failed to publish any significant articles in scientific journals. "The proof is in the pudding," Dr. Angell said. "Just show me the papers."

That may take some time. It will be three to four years, Dr. Straus predicts, before the current crop of clinical trials is complete. Still, in a recent interview, Dr. Straus came armed with two loose-leaf notebooks full of articles that had grown from NIH-financed research, some published in the respected *Journal of the American Medical Association*.

He acknowledged that the center "still has to prove itself." But, he said, "I predict it will."

For the American health care system, the implications of the new research will be vast, medically and economically. Health maintenance organizations are just beginning to cover some alternative therapies; Oxford Health Plans, for instance, offers coverage for acupuncture. If therapies being tested prove effective, patients will undoubtedly begin demanding coverage.

The new research could be a boon to manufacturers of herbs. Several manufacturers of dietary supplements are beginning studies of products such as ginkgo and Saint-John's-wort that could lead to their approval by the FDA, in the same way the agency approves prescription drugs, said Michael McGuffin, president of the American Herbal Products Association, a trade group.

The University of Pittsburgh, meanwhile, is joining Chinese scientists to develop herbal medicines as drugs. In addition, Dr. Steven DeKosky, who directs the university's Alzheimer's Disease Research Center, has also received a $3 million NIH grant to see if the ginkgo herb can prevent dementia. Two thousand elderly patients will be enrolled. If it works, he

ADDING IT UP

Other Therapies

Alternative medicine has grown into a multibillion-dollar industry.

THE BOOMING INDUSTRY

1998 ALTERNATIVE MEDICINE PROVIDERS

TOTAL $27 BILLION

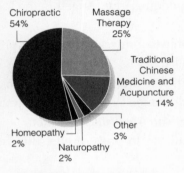

Chiropractic 54%
Massage Therapy 25%
Traditional Chinese Medicine and Acupuncture 14%
Homeopathy 2%
Naturopathy 2%
Other 3%

GOVERNMENT ALLOCATIONS

The National Center for Complementary and Alternative Medicine, part of the National Institutes of Health, has seen its budget grow substantially since it began.

FISCAL YEAR BUDGET, IN MILLIONS

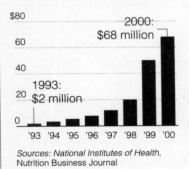

2000: $68 million

1993: $2 million

'93 '94 '95 '96 '97 '98 '99 '00

Sources: National Institutes of Health, Nutrition Business Journal

The New York Times

said, the next step will be to isolate the active ingredients and figure out how they work.

Some researchers, including Dr. Eisenberg of Harvard, say alternative therapies will not be truly accepted as mainstream until scientists can prove not just that they work, but how. But already, medical practice is opening up, said Dr. Marc C. Hochberg, the rheumatology professor at the University of Maryland who is an investigator in the acupuncture study.

In the year 2000, acupuncture was mentioned for the first time in the American College of Rheumatology's guidelines for medical management of osteoarthritis of the knee. "Our work has opened people's eyes," Hochberg said. "This used to be in the same ballpark as copper bracelets. I think we have taken acupuncture for osteoarthritis out of that realm."

Still, Dr. Hochberg said, an important question remains: Does the acupuncture really work, or is it just the placebo effect? Dr. Hochberg hopes to have an answer by 2002.

As for Mr. Katcoff, he is sold. He said he had been reading up on Chinese medicine, and had learned that even people who did not believe in it could benefit.

"I think I'm getting the real goods," he said recently. "I've been going twice a week, and this is my fifth week, and I can honestly say that the pains in the back of my legs are gone."

Sheryl Gay Stolberg, January 2000

FROM SCOTCH TO YOGURT, A WOLVERINE REPENTS

You can laugh at the array of little tinted bottles of arcane nutritional supplements that today's health devotees amass on their kitchen counters like a huddle of voodoo dolls. These worrywarts must see in these pills the magic of Lourdes.

But watch out. Should a nutriphile enter your life, these tinted attachments come, too. Such a person will be no more passive about your health than her own, and the effect may be that, having welcomed the nose into your tent, you now have the camel.

I am from Michigan. We are wolverines; we eat fiercely what we want. For me, meat, not fish; butter pecan ice cream as a vegetable; Scotch, mostly water after all, as part of the recommended six glasses a day. In my day, doctors advised that if you ate a balanced diet (i.e., different things), you needn't worry about the promotional urges of health-o-holics.

Into my life strides this person of firm body and rigid agenda, to be my girlfriend to the end of time. I am sixty. She, a decade younger, and looking a decade younger than that (a prime exemplar of her cause!), evolved in the 1960s, believing that one must take care of oneself. For the sake of togetherness, she wants me to live forever, which is a great idea, but requires more dietary dedication than I had in mind.

She launches an insidious assault on my assumed well-being. "Take a few Cs every day," it begins. "They've been proven." Bottled water because you can't trust the tap. Wash fruits. ("Don't you know what they spray?") Supper becomes kale and sardines and a little cairn of pills from the counter.

I argue that nutritional decay, if present in me, would be recognizable by now, and I am of course rebutted. It is: in creaky joints, slowed reactions, wheeziness. Her view is that "age" is a relative matter over which we have some control.

I am instructed to go without meat, sodas ("phosphates!"), sugar, alcohol—a list of everything I like. I bend only to hold her trust. I'll swallow her Cs but not buy a bottle for myself. I'll eat the salad and rush home to have a burger. I'll rinse an apple but not wash my food like a raccoon. Antioxidants? I am already rust-free. Everything of the Chinese ancients is extolled. But, I think, when they were cheerily living forever by their mysterious methods and herbs, there were available no Crunch 'n Munch or Buffalo wings.

She insists that she is just a loving woman who knows what's good for me. No absolute bans, just temperance. Like, nothing wrong with one Dewar's a month, say, or a T-bone in spring, another in autumn. But health takes no holiday. Inexorably, I lose my toehold. I recognize that in recent years my energy has flagged. I suffer malaise; concentration wanes, gums recede. I am declining before my eyes and hers, and she knows that I cannot live forever in this state of denial. And I, awakening to mortality, confronted by logic of fuel and body, am succumbing to her alluring conviction.

She persuades me to see a doctor. Not just any doctor, but her nutritional guru on Park Avenue. He puts me through every imaginable test just to confirm her diagnosis (I am older and more infirm than I need be) and affirm her program. He prescribes a start with four big bottles. I get CoQ10, L-Tyrosine, Antioxidant Formula, Siberian Ginseng.

Survival at stake, I have submitted, and there is no end to it. Everything I take into my body is now measured and inspected and fraught. My refrigerator is an earthy buffet of greens and browns—miso, tofu, oats and beans, gravelly black bread, venous garlic bulbs, ecru organic yogurt. There is flaxseed, pine-tree oil, aloe-vera gel. Everything I eat is washed to rid it of industrial goo and fingerprints.

On my counter is my own huddle of voodoo dolls, starting with As, going through Super Ginkgo Biloba, ending on Saint-John's-wort. There are new weapons every hour.

The other day, a friend treated me to a sirloin grilled over charcoal and a good glass of Johnnie Walker; I winced even as I savored. Once aware of the covenant between your corpuscles and your intake, you cannot easily sin again. I eat like a Trappist.

I am becoming secure in my conversion because, beyond the ordinary joys and trust of our partnership, I think I feel better than I otherwise would. It is impossible to be sure. When I sneak a bag of chips or a bar of Toblerone, I don't feel better. Maybe I'm just keeping a hand in, in case the currently discredited menus return to favor. Nutrition is an ever-shifting minefield. I must have the vigilance of a wolverine. Under her regime, so far we have both lived forever, you might say.

Richard Woodley, February 1998

THE MEDICAL ESTABLISHMENT SCRAMBLES
TO CATCH UP

As more and more Americans turn to herbal remedies, chiropractors and massage therapists, spending at least $27 billion a year on those and other forms of alternative health care, the medical profession is scrambling to catch up to the trend.

In November 1998, for the first time, an entire issue of the *Journal of the American Medical Association* was devoted to alternative medicine, and the association published sixty more articles on related topics in nine of its other journals.

Dr. George Lundberg, the journal's editor, decided the year before to take on the subject, in response to demand from doctors who wanted scientifically sound data on treatments and products that so many patients were asking about.

Of the seven research studies in the *Journal of the American Medical*

Association, three showed alternative treatments to be useless, but four identified treatments that seemed to work.

"In God we trust—all others must have data," Dr. Lundberg said at a news conference the association held in Washington, D.C., to present the findings. In an interview, he said the combination of positive and negative studies in the journal came about naturally, and not by the editors' design.

"That's just how it shook out," Dr. Lundberg said, adding that the editors had no stake in proving or disproving particular treatments. "We just wanted good science."

The journal's approach stands in contrast with that of the other leading journal in the United States, the *New England Journal of Medicine*, which during 1998 published a series of negative reports and editorials about various alternative treatments.

The *Journal of the American Medical Association* included a study by Dr. David Eisenberg, assistant professor of medicine at Harvard University and director of the Center for Alternative Medicine Research and Education at the Beth Israel Deaconess Medical Center in Boston. Dr. Eisenberg conducted a survey showing a sharp increase in the use of alternative medicine by Americans from 1990 to 1997.

Dr. Eisenberg's first survey on this subject was published in the *New England Journal of Medicine* in 1993. In the newer survey, Dr. Eisenberg and his colleagues define alternative medicine to include chiropractic, acupuncture, massage therapy, biofeedback, megavitamins, homeopathy, relaxation techniques, guided imagery, spiritual healing by others, self-help, commercial diets, folk remedies, hypnosis, diets like those based on vegetarianism or macrobiotics, herbal remedies and forms of "energy" healing that involve touch, magnets or other devices.

In the studies published in the *Journal of the American Medical Association*, researchers found good results using Chinese herbs for irritable bowel syndrome; saw palmetto, an herbal product, for bladder symptoms caused by prostate enlargement; yoga for the wrist problems caused by carpal tunnel syndrome, and an acupuncture-like treatment for encouraging fetuses in the breech position to turn in the womb.

The studies found no benefit in using chiropractic manipulation for tension headaches; herbal supplements containing Garcinia cambogia for weight loss, or acupuncture to control pain from nerve damage caused by HIV, the virus that causes AIDS.

In 1990, 61 million Americans were estimated to have used some form of alternative medicine. By 1997, the figure had risen to 83 million. Visits to practitioners of alternative medicine also rose sharply, to 629 million in 1997 from 427 million in 1990. Those figures stand in marked contrast with visits to establishment doctors, which dropped to 386 million in 1997 from 388 million in 1990.

Chiropractors and massage therapists accounted for half of all the visits to alternative practitioners. And the most frequent users were people age thirty-five to forty-nine with college educations and annual incomes of over $50,000. Noting that the group includes baby boomers, Dr. Eisenberg predicted that their demand for alternative treatments would increase over the next twenty to thirty years.

Yet the figures do not mean that people are abandoning traditional medicine, Dr. Eisenberg said.

"On the contrary," he said, "the overwhelming majority who are using alternative therapies are also seeing their medical doctors."

Over half the alternative remedies were used not to cure illness but to prevent it, the survey said.

One figure that worries him, Dr. Eisenberg said, is that few people tell their doctors what alternative therapies they are using, and such reticence may lead to harmful interactions with prescription drugs. Dr. Eisenberg urged doctors to ask patients in a nonjudgmental way about all remedies and treatments that they might be trying.

Another concern, he said, is that people with serious illnesses like cancer will try to take care of their own symptoms with drugstore or herbal potions, losing precious time and letting the disease advance.

In a decidedly unorthodox report, at least by Western standards, the journal reported a study of a treatment involving the burning of a cigar-shaped roll of herbs near an acupuncture point on either little toe of a pregnant woman whose fetus was in the breech position. The purpose was to stimulate the fetus to turn around for a normal, headfirst delivery. The smoldering plant, *Artemisia vulgaris*, also called mugwort, or, in

Japan, moxa, is held as close to either small toe as a woman can tolerate without her feeling pain.

The technique, moxibustion, has been used in China to turn breech fetuses "since ancient times," said the authors of the report, Dr. Francesco Cardini, a physician in private practice in Verona, Italy, and Dr. Huang Weixin, of the Jiangxi Women's Hospital in Nanchang, China.

The treatment is thought to make the fetus more active somehow, and more likely to somersault into the right position for birth.

To test the theory, Dr. Cardini and Dr. Huang studied 260 women at two hospitals in China in the thirty-third week of their first pregnancy, after ultrasound scans showed their fetuses to be in the breech position. In a woman pregnant for the first time, if a baby is breech by the thirty-third week, the odds are high that it will stay that way. Breech fetuses can be injured during birth, and in the United States they are often delivered by cesarean to avoid the risk.

In Dr. Cardini's study, women were picked at random to receive either moxibustion or no treatment. The treated women would sit or recline, and their husbands would burn the mugwort sticks near their little toes at a location called acupoint BL67, or Zhiyin, for thirty minutes at a time once or twice a day for one or two weeks.

After two weeks, 75.4 percent of the babies in the moxibustion group had turned, compared with 47.7 percent in the untreated group. Later, 75.4 percent in the moxibustion group were born headfirst, and the figure in the other group rose to 62.3 percent, but only because doctors turned some of the breech fetuses manually just before birth.

Dr. Cardini said it was impossible to tell whether the effects had come from the sensation of heat to the toes, or the fumes from the mugwort. But since moxibustion is cheap, easy and harmless, it is worth trying, he said. If it fails, Dr. Cardini said, doctors can always try to turn the baby before delivery.

Following are some alternative remedies reported to work in the medical association's journal:

- A mixture of twenty or more Chinese herbs used for irritable bowel syndrome, a hard-to-treat condition

that affects millions of people and can cause severe
abdominal pain and constipation or diarrhea.
- Yoga, for the wrist pain and other problems caused by
carpal tunnel syndrome, a disorder brought on by
typing and other repetitive motions.
- The herbal remedy saw palmetto (*Seronoa repens*) for
bladder problems caused by enlargement of the
prostate gland.

The treatments found not to work included chiropractic manipulation for tension headaches, the popular herb Garcinia cambogia for weight loss and the use of acupuncture to control pain from nerve damage caused by HIV. But researchers cautioned that these studies were the beginning of scientific investigations into alternative treatments.

"We have an obligation medically to determine whether these things are effective," said Dr. John McConnell, chairman of the department of urology at the University of Texas Southwestern medical school.

Dr. McConnell questioned some of the positive studies on saw palmetto, because it was found to work as well as a drug that itself does not work in many patients. In addition, he said, there are so many different saw palmetto formulations on the market that it is hard to know which one might work, or why.

"When patients ask me about it I tell them I think from the data that the agent is quite safe, and if they want to take it as an alternative approach that might provide some partial improvement, I don't object," Dr. McConnell said.

What worries him is that some men will unknowingly take saw palmetto for symptoms caused by tumors of the prostate or the bladder.

"We have a great fear of men going to the supermarket for two years straight and getting their saw palmetto and not realizing they have a growing cancer," he said.

Denise Grady, November 1998

VOODOO PRIESTS, BOTANICAS, HERBS
AND AMULETS

When in August of 2000 investigators shuttered a large, unlicensed medical clinic in Flushing, New York, that they said offered Chinese and Western remedies, they provided a glance behind a curtain that shrouds an expansive underground health care system serving hundreds of thousands of the city's immigrants.

While the clinic, the New York Beijing Hospital of Traditional Chinese Medicine, may have been more brazen than other centers—it advertised in a local Chinese paper and ran a Web site promising care for a variety of ills—it is only one of perhaps thousands of clinics, herbalists, spiritual centers and makeshift medical offices where many of the city's immigrants go for medical care.

Stymied by a lack of health insurance, fearful of the medical centers' potential connections to immigration authorities and longing for familiar remedies dispensed by someone who speaks their language, many of the city's immigrants have been driven to create their own complex methods of getting health care.

The landscape of their alternative medical sources is as vast and textured as the city's immigrant population, comprising herbal healers used by many people from the Caribbean and South and Central America, voodoo priests frequented by some Haitians, pharmacists who double as internists and doctors, from regions ranging from Russia to India to Poland, who lack an American license but set up shop offering some form of care to those who seek them.

"There is a whole unregulated sector of medicine at work in New York," said Dr. Francesca M. Gany, the executive director of the New York Task Force on Immigrant Health.

About 65 percent of the hundreds of immigrants in Queens who responded to a survey said they used an alternative source of care in addition to or instead of the city's larger health care system, Dr. Gany said. She added that she believed the same held true for the city's broader immigrant population.

And the treatments doled out by these centers vary: herbal remedies used to treat stomachaches and cradle cap; exorcisms for patients with chronic stomach pain; amulets attached to babies to ward off evil spirits; and antibiotics that are dubiously obtained and unwisely administered.

Most often, patients who are new immigrants mingle in two medical worlds, the city's vast array of hospitals and clinics, and a second sphere, where folk remedies are obtained. A few avoid the American medical system entirely, believing they cannot afford it or fearing the doctors, and rely totally on other healers. Others get no health care at all, relying on home remedies until they become terribly ill and end up in a hospital emergency room.

Maria Sambrano, an immigrant from Honduras, said she inhabited both worlds, depending on her needs. "I think some plants work better than medicine," said Ms. Sambrano, who was waiting to meet with a spiritualist at Botanica Santa Barbara in Washington Heights last week.

While many doctors say some folk treatments like herbs are harmless or even beneficial, health care experts are concerned that vast swaths of immigrant groups lack access to conventional health care, and that more centers like the one in Queens may be offering wholly unregulated medicine that they are ill equipped to provide.

And patients may end up paying more for some care than they could be getting at city clinics that charge on a sliding scale based on income.

"In the minds of our patients, alternative medicine is the standard of care and what we do is alternative medicine," said Dr. Guillermo Santos, the medical director of Betances Health Unit, a community health center on the Lower East Side.

"This poses two problems," Dr. Santos said. "People may have serious illnesses they may be trying to cure at home. Or they don't tell providers what they are using out of fear." The center's doctors try to stay current on the herbs that patients tend to use, and have worked with neighborhood shamans, showing them how to spot the basic symptoms of diseases like tuberculosis.

Dr. Jackson Kuan, the assistant director of gastroenterology at Flushing Hospital, said he occasionally saw patients who had misused herbs on the advice of alternative healers. He said he recently saw a Korean patient who had been given an herbal concoction that led to fatal liver failure.

And health care workers have been alarmed in recent years by the increased use of mercury among Caribbean residents, especially in the Crown Heights section of Brooklyn.

Illegal centers usually operate far below the radar screen of law enforcement, advertising mostly by word of mouth or through subtle marketing in the language of their intended customers, an increasingly diverse group.

"It is hard just to become aware of the various services that are being provided," said Wayne M. Osten, director of the State Department of Health's Office of Health System Management. Mr. Osten said the department closes twenty to twenty-five unlicensed medical centers a year. "We are looking to hire staff with those skills to better police it, because as you get more and more communities it does become a tougher problem to monitor."

Yet many healers operate legally, if on the fringes. For instance, according to Dr. Gany and other experts, some of the centers serve as entrees to the larger medical world, where new immigrants are directed to clinics and hospitals and assured that immigration officials will not be notified if the immigrants are patients.

Further, understanding how immigrants use alternative centers helps doctors better treat patients who do not share their language and culture. "I don't think these places are necessarily an impediment to care," said Dr. Mary McCord, a pediatrician in Washington Heights who had an intern conduct a study of her patients' herbal use.

"If we can get people to tell us what they are doing, we can negotiate, because people do make choices," Dr. McCord added. "They might say, 'I have asthma but I have heard bad things about those medicines so let me try honey and onions.' So maybe we can get them to use honey and onions and something else. One skill in being a doctor is to accept where people are coming from and to be willing to negotiate according to their beliefs."

The folk healers range greatly from group to group, neighborhood to neighborhood, with much overlap. Hispanics, Russians and people in the

Caribbean alike use herbal medicine, although often in different preparations. Russians, according to health care workers, lean more toward
vitamins. Shamans have different functions, sometimes performing
voodoo ceremonies for Caribbean clients, or doing what they say is healing work with their hands.

The Chinese gravitate toward herbal treatments and acupuncture, as
do some Koreans. Southeast Asians often practice yoga and use medicines from their countries.

Each nation offers its own folk remedies, herbs and medical concoc-
tions—rose water for nerves; shark oil for various flu symptoms; cordial de
monell, a sedative mixed with oil, for teething; and anise for nausea, to
name just a few. These treatments are most often purchased at botanicas,
stores that specialize in herbal medicines, oils and religious wares. At
Botanica Santa Barbara, one can find fresh rosemary, dozens of oint-
ments, creams and oils to keep away evil spirits, ignite romance or invite
prosperity.

Lisa Garcia, a card reader, helps customers with personal problems
and says she removes pain with her hands.

"Sometimes people go to the doctor and when it doesn't work, come
here," said Antonio Mora, the store's owner.

But while many immigrants prefer many folk or home remedies to
conventional medicine, far too many are shut out of the health care system because they lack insurance or are unaware of what is available to
them cheaply, experts said. About 40 percent of legal immigrants are
uninsured, said David Sandman, a program officer at the Common-
wealth Fund, a private philanthropic organization in New York. Among
illegal immigrants, the number is far higher, he said.

And then there is the intense distrust many immigrants feel toward the
medical establishment. Dr. McCord said that many of her Dominican
patients had negative notions about asthma medicine. Dr. Santos said
many Jamaican patients shunned hypertension medicine, preferring
herbs. And some Asians are afraid to have blood drawn because they
think it will only weaken them, said Dinah Surh, the administrator of
Sunset Park Family Health Center in Brooklyn.

Her center, with its diverse staff, has gone to great pains to attract many immigrant groups. It set up a mosque for Muslim patients to pray in. It offers acupuncture—now used by patients around the world—as one way of attracting Chinese patients.

The center went for other touches, Ms. Surh said. "We wanted to have a fish tank. Some Chinese groups said we need gold-colored fish for good luck, so we added those. But the tank is right below a skylight, and they told us the good luck would go out of the skylight. So we put a shade there."

Many doctors said that thousands of years of herbal medicine are nothing to sneeze at, and pointed to a highly increased interest among American patients in Eastern techniques like yoga and acupuncture. Indeed many large hospitals have adopted these types of practices in recent years.

And conventional doctors have a few tips to learn from folk and traditional healers, some experts concurred, like advertising in various languages and getting the word out through community groups. But still, many, many immigrants will always rely on a mix of services.

"I use conventional medicine," said Ray Gongora, who immigrated from Cuba in the 1960s and often turns to herbs. "But emotionally I don't get what I need. They give you a blood test and send you on your way, but if you're not prepared mentally, you get depressed."

Jennifer Steinhauer, August 2000

HOSPITALS DISCOVER THEIR INNER SPA

A smiling concierge in the lobby directed Debra Paget toward the eighth-floor lounge, a sumptuous room, where she plunged into a cushy banquette. Sitting with a friend amid fountains, pink orchids and filigreed screens, she might have been at the Four Seasons Hotel, waiting for a waiter to bring her a cocktail. In fact, Ms. Paget was waiting to see her gynecologist, whose office was tucked at the rear of the lounge behind a high ash-panel wall.

This was the reception room at the Laurance S. Rockefeller Pavilion, a satellite clinic built last year by Memorial Sloan-Kettering Cancer

Center. The pavilion offers diagnosis and treatment for cancer in a setting that is part luxury hotel, part Zenlike retreat. And for Ms. Paget it represents a marked improvement over Sloan-Kettering's main hospital cluster half a mile uptown, where she was treated last year for ovarian cancer.

Sloan-Kettering, with its narrow corridors and shabby furniture, was "like a bad scene from a 1950s movie," she recalled with a shudder. Each time she visited, her blood pressure spiked. Now, when she arrives at the pavilion waiting room for her quarterly posttreatment checkup, the roar in her head has subsided to a hum.

Of course, a fancy waiting room, even one with haiku engraved on the walls, does not quite alleviate the stress of being treated for cancer.

"You know what you're here for, and no amount of design will ever get your mind past that," said Ms. Paget, forty-five, a program manager for IBM.

Even so, more and more medical centers are keeping step with the Rockefeller Pavilion, revamping their decor and introducing luxury services to bolster the spirits of patients and give them a sense of well-being. In recent years, doctors and hospitals have integrated alternative and Eastern-influenced treatments with conventional Western medicine. Now, they are extending that holistic approach to the look and feel of the clinical environment.

Think of it as the aesthetic equivalent of acupuncture. In the New York City area, health care institutions and a spate of wellness centers are wooing patients with amenities like on-the-site hair salons, Zen tearooms and lavish kimonos, which make chilly clinics and consulting rooms seem as dated as high-button shoes. Efforts to warm the atmosphere vary from place to place. But at wellness resorts and even in traditional hospitals, patients find the mellow lighting, waterfalls, vanilla-scented candles and sea grass common at a New Age spa.

Even uniforms have been made over with cheery patterns and bright colors, reinforcing the impression that the hospital staff is as friendly and accessible as, say, one's favorite hairdresser.

To hear it from some physicians, medicine's new emphasis on style is long overdue. Among the leading proponents of soul-soothing decor is

Mehmet Oz, a cardiothoracic surgeon and an outspoken champion of healing through design.

"There is no question that in the past we have undervalued the aesthetics of care," said Dr. Oz, whose office at New York Presbyterian Hospital is furnished with Oriental carpets and wood paneling. "I wanted my patients to feel they were in my house," Dr. Oz said. "If I could put a fire in the corner, I would." New Age chimes tinkle on the sound system, and the scent of coconut wafts from the corridors into the consulting room, where patients can gaze out at the Hudson River.

The Integrative Health Center at the Rockefeller Pavilion is similarly airy, offering acupuncture and massage as well as chemotherapy in a room painted with blue skies and scudding clouds. Other clinics have an earthier feel. Natural materials like slate and silvered wood cover almost every surface at the SoHo Integrative Health Center on Crosby Street in Manhattan, which opened this month. Run by Dr. Laurie Polis, a dermatolgist, the center is filled with the reassuring sights, sounds and scents of nature.

"I wanted to dispel anxieties that rise from memories of walking down a sterile hallway, a nurse in white shoes coming at you with a syringe," Dr. Polis said.

Determined to create an anticlinical environment, she commissioned Clodagh, an architectural designer known for her woodsy spa interiors and stores, to create a setting that evokes a Zen garden and a rain forest. Its focal point is a twenty-seven-foot wall of water that plunges from the upper floors to the lobby.

Patients awaiting the removal of skin lesions or a consultation with the house internist or ophthalmologist can steady their nerves with a facial, a seaweed wrap or a visit to Steven Dillon, the center's own hair guru. Cocooned in sand-color terry-lined robes, the patients, who are called "clients," sit in the waiting area sipping iced green tea and inhaling the house fragrance, a blend of ginger and passion flowers.

A similar hush pervades the Continuum Center for Health and Healing, an outpatient clinic of the Beth Israel Medical Center in New York. Opened in June 2000 at Fifth Avenue and Twenty-eighth Street, the center offers traditional Western medical treatments alongside Eastern therapies in an environment that looks like a Hong Kong hotel.

Tibetan carpets, rough-hewn wooden benches and a weeping fig tree, among other features, were installed at the suggestion of Alex Stark, a New York feng shui specialist. Chinese cabinets, fountains and a limestone corridor make the reception area feel like a sanctuary, compelling visitors to lower their voices.

Across the Hudson, at Hackensack University Medical Center, Suzen Heeley, the hospital's designer, was so infatuated with the spa concept that she installed a health resort on the premises. Hackensack's Beyond day spa, which she says is the first spa inside a hospital, opened in June. It borrows liberally from the Asian design themes and the treatment menus of upscale health resorts like the Peninsula and Bliss in Manhattan. As its news release perhaps too chipperly announces, "Here is a place where women can schedule a morning massage and manicure, and an afternoon mammography."

She can also retreat to the Shangri-la–style meditation room to sip rosebud tea through a silver straw and sample a sugar bath with litchi, one of the bath products offered by brands like Fresh, Lazar tigue and Creed.

Some of the services are extended to patients in the adjacent hospital building. Those who cannot get to the Beyond Day Spa can enjoy a bedside facial while watching seascapes and sailboats on television sets tuned to the Relaxation Channel.

Medical chic has found its way around the country, too. At Northwestern Memorial Hospital in Chicago, picture windows with lakefront views are among the luxurious features that were built into each room when the hospital was redesigned last year. Other comforts include corner shelves to hold cards and flowers, carpeted corridors, $30,000 patient beds that convert to easy chairs, and plush window seats that fold out for family members who stay the night. The hospital says the cost of such features, which are partly paid for by benefactors, will not be passed on to patients.

When Northwestern's Women's Hospital, part of a $580 million hospital development project, opens in 2004, painted landscapes will decorate the ceilings in patient rooms. "Research has shown that patients who look at boats and beaches in pre-op do much better in surgery," said Alice Domar, director of the Center for Women's Health at the Mind Body Medical Institute of Harvard University. Dr. Domar consulted with architects on the hospital's design. "Women especially are conscious of aesthetics," she said. "If the room looks good, it makes them feel more confident in the hospital."

It also makes them feel at home. Hoping to create an aura of cozy domesticity, designers at Roosevelt St. Luke's Hospital on New York's West Side decorated the labor rooms in the childbirth center in festive chintz. The flower-pattern curtains and bedspreads, winged chairs and rockers look better suited to a bed-and-breakfast in the Cotswolds than to a delivery room.

In lieu of hospital gowns, St. Luke's maternity patients are encouraged to wear their own nightclothes. At most hospitals and clinics patients must still wear shapeless gowns in dispiriting shades of teal and gray.

Hackensack hospital has commissioned Nicole Miller, a designer known for animated prints, to give the classic gown a makeover. Ms. Miller's breezy trousers, shorts and kimonos are patterned with needles and stethoscopes. Not exactly calming but more uplifting than standard-issue hospital blue.

By far the most animated looks in hospital halls are uniforms, which are turning up in a giddy explosion of colors. "Five years ago, my sales reps around the country were only selling teal blue and misty green," said Alan Kay, the president of Howard Uniforms, a distributor of hospital scrubs. "Now, there are twenty or twenty-five colors, and there must be a hundred prints."

Hot orchid and flamingo pink have lately turned up as alternatives to washed-out pastels, which were originally designed to help patients distinguish nurses from X-ray technicians. Companies with names like Feel Good Scrubs Wear and Crazy Scrubs show products on the Web, selling colorful uniforms and manic prints, including tie-dye designs and Hawaiian florals.

"These things are done mostly for the patient," Mr. Kay said. "Bright uniforms cheer them up and make them feel more comfortable."

The health care industry's new emphasis on more stylish settings also has a profit motive. To lure and keep clients who might otherwise have defected to one of Manhattan's tonier wellness centers, Jack Ferguson, the president of Hackensack University hospital, keeps one eye fixed on image, the other on the bottom line.

"We want to do everything with style and class, from installing mahogany paneling in the hospital's main lobby to providing high-quality products at the spa," he said.

He expects his efforts to pay off and thinks the spa will clear $50,000 in its first year. The funds are funneled back to the hospital to pay for new facilities, Mr. Ferguson said.

Clients at Hackensack and elsewhere around the country readily pay for small luxuries like a reiki massage ($45) at the Rockefeller Pavilion or a warm cream pedicure at the Beyond Day Spa in Hackensack ($35), where the price of a single room is $1,600 a day.

Marie Tortoriello, who spent a week with her husband, William, at Northwestern Memorial Hospital, where he had surgery, seemed enchanted with their $950-a-night room. "We felt like we were in a hotel," she said. Among the features that impressed her were deep picture windows and a wing chair with an ottoman. "It was as though they were part of a Victorian parlor," she said. "It wasn't the hospital look at all, and that makes such a difference."

Ruth La Ferla, August 2000

ACUPUNCTURE FOR FIDO

The stagger in his gait and pleading in his eyes said it all. Al had taken everything that a greyhound could be expected to, and then he had taken even more.

Once he had been a racer, sleek and fleet. Then came abandonment on the beaches of Brooklyn. Mercy arrived in the form of a new owner and a home in the New Jersey suburbs, but at age eight, Al's back gave out. Two painful surgeries and more than $6,000 later, he still wasn't the dog he used to be.

His journey into Manhattan on a Saturday morning was a pilgrimage of stubborn hope. There, in a backyard in Murray Hill, Al dipped into his own Lourdes, a circular pool of heated water that might do what the operations, acupuncture and Bach flower essences had not: heal him. With Jodi Richard, a trained canine hydrotherapist, holding tight to his rump, Al paddled and paddled, going nowhere fast, his gimpy back legs freed from gravity so they could get the exercise they sorely needed.

His owner, Jackie Wright-Minogue, rushed to him as soon as he left the pool to rest under a pink towel on the cushion of a lawn chair. "I want him to get well," she said, articulating the simple wish that had wrought such complicated ministrations. "I want him to have a good life."

That desire, seemingly boundless among many pet owners, has ushered in a whole new era in animal care. Ms. Richard's business, Bonnie's K 9 Swim Therapy Center, named for her German shepherd, is but one example. Elsewhere around the New York region, veterinarians are hooking dogs and cats to electric acupuncture machines, dosing them with homeopathic remedies, placing putatively therapeutic magnets beneath their beds, even spraying the air around them with lavender, lemon or eucalyptus in the name of aromatherapy.

All this is perhaps the inevitable outgrowth of a culture blissed out on Saint-John's-wort and mesmerized by Andrew Weil. It is also the ultimate illustration of the degree to which many Americans insist on sharing their own habits and extravagances, from summer camp to spa treatments, with the four-legged members of their families.

Dr. Gerald M. Buchoff, a veterinarian in North Bergen, New Jersey, has performed acupuncture on iguanas with brittle bones. Dr. Marcie Fallek, who has offices in Greenwich Village and Fairfield, Connecticut, has administered homeopathic treatments—solutions with minuscule traces of special plant or mineral ingredients—to a pet raccoon that was seemingly depressed over a canine companion's death and had stopped using its litter box.

The raccoon's owner, fearful that law enforcement authorities would learn that she was keeping a wild animal, declined to be interviewed for this article, even anonymously, Dr. Fallek said. "Her psychic told her there might be trouble," Dr. Fallek explained. "Plus, Mercury's in retrograde and, well, you know."

Which raises the obvious question: How much of this is pure quackery? As it turns out, less than one might think.

Dr. Richard Swanson, president of the American Veterinary Medical Association, said that the legitimacy of acupuncture, at least on mammals with skeletal structures similar to people's, was beyond doubt, and that hydrotherapy and chiropractic were probably effective.

But Dr. Swanson cast a more skeptical eye on homeopathy, Bach flower essences and the like. "That's really getting on the fringe," he said, adding that a lack of rigorous scientific study into such treatments undercut the sunny testimonials of some veterinarians and their clients. "The world is made up of a lot of very vulnerable and gullible people," he cautioned.

The newfangled treatments that come under the rubric of alternative or holistic veterinary medicine certainly are not cheap. In New York City—where, granted, prices for most things tend to be highest—half an hour of acupuncture generally costs $50 to $75; an hour's worth of immersion in Ms. Richard's healing waters costs $75. Because treatments are usually repeated over the course of several weeks, the final bill can run into the high hundreds.

The American Holistic Veterinary Medical Association, which was founded in 1982, reports a membership of 1,000 veterinarians. The International Veterinary Acupuncture Society, founded in 1974, reports 1,500 members, up from 500 five years ago, though that is still a small fraction of all veterinarians.

Donna Watkins, a spokeswoman for the society, said veterinary acupuncture has been around long enough that it is now being ventured on a wide variety of animals in addition to horses, cats, dogs and parrots.

"A friend of mine in California regularly does turtles—well, not the shell," she said. "I know a guy in San Diego who is doing a dolphin."

Although pets being given alternative treatments are often following their owners' leads, the inspiration sometimes works the other way.

"I started going to an acupuncturist for stress because I saw how well it worked for Lola," Liz Santander, an interior designer from Chappaqua, New York, said of her 150-pound Great Dane as the dog awaited her latest treatment the other morning in the offices of Dr. Phillip

Raclyn on the Upper West Side. It was a busy, busy day. While Lola, who was bouncing back from a stroke, cooled her paws in the lobby, Ike, a partially lame shepherd mix, received massage therapy in an examining room.

Meanwhile, in the examining room next door, Dr. Raclyn inserted an acupuncture needle into the forehead of Spike, a female cat with kidney problems. For a few seconds, Spike looked like a unicorn; then another dozen needles went in, and she looked like a pin cushion. Relaxed rather than bothered, she nearly fell asleep.

Frank Bruni, August 1998

[2]

Offerings Many, Rules Few

*The Booming Alternative Industry and Its
Frustrated Regulators*

Without a doubt, the greatest boon ever to the makers of vitamins, miner-als, herbal products and other so-called natural remedies was the Dietary Supplement Health and Education Act, passed by the 103rd Congress in 1994. Basically, DSHEA treats those products as if they are foods rather than drugs, meaning that manufacturers, unlike drug makers, do not have to prove safety or effectiveness and that the products do not have to be approved by the Food and Drug Administration. Normally, the studies and testing in humans required to get a drug through the FDA approval process cost several hundred million dollars; DSHEA allows supplement makers to circumvent that process, and the supplement industry has grown consider-ably since the act was passed, by about 20 percent a year to its current level of about $14 billion a year.

Supporters of DSHEA say it gave the public freedom to choose among all sorts of herbal and nutritional products that had not been widely avail-able before. Marketers of those products argued that they included many folk remedies that had stood the test of time and did not need extensive testing; in addition, many supplement makers say they cannot afford the full-blown approval process, especially since products like herbs and vita-mins are not patentable, making it difficult or virtually impossible for them to recover the costs of testing.

But DSHEA has significant drawbacks. The failure to require proof of safety and effectiveness means an unscrupulous company could get a dan-gerous or useless product onto the market, and nothing would be done about it until after someone got hurt or the product was proved to be inef-fective. By that time, many people would have taken it, wasting countless amounts of money, risking injury and possibly missing out on legitimate treatments. The lack of regulation also means there are no outside stan-dards for quality control imposed on the supplement industry. Products may not contain the dose printed on the label; indeed, testing has found that some supplements do not contain any of the stated ingredient at all.

DSHEA also created a whole new world of labeling that borders on the absurd. Because supplements are not drugs, their makers cannot make druglike claims for them: that is, they cannot say that the products will pre-vent, treat or cure diseases. What they can make are vague, odd-sounding statements of "nutritional support" and claims about the products' effects on the "structure and function" of the body. Here, for example, is a structure-function claim from a bottle of vitamin E capsules: "contributes to a healthy heart and enhances the immune system." But a claim to prevent heart disease or infections would not be allowed. Saint-John's-wort labels can say the herb promotes emotional well-being but not that it can treat depression. Labels for other products that cite studies showing specific effects, like lowering cholesterol, bear this disclaimer: "This statement has not been evaluated by the Food and Drug Administration."

Critics of the law say it has given consumers access to products—but prevented them from finding out what the products are for.

Some researchers have suggested that a separate approval process and special criteria be established for herbal products and other supplements, taking into account that many of the products have been around for a long time and showed no evidence of harm. Relaxed rules would allow strong proof of safety and "reasonable" proof of efficacy, which could be accom-plished for a few million dollars rather than hundreds of millions. But such a change could be accomplished only by an act of Congress.

In the meantime, in some cases where the FDA is essentially hamstrung, the Federal Trade Commission has stepped in and taken action against companies making outrageous claims for their products. The FTC requires that advertising not be misleading or deceptive, and can bring injunctions against companies making unsubstantiated claims, and in some cases confiscate ill-gotten profits.

REAL MEDICINE, OR MEDICINE SHOW?

The makers of herbal supplements are in the business of selling stamina and serenity in a bottle. But as the public's appetite for such products as Saint-John's-wort and echinacea has grown stronger, the business itself has become anything but serene.

Once largely the province of obscure manufacturers with limited distribution, the pills and powders that supposedly sharpen the mind and lift the spirit are no longer consigned to a spot next to the bee pollen at the local health food store. Now they carry trusted brand names and command premium shelf space in supermarkets, drugstores and mass retail chains throughout the country.

With billions of dollars in sales up for grabs, the battle for market share has become intense, pitting large drug companies and consumer products makers against one another in a race to put their brands on formulas that they say promote everything from mental focus to a healthy prostate.

At the same time, questions about the value of all those pills and powders have become more pointed, courtesy not only of government regulators and consumer advocates but also of drug companies that have opted to stay on the herbal sidelines.

The big new makers and retailers of the supplements argue that they are simply providing natural solutions for good health in an age of self-medication—and that they are drawing criticism in part because their products are seen as cut-rate competition for high-profit pharmaceuticals.

Products like Saint-John's-wort, whose fans see it as an alternative to Prozac, and echinacea, which is promoted as effective in bolstering the immune system, are plant-based substances whose properties can help to alleviate everyday ailments, their manufacturers say. They are also quick to note that the substances have been used for centuries in Asia and Europe and are increasingly being accepted as an adjunct to Western medicine.

But industry critics say the manufacturers' motivations are anything but wholesome. The critics say that manufacturers, like clothing designers who slap their labels on jeans, are simply seeking to cash in on the latest fad that has turned mainstream. The difference, they add, is that putting respected names on herbal pick-me-ups lends undeserved credibility to a loosely regulated industry of products with often questionable safety and efficacy.

Whatever the motivation, the competition to establish leading brands is intensifying. Celestial Seasonings Inc., known for its teas, is counting on its earthy image to sell a line of herbal supplements. The products include a formula containing Saint-John's-wort called Mood Mender, which the company says is useful for a positive outlook.

The American Home Products Corporation, which makes Centrum vitamins, is seeking to capitalize on that brand by extending it to herbal remedies. The Bayer Corporation, maker of One-A-Day vitamins and minerals, has entered the market with a line of products that combine vitamins and herbs. They include formulas for "a healthy emotional balance" which contain Saint-John's-wort and a second supposedly mood-enhancing ingredient, kava, and another containing ginkgo biloba, an herbal substance that "helps support memory and concentration."

Even Wal-Mart has gotten into the act with private-label supplements sold under the name Spring Valley.

What has all these companies suddenly hopping on the herbal bandwagon is greater consumer demand, particularly among aging baby boomers, for products that offer the hope of staying youthful. A frustration with traditional health care is also a factor.

"What we are trying to do is respond to what the customer is asking us for," said Paul Beahm, a divisional merchandising manager at Wal-Mart. "More and more, the public is focused on prevention and health care needs, and the vitamin and nutritional supplement category is one they've been asking for."

Moreover, a law that watered down the Food and Drug Administration's regulatory authority over dietary supplements, including herbal products, has made the industry much more palatable to retailers and marketers.

As a result of all this, retail sales of the supplements have increased sharply, growing by 18 percent in 1997, to $3.6 billion, and 75 percent in all since the regulatory changes were adopted in 1994, according to the *Nutrition Business Journal*, a trade publication.

"The increase in consumer confidence in these products is indicative of the overall explosive growth in this category," said Steve Hughes, president and chief executive of Celestial Seasonings. "As the major brands and more established companies come into this category, it's going to segment the category into premium brand and the others, and every major mass retailer and drug retailer is looking at private label."

But not everyone sees the trend as a healthy one for consumers.

"It's important to understand that this is not about health and this is not about well-being; this is about money and jumping on a bandwagon," said David A. Kessler, a former head of the FDA who is now dean of Yale University's medical school. Dr. Kessler waged a vigorous but unsuccessful battle against the law that virtually stripped his former agency of its authority to regulate herbal and other dietary supplements.

For healthy people, most of the products pose little or no risk, and some, containing garlic and ginseng, may even be helpful, Dr. Kessler said. The danger, he said, is that some people with potentially life-threatening illnesses will use the products in place of standard medical treatments. That has always been a risk, but the marketing giants now pushing into the industry can pitch these formulas to more consumers, he said.

"The way they are positioned in the marketplace can lead people down roads to ineffective treatments," Dr. Kessler said, pointing to products whose names, he argued, could cause consumers to think they could be used instead of prescription drugs. "If you promote a product as Mood Mender, you have a responsibility to that person who is depressed, and if that product doesn't work you are doing harm.

"People with specific illnesses look at these products a different way than the healthy person," he added, "and it is through their eyes that the marketplace must be judged."

In some cases, critics say, the supplements can be quite dangerous indeed. The FDA, for example, is attempting to rein in the use of the herbal stimulant ephedra, which is sold by various companies under different names. The formula, which manufacturers say is safe, has been linked to more than a dozen deaths nationwide. Marketers promise that the pills provide an amphetamine-like rush, aid in weight loss and even increase sexual sensation, but medical experts say they can cause heart attacks, strokes and seizures.

The big-name herbal pill dispensers now entering the market say they are sticking to more "mainstream" substances and argue that those formulas are safe and effective when taken by healthy people in recommended doses. Besides, they say, unlike the little-known manufacturers that once dominated the industry, they have the research and development budgets and purchasing power to ensure product quality.

"We spend tens of millions of dollars putting together manufacturing and quality control processes," said Elliot Friedman, chairman and chief executive of Pharmaprint Inc., which produces supplements that American Home Products markets under the Centrum name. "The big companies are very protective of their brands."

That may be, but the critics say consumers have a false sense of security about the regulatory oversight of supplements. They mistakenly assume, the critics contend, that the supplements are subject to the same scrutiny as toothpaste, cough drops and other seemingly benign products under the FDA's watch. The agency requires those goods to carry general cautionary labeling and dosage information and it imposes limits on the claims that can be made in marketing.

Herbal supplements, however, are regulated by a looser set of standards. Before the passage in 1994 of the Dietary

Feeling Good

Herbal remedies are gaining in sales and acceptance, and Saint-John's-wort is soaring.

Top herbal remedy sales in the U.S., in millions of dollars; percentage change from 1995 to 1997

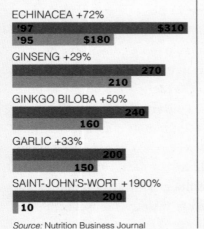

ECHINACEA +72%
'97 $310
'95 $180

GINSENG +29%
270
210

GINKGO BILOBA +50%
240
160

GARLIC +33%
200
150

SAINT-JOHN'S-WORT +1900%
200
10

Source: Nutrition Business Journal

Supplement Health and Education Act, manufacturers were prohibited, for instance, from making claims about the potential benefits of their products. But the revised guidelines allow companies to advertise the health effects of herbal supplements—without having to conclusively prove their effectiveness—so long as the wording does not suggest that the products prevent, treat or cure disease.

That gives companies much greater range in making product claims than manufacturers of, say, mouthwash. While a company cannot claim an herbal supplement cures cancer or relieves depression, for example, it can say that it "promotes prostate health" or "aids in mental focus."

Critics also worry that pharmaceutical companies will attempt to classify some products as herbal supplements instead of as drugs to skirt the rigorous process required to bring a drug to market.

Meanwhile, as other drug makers begin producing herbal pills, the FDA is struggling to find a way to exercise its limited oversight authority.

American Home Products declined to provide an executive to discuss its supplements business beyond issuing a statement through a public relations representative saying that "herbals represent a large and growing market with increasing consumer acceptance."

"Consumers are looking for a name they trust and, to be honest, that's why we went with Centrum," Mr. Friedman said. "Pharmacists know it, doctors know it, and consumers know it. That is the edge in bringing these new people into the fold."

Dana Canedy, July 1998

RED YEAST RICE REDUX

In a factory in Farmington, Utah, a region that is the heart of the nation's herbal and vitamin industry, a stainless-steel contraption was hard at work, spitting out clear plastic capsules at the rate of ninety thousand an hour. Each contained precisely 600 milligrams of a fine, brick-colored powder that federal health officials were trying to ban.

The powder, a pulverized strain of rice fermented with red yeast, is imported from China, where it has been consumed for two thousand years, as an herbal remedy (it is thought to improve blood flow) and a food (it spices up tofu and makes a tasty marinade for duck and pork). Then in 1993, William McGlashan Jr., a young California venture capitalist, learned that scientists in Beijing were studying red yeast rice for another reason: it seemed to lower cholesterol.

From 1996 through the first half of 1998, Pharmanex, Mr. McGlashan's company, was selling the encapsulated red powder under the trade name Cholestin in thirty-seven thousand American stores, from health food outlets to the giant Wal-Mart chain. Mr. McGlashan called Cholestin a dietary supplement. Officials at the Food and Drug Administration called it something else: an illegal, unapproved drug.

On June 15, 1998, in the gray-stone federal courthouse in Salt Lake City, United States District Judge Dale A. Kimball was asked to determine who was correct. The case was watched as a pivotal battle between the agency, chafing at a 1994 law that left it almost powerless to regulate vitamins and herbal products, and the dietary supplement industry, which had grown wildly since the law was passed.

At issue was not whether Cholestin was dangerous; no one argued that it was. Rather, the agency contended that Cholestin had crossed the increasingly murky boundary that separates dietary supplements from drugs, because it contains an ingredient, lovastatin, that is the key component of a cholesterol-lowering drug. Pharmanex said lovastatin occurred naturally in the rice and that Cholestin was more akin to a food than to a drug.

Aside from the turf battle between the supplement industry and regulators, the dispute raised crucial questions: Is there a distinction between these herbal products, which may contain naturally occurring chemicals as potent as those in any drug, and the drugs themselves? Must products like Cholestin be subjected to the rigorous testing that drugs undergo?

"You see more and more dietary supplements sold right next to over-the-counter drugs," said William B. Schultz, the FDA's deputy commissioner for policy. "There is a risk that the line will blur."

Indeed, it is already blurry. "Foods are medicines; medicines are foods," said Loren Israelson, executive director of the Utah Natural Products

Alliance, a trade group based in Salt Lake City that represents ten of the nation's biggest supplement manufacturers. "If you drink coffee in the morning, why are you drinking coffee? You're looking for the caffeine, a stimulant. That same caffeine is sold over the counter as No Doz. That's a drug when it's in a pill form, and it's a food when it's in coffee. Why is that?"

The Food and Drug Administration struggled with such questions for decades. But with the passage of the 1994 Dietary Supplement Health and Education Act, the law under which the Cholestin case was to be decided, the agency's task grew even more vexing.

The new law moved dietary supplements out of the underground and into the mainstream, giving manufacturers like Pharmanex the long-sought right to advertise the potential benefits of herbs, even if the evidence for those benefits was sketchy. Unless the FDA can prove the product is unsafe, companies can say what they wish, so long as they do not claim their products can prevent, treat or cure disease. Thus, Mr. McGlashan could advertise that Cholestin "promotes healthy cholesterol," but not that it "prevents heart attack or stroke."

"For the first time," he said, "we can educate the American consumer about what the product does. We don't have to rely on a person in a health food store to explain it."

By 1998, the agency had received about 2,300 notifications from manufacturers intending to make claims about their products, and had objected to about 150 of them. It had also proposed a rule that would restrict, but not eliminate, the manufacturers' ability to use the herbal stimulant ephedra, which had been linked to more than a dozen deaths nationwide. It had banned one ephedra-based product and it was now trying to ban Cholestin.

Agency officials said the 1994 law, restrictive though it is, gives them the authority to take Cholestin off the market because it bars companies from bringing dietary supplements to market if they contain the same active ingredients as previously approved drugs. In passing the Dietary Supplement Health and Education Act, Mr. Schultz says, Congress did not intend for companies to skirt the drug-approval process by selling medicines under the guise of dietary supplements.

Lawyers for Pharmanex, however, contended that Cholestin fell squarely within the intent of the 1994 law.

"This product was specifically developed to be a dietary supplement," said Daniel Kracov, a company lawyer. "What the FDA objects to is the fact that this product has a drug substance in it, in their view. You may object to that, but our response is: If you don't have a safety issue, don't go after these products."

Whatever the outcome, Dr. David A. Kessler, the former Commissioner of Food and Drugs, said the agency's action would hardly make a dent in the rampant proliferation of herbal remedies that he says are ineffective at best and unsafe at worst.

"Just walk into your pharmacy; it's out of control," said Dr. Kessler, who waged a bitter, unsuccessful battle against the 1994 law as commissioner. "Efficacy is now defined as what sells off the shelves. The agency is powerless."

While the law was a disaster for regulators, it was a windfall for makers of dietary supplements and vitamins. After the act was adopted, annual sales of dietary supplements in the United States skyrocketed, jumping to nearly $12 billion in 1997 from more than $8 billion in 1994, according to the *Nutrition Business Journal*, a trade publication.

The furious growth led some of the biggest pharmaceutical companies to begin developing their own herbal products. That worried Mr. Schultz, the FDA deputy commissioner for policy. "If companies that would have tested their products and sold them as drugs are now going to not test them and sell them as dietary supplements," he said, "then we have lost information about the safety and efficacy of those products."

Among the law's beneficiaries was Mr. McGlashan, a thirty-four-year-old Stanford University business school graduate who studied Chinese history. With the aging of baby boomers, Mr. McGlashan saw a growing demand for natural medicines the Chinese have used for centuries.

Mr. McGlashan says he had a vision for his business; he wanted to apply "pharmaceutical rigors" to the dietary supplement industry, using research to persuade consumers that Eastern therapies worked. In early 1994, he met Michael Chang, a former pharmaceutical industry researcher who had set up a plant to produce herbal medicines in Huzhou, China, near Shanghai.

Dr. Chang scoured Chinese research for promising herbal products; identifying five thousand, the list was narrowed to thirty. By early 1995, Pharmanex was born, with headquarters in Simi Valley, California. Red yeast rice, called hong qu, was one of its most promising projects.

"We know hong qu has been used for centuries, but we don't know why it lowers cholesterol," Dr. Chang said. "We need to find out."

The 1994 law, Mr. McGlashan said, made it worth investing in science. The company introduced Cholestin at the end of 1996, after nearly three years of study. Soon after, Pharmanex enlisted Dr. David Heber, director of the Center for Human Nutrition at the University of California at Los Angeles, to study the effects of Cholestin in adults with moderately elevated cholesterol.

The study, financed by Pharmanex, compared the cholesterol levels of forty-two adults who took 2.5 grams of Cholestin every day for three months with the levels in forty-one adults who were given placebos. Dr. Heber said the total cholesterol counts of those who took the supplement dropped, on average, from 250 to 210.

Dr. Heber dismissed the contention that red yeast rice is a drug; instead he called it "a functional food." The same cholesterol-lowering ingredient in lovastatin, he noted, occurs in even higher concentrations in oyster mushrooms, commonly used in Asian cooking. And nobody, he said, was trying to ban mushrooms.

However, Dr. Richard A. Friedman, director of psychopharmacology at New York Hospital–Cornell Medical Center, contended that the current distinction between dietary supplements and drugs was based on semantics, not biology, and that both should be carefully regulated.

"If there is a biologically active component in the supplement, to say it is not a drug is illogical because it will have a similar effect," he said. Companies like Pharmanex, he added, "want to be able to implant the idea in the public that the drug is medically beneficial" without the rigorous research.

That kind of science, Mr. McGlashan admits, would cost far too much for a small company like his. Yet with a decent body of research behind Cholestin, he said, he at one time envisioned himself becoming the FDA's model for good behavior.

Instead, he received a visit from FDA investigators in 1997; the agency had received complaints that Cholestin contained lovastatin, both from a pharmacist and from Merck & Company, which makes Mevacor, the cholestorol-lowering drug, known generically as lovastatin.

Shortly thereafter, federal authorities impounded ten tons of red yeast rice. Then in May 1998, the FDA notified Mr. McGlashan that it considered Cholestin illegal, a move that led the company to ask for a hearing before Judge Kimball.

"This case is going to determine the extent to which companies can imitate prescription drugs," said Mr. Schultz of the FDA, "and avoid the approval process."

But Mr. McGlashan contended that the dispute was an economic one. Cholestin, he said, was intended for use by people who are too healthy for Mevacor. Merck, he said, was trying to push Cholestin off the shelves—a charge denied by Jan Weiner, a company spokeswoman.

While the court case is pending, Mr. McGlashan said, sales of Cholestin are booming. Even his mother called, he said, asking, "How am I supposed to get my Cholestin?"

Mr. McGlashan had no answer. Standing outside the low-pressure room where the encapsulating machine was spinning, a lab coat covering his royal blue shirt and Hermès tie, he looked a little wistful. The fine red powder being packed into the capsules, he said, was the last of his supply.

Sheryl Gay Stolberg, June 1998

In February 1999, Judge Kimball ordered the FDA to lift its ban on importing red yeast rice powder. His ruling said that Cholestin met the definition of a dietary supplement, and allowed Pharmanex to continue importing the powder and marketing its capsules.

IS IT A DRUG? IS IT A FOOD?
NO, IT'S A SUPPLEMENT

John Kovarik got a rude shock when he went to his pharmacy to fill a prescription: his insurance company refused to pay for it.

"I was flabbergasted," said Mr. Kovarik, a lawyer in South Palm Beach,

Florida, with a life-threatening genetic disorder known as Wilson's disease. To fight its symptoms, Mr. Kovarik needs an effective treatment to keep copper from accumulating in his body and destroying his vital organs.

He had been taking a drug that could have caused irreversible and sometimes lethal side effects. So, Mr. Kovarik said, he negotiated the maze of his health maintenance organization to find a doctor who would prescribe a newer and safer drug, Galzin. But when his insurance company, Humana Inc., refused to pay for Galzin, Mr. Kovarik angrily called the company from the pharmacy counter.

"I was telling them that I have this life-threatening disease," Mr. Kovarik said, "and that this drug is life sustaining. I told them that the drug I was using was having deleterious side effects. I told them that Galzin is FDA approved." Later, he wrote letter after letter, to no avail.

The problem is that Galzin is zinc acetate, and zinc acetate is sold both as a prescription drug and over the counter as a food supplement. The supplement and the drug are supposed to be the same, but the supplement is not licensed by the Food and Drug Administration, so its manufacture is not regulated and there is no guarantee that the dose on the package is correct.

Humana questioned why it should pay for a prescription drug when the supplement was available. A month's supply of Galzin costs $95, Mr. Kovarik said. If he bought the supplement, it would cost $10 to $15, he said.

"We do not cover nutritional supplements," said Valerie Kennedy, a Humana spokeswoman.

But cost is not the crucial issue, said officials at Teva Pharmaceuticals USA of Sellersville, Pennsylvania, which makes Galzin. "The real issue here is the safety of the patient," said Dr. Carole Ben-Maimon, a senior vice president. "The patients taking a prescription product know what they are getting and how it was made."

A product can be a drug if a company tests it for safety and efficacy, receives approval from the Food and Drug Administration and makes the product according to federal standards. But under current rules, many of the same products can be sold as supplements if they do not make drug claims.

"The boundary between food and drugs is by no means clear and sharp," said Dr. John Hathcock, the director of nutritional and regulatory science for the Council for Responsible Nutrition, which represents the supplement industry. "It is perfectly legal and, I believe, also legitimate for some products to be on the market both as supplements and drugs."

Patients who need products to treat diseases can take the drugs if their doctors prescribe them, Dr. Hathcock said, while others can buy the supplements.

But patients, their advocates, and companies that try to sell drugs like zinc acetate say it is not that simple. Because a substance sold as a supplement is not regulated by the FDA, there is no guarantee that it will contain the product on its label or that the dosage stated on the label is accurate. Although only a few products are sold as both drugs and supplements, some are vital to patients, especially those with rare disorders who must take them regularly and in fixed amounts.

"It's a big problem," said Abbey Meyers, the executive director of the National Organization for Rare Disorders, an advocacy group based in Fairfield, Connecticut. "If your life depends on one of these products, you can't take a chance on buying an over-the-counter supplement that may contain no ingredient or half the ingredient or two or three times more of the ingredient."

Ms. Meyers said her group financed a study in which Duke University scientists analyzed over-the-counter L-carnitine supplements from a variety of companies. They found that doses varied markedly, even in pills coming from the same bottle, with some pills containing no carnitine, others containing more than the label specified and most providing less than 60 percent of the dose promised on the label.

And yet, said Lynn McHenry Morgan of Concord, California, when she changed insurance companies, her new insurer, Blue Shield, told her it would not pay for prescription L-carnitine for her two children, who need the drug to treat a rare and debilitating disorder involving the mitochondria, which provide energy to cells.

Ms. Morgan said she lobbied Blue Shield for three months before the company agreed to pay.

Dr. Nancy Stalker, the director of pharmacy services at Blue Shield of

California, said the company wanted patients to get the care they needed, but had a policy restricting payments for drugs that also were nutritional supplements.

Doctors who treat patients in similar circumstances say they often end up imploring insurance companies to pay for the prescription drugs. Dr. Susan Winters, a geneticist who treats children with rare metabolic disorders, said she aggressively fought for insurance coverage for drugs like L-carnitine, but said she did not always win.

Ms. Meyers said that drug companies realized that testing a drug and getting the FDA's approval to market it might not be worthwhile if the drug could also be sold as a supplement. With zinc acetate, she said, her group actively sought a company to sell the product as a drug. "Nobody would do it," Ms. Meyers said. "Who wants to put the money into making a pharmaceutical-grade zinc when you can buy zinc over the counter?" Finally, she said, Teva agreed to do it.

But the situation can be different when a drug is not urgently needed for patients with an otherwise lethal disease. Dr. Richard J. Wurtman, a cofounder of Interneuron, a small drug company in Lexington, Massachussets, was convinced that melatonin worked as a sleeping pill if the dose was correct. He wanted to test and market it as a drug. But when he urged this course on his company, he said, he was met with "absolutely zero interest."

"The problem is convincing a company in this country to invest the tens of millions of dollars to get the drug on the market and then have it come out and compete with a supplement," Dr. Wurtman said. "As long as something is available as a dietary supplement, no company will invest in it."

And so Interneuron joined the supplement makers. It is marketing melatonin as a supplement that can induce sleep, through a subsidiary called InterNutria.

Gina Kolata, February 1999

CURES CANCER! PREVENTS AIDS! IMPROVES SEX! SORRY, YOU CAN'T SAY THAT

For the first time, in November 1998, the Federal Trade Commission issued advertising guidelines aimed specifically at the nation's booming dietary supplement industry.

The guidelines were the commission's second action within a week on claims by the industry, which earned nearly $12 billion in 1997 and is growing at about 20 percent a year. A week earlier, the commission sent E-mail warnings to 1,200 Internet sites that it said had made "incredible claims" for drugs, devices and dietary supplements, including herbal remedies that purported to ward off AIDS or cure cancer.

In addition, the commission has taken legal action against seven supplement manufacturers over advertising claims for various products, including an impotence remedy called Vaegra—a clear effort to cash in on Pfizer's approved impotence drug, Viagra—and a shark cartilage product that supposedly cured cancer, rheumatism, arthritis, diabetes, fibroid tumors, bursitis, circulatory problems and cysts. Several weight-loss potions have also been made targets of the commission.

The guidelines, which were posted on the commission's Web site and sent to trade associations for the supplement industry, did not amount to any change in policy, said Michelle Rusk, a lawyer for the commission. Basically the FTC requires that advertising be truthful, that it not be misleading and that advertisers be able to back up their claims. The new guidelines explain how those requirements apply to the supplement industry and spell out the kinds of claims that supplement manufacturers can and cannot make.

Jodie Bernstein, director of the FTC's Bureau of Consumer Protection, said that in recent years the commission had issued similar guidelines to define "low fat" for the food industry and terms like "recycled" and "recyclable" for other producers.

The new supplement guidelines were prompted by the tremendous growth of the industry, Ms. Bernstein said, and by confusion among manufacturers about what was allowed in advertising.

"There are a lot of new players," she said.

In addition, the Dietary Supplement Health and Education Act of 1994 limited the authority of the Food and Drug Administration to regulate supplements—vitamins, herbs and other food-based products, as opposed to drugs—and that change left the public and many manufacturers wondering what the rules were.

Ms. Bernstein said the commission had worked with industry and consumer groups for a year to develop the guidelines.

Response from the industry was favorable. Alan Raul, a lawyer at Sidley & Austin, a Washington law firm that represents the National Nutritional Foods Association, said: "The FTC has really reached out to the dietary supplement industry to provide assistance and guidance in the sort of advertising claims on dietary supplements that are appropriate. It looks like a thorough, helpful piece of guidance that will be useful to the public and to the industry."

Dr. Annette Dickinson, director of scientific and regulatory affairs for another trade association, the Council for Responsible Nutrition, said, "We think it's a very good idea, and a useful guide."

The guide, a twenty-six-page document, explains that the Food and Drug Administration is responsible for claims on labeling, and the FTC for advertising claims, including those on the Internet. It provides thirty-six hypothetical examples of advertising claims, and explains how the law would apply to them.

Advertisers are responsible for implied claims as well as expressly stated ones, the guide says, so that if an advertisement cites "university studies" in support of a product, the studies must not only exist but also deliver on the implied message, which is that they are reliable.

Similarly, if an advertisement says that 90 percent of cardiologists take a certain product, the manufacturer must be able to demonstrate not only that fact but also the implied claim that the product is good for the heart.

Unlike FDA labeling rules, which forbid claims that supplements can treat or prevent disease, the FTC guidelines allow such claims in advertisements, provided that the manufacturer can substantiate them. What qualifies as substantiation is also explained in the guidelines: "competent and reliable scientific evidence," including tests, analyses and research conducted and evaluated by qualified professionals.

But advertisers cannot, by picking and choosing among studies, present only those that back their claims. The guidelines say the advertisements must reflect "the totality of the evidence."

The commission also requires that advertisers disclose, clearly and prominently, "qualifying information" like side effects or the fact that a weight-loss product works only if the consumer also diets and exercises.

Companies must also disclose whether a person who endorses a particular product is being paid for the endorsement and whether the person is qualified to make such an endorsement. If, for example, a person identified as "Dr. Jones" speaks on behalf of vitamins but is a doctor of Romance languages rather than of medicine, the advertising is not acceptable.

Advertisers are also barred from implying that any food supplement has been approved by the FDA, which has no authority to regulate supplements unless they violate its labeling rules or become implicated in consumer illness.

Denise Grady, November 1998

WHAT'S *REALLY* IN THOSE PILLS?

A chemist took a dozen pills from plastic sandwich bags, dissolved each in water, poured the solutions into tiny test tubes and placed them on a machine attached to the computer. A robotic arm then picked up each small vial and moved it into position, while an automatic needle drew out several drops of solution for the computer to analyze.

The computer at the Alpha Chemical and Biomedical Laboratories in Petaluma, California, tested various brands of glucosamine and chondroitin, popular pills sold without a prescription to relieve arthritis pain. The results of these and other lab analyses: nearly one-third of the brands tested did not contain what their manufacturers claimed.

Americans spend $14 billion annually on dietary supplements, which include vitamins, minerals, herbs and other "natural" remedies, for a whole range of ills, like joint pain, difficulty urinating, memory loss and depression.

But it is next to impossible for consumers to know exactly what is in most of the pills and capsules they are buying, or what effect they are likely to have.

The Food and Drug Administration does not require manufacturers to prove the safety or efficacy of supplements before putting them on the market. Dosages are not standardized. And, unlike prescription drugs or over-the-counter medicines like aspirin, there is no federal quality control to make sure that what is on the label reflects what is in the bottle.

To fill the gap, a new private company, ConsumerLab.com of White Plains, New York, is testing various products for quality and potency at independent laboratories across the country, including Alpha Chemical. The magazine *Consumer Reports* and the Good Housekeeping Institute, which tests products for *Good Housekeeping* magazine, have also begun evaluating dietary supplements.

ConsumerLab.com, founded by a physician-turned-businessman and a research chemist formerly with the Food and Drug Administration, is posting the results of its tests on its Web site. It is also licensing a seal, similar to the Good Housekeeping Seal of Approval, for products that meet its standards. The company hopes to make money by selling its seal to producers and its information to third parties on the Internet, like health care Web sites and online retailers.

"This is not a well-regulated area—some would say it's not regulated at all," said Dr. Tod Cooperman, ConsumerLab.com's founder and president, and a physician. "People are throwing their money out the window with some of these products."

The results of the tests conducted so far show a wide variation in quality among some of the most popular supplements. All ten glucosamine products tested contained what the manufacturers claimed. But nearly half the combined glucosamine-chondroitin tablets flunked the test. Some had only 25 percent of the ingredients that their labels claimed. Glucosamine, made from crab shells, and chondroitin, made from cow, pig or shark cartilage, are both sold to treat arthritis in the knee. They are among the fastest-growing dietary supplements.

ConsumerLab.com found fault with ten of twenty-seven brands of saw palmetto, an extract of palm tree berries marketed to reduce the frequency and urgency of urination in men with enlarged prostates. "One had only half of what it was supposed to have," Dr. Cooperman said.

The laboratories found that one-quarter of the thirty brands of ginkgo biloba, an herbal extract used to enhance memory, did not have adequate levels of the active ingredient listed on the label.

When the Food and Drug Administration considered regulating these products in the early 1990s, manufacturers and health food stores orchestrated a massive letter-writing campaign to oppose stricter controls.

Congress listened to the industry, and the result was the Dietary Supplement and Health Education Act of 1994, which created a new category called dietary supplements, subject neither to the regulations for drugs nor to the manufacturing standards of foods.

Since then, the sale of dietary supplements has boomed to $14.1 billion in 1999 from $8.3 billion in 1994. Once sold largely in health food stores, herbal preparations like ginseng, ginger, ginkgo biloba and garlic now take up whole aisles of drugstores. Pharmaceutical giants like Bayer have joined the small, little-known companies in developing and marketing some of these products.

Industry officials may quibble with particular testing methods, but they acknowledge that some companies' sloppy manufacturing practices make it difficult for consumers to know what is in the pills they are buying.

"This is not a good situation," said John Cardellina, vice president for botanical science at the Council for Responsible Nutrition, a trade organization of one hundred companies that sell herbal remedies and other dietary supplements. "The industry has to do something to lift the quality of the products."

Currently, the Food and Drug Administration may pull a product from the market only after it has been shown to be dangerous. The burden of proof is on the agency to show that it is harmful, rather than on the manufacturer to show that it is safe.

The food and drug agency is also charged with establishing "good manufacturing practices" for companies to follow when making dietary supplements. An agency spokeswoman acknowledged that it had been slow to draw up those standards but said they would be out by the end of 2000.

An Office of Dietary Supplements has also been established within the National Institutes of Health to assemble fact sheets on various vitamins, minerals and herbal supplements that will summarize what is known about the safety and effectiveness of each product. The National Institutes of Health also is conducting long-term placebo-controlled clinical trials to determine the efficacy of some of the most popular remedies.

The United States Pharmacopeia, the nonprofit organization that sets standards for potency and dosages of drugs in coordination with the Food and Drug Administration, is developing standards for herbal remedies.

In the meantime, tests by ConsumerLab.com and others are a useful effort to fill the information gap, said senior researchers at the United States Pharmacopeia and the institutes.

"Any testing will certainly be useful," said Dr. Srini Srinivasan, who directs the dietary supplement division of the United States Pharmacopeia. "Whether something works or not is another matter. But you should at least be getting what the label says."

ConsumerLab.com's results are consistent with those found by *Good Housekeeping* and *Consumer Reports*. "It's kind of the wild, wild West out there," said Ronni Sandoff, health editor of *Consumer Reports*.

Chemists at the Good Housekeeping Institute analyzed eight brands of SAMe, an herbal preparation marketed as a "natural Prozac" to treat depression, and found that two had only half the active ingredient promised on the label. One had none at all. On the other hand, the Good Housekeeping Institute gave its seal of approval to several supplements that met the standards of quality, safety and efficacy required of the magazine's advertisers.

Consumer Reports, for its part, tested ten brands of ginseng, an Asian root marketed to build energy and endurance. Several were found to have almost none of the active ingredient listed on the label.

Clara Hemphill, June 2000

TAPPING THE MARKET IN MORNING SICKNESS

The makers of vitamins, herbs and dietary supplements may market products for natural conditions like morning sickness, hot flashes and memory loss in aging without proving they are safe or effective, the Food and Drug Administration announced in January 2000.

The decision, which reverses an earlier proposal, is just one in a series of legal and regulatory victories for the dietary supplement business, which has been growing by leaps and bounds since Congress passed a law in 1994 that severely restricted the FDA's authority to regulate the industry.

The move enraged and startled consumer advocates, who said it would weaken patient protections.

"This is a snake-oil exemption," said Dr. Sidney M. Wolfe, director of the Public Citizens' Health Research Group in Washington. "It's a complete cave-in to the industry."

But drug agency officials said the new rule was an important part of their ten-year strategy to increase consumer confidence in the safety, composition and labeling of vitamins, herbs and other nutritional aids that have become an integral part of the lives of millions of Americans.

"This is not a free-for-all," said Peggy Dotzel, the associate acting commissioner for policy at the FDA. "What the agency is doing is faithfully carrying out the intent of Congress in passing the law."

The law is the Dietary Supplement Health and Education Act, which distinguishes between products that makers say "affect the structure or function of the body" and those that are said to prevent, treat or cure disease. The law allows supplement manufacturers to sell products without FDA approval—and therefore without the rigorous safety and efficacy review that is required of drugs—as long as they make only structure or function claims, and not claims related to disease.

But the law was not specific. So the FDA decided it needed a new regulation to clarify its authority and to delineate which claims fall into which category.

The new rule was first proposed nearly two years ago, in April 1998. At the time, the agency said that while natural states like aging, pregnancy, menopause and adolescence were not diseases, they could be associated with abnormal conditions—like morning sickness or premenstrual syndrome—that are diseases. Products intended for those conditions would then have required FDA approval.

But after reviewing thousands of public comments from industry representatives, consumers and others, Ms. Dotzel said, "the agency was convinced that these, in fact, are not diseases."

"These are normal, common conditions that are associated with the different stages of life," she said. "So claims about these conditions are not disease claims."

However, the rule states that uncommon or serious conditions associated with these life stages will still be treated as diseases. So a company may market a dietary supplement for teenagers who have acne, but not for acne so severe that the symptoms include cysts.

Industry representatives said they had not had time to review the new rule, which is 281 pages long, and could not comment on it in detail. But Corinne Russell, a spokeswoman for the Consumer Healthcare Products Association, a trade group representing eighty manufacturers of over-the-counter drugs and dietary supplements, said her organization was "cautiously optimistic" about the way the regulation had narrowed the definition of what is a disease.

"We thought the proposed rule was way too broad," Ms. Russell said.

The final rule precludes manufacturers from making what the FDA describes as express disease claims or those that are implied. For instance, manufacturers cannot state that a product "prevents osteoporosis," or even that it "prevents bone fragility in postmenopausal women," without obtaining FDA approval. But a company could say its product "maintains a healthy circulatory system" or that it promotes relaxation.

One academic expert said today that it was a tricky business to draw distinctions between diseases and natural life passages.

"If they are going to make a distinction between diseases and normal states, they are on a slippery slope," said the expert, Dr. Richard A. Friedman, director of the psychopharmacology clinic at the Weill Medical College of Cornell University.

For instance, Dr. Friedman said, there is no laboratory test for dementia, so a person who takes the herb ginkgo for memory loss due to aging might in fact be in the early stages of Alzheimer's disease. And he cautioned that just because a product was natural did not mean it was necessarily safe. Dr. Friedman and others were especially worried that, under the FDA's interpretation of the law, a pregnant woman might endanger her fetus by taking an herbal product for morning sickness.

"It doesn't make any difference whether a product is synthetic or found in a plant," Dr. Friedman said. "It can be just as potent biologically."

Legal experts said the FDA had little choice but to act as it did.

"FDA has not done well in this area," said Robert G. Pinco, a food and drug lawyer who, in the 1970s, ran the agency's division for regulating over-the-counter drugs. "Every time they have gone into court to try to limit one of these claims, they have lost. It's because Congress has really changed the paradigm."

Sheryl Gay Stolberg, January 2000

The proposed rule quickly came under fire from experts on birth defects, who said that unborn babies would be put at risk if supplements, which had undergone little or no scientific study, were marketed to pregnant women as remedies for morning sickness and puffy legs. The experts cited the example of thalidomide, prescribed in other countries during the 1960s for morning sickness, which led to limb deformities and other birth defects in ten thousand babies. The drug had never been approved in the United States, because FDA officials questioned its safety.

In February 2000, a month after announcing the rule, the FDA reversed itself, withdrawing the provisions that allowed "claims related to pregnancy."

HUMAN NATURE: A MAN WITH A GARDEN
THAT'S A MEDICINE CABINET

One day in September, in Fulton, Maryland, I stopped by Dr. Jim Duke's garden to check out the little six-acre spread he calls Herbal Village. Fulton is one of those little burgs off the interstate, where the farms have given over to ranch houses, with guys out on their power mowers every Saturday, riding herd on their lawns.

But Dr. Duke's place is as different as the man himself, who looks more like a sixty-nine-year-old hippie, standing barefoot by his kudzu vine, than an eminent botanist, with twenty books and two hundred scientific papers under his belt (if he wore one with his cutoffs).

"My neighbors think I'm crazy for putting in kudzu, but it has more genistein than soy," said Dr. Duke, who is a doctor of botany, as he stood in the plot labeled APHRODISIA. "Genistein is what everybody's promoting soy for, to help prevent breast cancer."

With the help of a few friends, Dr. Duke had planted about two hundred medicinal herbs, in eighty plots, each devoted to some disease or ailment. I had a hard time not making a beeline for the WRINKLES garden, but APHRODISIA wasn't bad. Since when is this an ailment?

"Well, we didn't like the word *impotence*, and nobody liked the word *frigidity*," Dr. Duke said in the slow, easy voice of a southerner, fingering the big leaves of the vine that ate Alabama, his home state.

The Agriculture Department imported kudzu from China years ago, for erosion control, and it has since climbed over cars and houses all over the South. Its purple blossoms, which smell like grape soda, strike fear into the hearts of agricultural extension agents. But both men and women may want to graze on it, since studies indicate that genistein may help guard against prostate as well as breast cancer.

"I make tempura with the leaves, and it tastes like deep-fried anything," he said. He makes Jell-O out of them, too. (Dr. Norman Cragg of the National Cancer Institute, however, cautions, "People should be very careful before going into their yards and harvesting plants for which there is no toxicity data.") The same vine is helping alcoholic hamsters at Harvard University. When the research scientist Dr. Wing-Ming Keung gave the rodents an extract of the Chinese herb, it cut their drinking in half.

Epimedium, known as horny goat weed in the folk literature, grows in APHRODISIA, too. "I'm not responsible for that nomenclature," he said. "But the people looking for herbal Viagra like it."

Dr. Duke recently retired from thirty years of researching plants for the Agriculture Department. Over the years, he has roamed the jungles of Central and South America, learning from folk healers and collaborating with the National Cancer Institute to identify plants that could prevent or treat cancer and other diseases.

"He's a genius," said Michael J. Balick, the director of the Institute of Economic Botany at the New York Botanical Garden in the Bronx. "He maintains the highest levels of scholarly research. To top it off, he writes poetry and composes music. And he's a hell of a nice guy."

When Dr. Duke isn't sampling vines in the Peruvian jungles, he's lecturing about the plants that are the origins of drugs. Or weeding his herbal "farmacy," which is open to the public by appointment (301-498-1175). Nothing is for sale; the plants are there to educate.

The plantsman spent years compiling *Dr. Duke's Phytochemical and Ethnobotanical Databases* for the Agricultural Research Service (www.ars-grin.gov/duke/), where you can surf for everything from folklore to scientific studies to the chemical compounds of a particular plant. And his latest book, *The Green Pharmacy* (Rodale Press, now a St. Martin's paperback), is a chatty guide to natural remedies.

He speaks to an eager audience. In 1997, sales of dietary supplements and herbal products totaled $3.6 billion. Sales of echinacea were $310 million; ginseng, $270 million; ginkgo, $240 million, and Saint-John's-wort, $200 million.

"A lot of people who take an herb for an ailment never see the herb growing," Dr. Duke said, moving on to a giant ginger plant, thriving in the ARTHRITIS garden. "But if they do a little weeding or pruning, they can bond with their plants."

Dr. Duke talks in a rambling way that harks back to the Alabama hills. "By five," he said, "I knew where my temple was—the forest." He led the way to a shady little ravine full of maples, oaks, black gum and ash. A lone ginseng was growing beneath a giant tulip poplar. In spring, May apples carpet these woods. The May apple is the source of a compound called etoposide, which has been isolated and synthesized to treat lung cancer. Wild yam grows here, as well, and its tuber is the source of diosgenin, a compound used to produce synthetic steroids and hormones.

Imagine the healing powers in the Peruvian rain forest, which has fifty times the diversity of this eastern deciduous forest. "These are the plants we've co-evolved with for twenty-five thousand years," Dr. Duke said, meaning that's how long people have grazed on plants in the New World, which is an eye blink, compared to Africa, where humans have been grazing for 3.5 million years.

Back up the hill, in the DEPRESSION garden, we stared at a floppy little wildflower, called Saint-John's-wort. "A lot of times, to my surprise, my lectures are to doctors," he said. "Most of them hate it, but their patients are taking these things, so they've got to learn. But if I can get ten physicians, I can usually get one to say: 'You're right, Duke. I don't know for sure that Prozac is better than Saint-John's-wort.' Then I can say, 'Well, if you're not sure, who is?'"

Dr. Duke would love to see controlled studies of these herbs. As a botanist, he believes that the whole plant is better than a "silver bullet" from one of its compounds. "Through our co-evolution with these natural compounds, your body has learned to exclude the bad and grab the good," he said. "When you give it a silver bullet, you don't give it a menu of things. When you give it a whole herb, you're giving it thousands of compounds, which it already knows and has mechanisms for utilizing or excluding."

Which is why this botanist and gardener trusts Saint-John's-wort more than Prozac.

So do you make a tea with it?

"I ain't depressed," Dr. Duke said, sounding as peaceful as an Alabama woods.

Ann Raver, October 1998

[3]

Some Help, Some Harm, Many Remain Mysterious

Herbal Remedies

Anyone who doubts that powerful medicines can come from plants might want to reconsider that notion after a look at the following list, which includes just a small fraction of the drugs derived from bark, flowers or other plant parts: aspirin, the heart drug digitalis, the malaria remedy quinine, the cancer drug taxol, cocaine and of course opium and its derivatives, including morphine and heroin.

In his book, The Best Alternative Medicine *(Simon & Schuster, 2000), Dr. Kenneth Pelletier, of Stanford University, says that "about one quarter of all U.S. prescription drugs are derived from herbs." And he also notes that 1,500 herbs are sold in the United States, a market of $3 billion a year.*

Several things set herbs apart from conventional medicines. Whereas most mainstream drugs rely on concentrated doses of one or just a few active ingredients, herbs by their very nature are mixtures of many ingredients, some not even identified, generally in minute quantities. Mixing two or more herbs, as is done in traditional Chinese medicine, may actually amount to mixing hundreds of components. When taken in small doses, herbs are generally thought to have more subtle effects, and far milder side effects, than conventional, single-ingredient drugs. And therein lies their appeal to many people.

Herbal remedies, unlike man-made ones, may be quite variable, depending on where the plants grew, what the growing season was like, which parts of the plant were used and how they were processed. Experts say that some of the uncertainty from batch to batch can be eliminated by "standardizing," that is, ensuring that a measured amount of a known active ingredient is present. But standardizing for one component does not take into account varying levels of others that may have biological activity.

In addition to variations in the herbs themselves, the products containing them are also prepared in many different ways. They may be sold as whole herbs, teas, powders or extracts dissolved in water, oil or alcohol. Medicinal herbs may be added to teas, fruit juices, diet drinks and even soda pop. Because the industry is largely unregulated, consumers cannot be sure just what they are buying.

But matters of dose and formulation are secondary to the fundamental question: Do herbal remedies work, and are they safe? Many of the popular books and articles have to be taken with a grain of salt, because they simply recycle the same folklore, anecdotes and unproved theories. Scientific studies have been conducted on some herbs, and more are sure to come, though drug makers have had little incentive to conduct such research, because it is expensive and the substances being tested are generally not patentable, which means that the research costs will be difficult or even impossible to recover.

AMERICANS GAMBLE ON HERBS AS MEDICINE

Herbal medicine, the mainstay of therapeutics for centuries before modern purified drugs relegated it to the status of near-quackery, has in the late 1990s emerged from the fringes of health care with an astonishing flourish and now shows clear signs of joining the medical mainstream.

Despite many cautionary tales about adulterated and even dangerous products, herbs formulated as capsules, tinctures, extracts and teas—and increasingly as additions to common foods like potato chips and fruit drinks—are now routinely used by a third of American adults seeking to enhance their health or alleviate their illnesses. Each day the herbal realm wins new converts, particularly among those who have become disillusioned with the cost and consequences of traditional drugs, distrustful of conventional physicians and convinced that "natural" equals "good."

Yet, because herbal products are classified as dietary supplements, not drugs, and face none of the premarket hurdles drugs must clear, consumers have no assurance of safety or effectiveness. Indeed, scores of products sold in the United States are listed by European and American authorities as ineffective, unsafe or both, and manufacturing standards to assure high quality have been proposed but are not yet in force.

Thus, countless consumers are wasting their money on useless products or jeopardizing their health on hazardous ones. Among the serious side effects that have been linked to herbal remedies are high blood pressure, life-threatening allergic reactions, heart rhythm abnormalities, mania, kidney failure and liver damage. A few widely available products, including sassafras and comfrey, contain known carcinogens.

At the same time, according to a report last year in the journal *Psychosomatics*, unsuspecting consumers "have used herbal remedies with good results only to discover that the benefit was actually derived from the presence of undisclosed medicines," including steroids, anti-inflammatory agents, sedatives and hormones.

"The lack of quality standards is the number-one problem in the whole industry," said Dr. Varro E. Tyler, emeritus professor of pharmacognosy (the study of active ingredients in plants) at Purdue University. Dr. Tyler, a leading expert on herbal medicine, has no equity interest in any herbal manufacturers, though he has acted as a paid consultant and lecturer to the industry. He said: "I feel sorry for the typical consumer. How is he or she to know what is best, what products are reliable and safe? Even when a label says the product has been standardized, the consumer has no way to know if it actually meets that standard." But even if an herbal product has been standardized—reliably made in some standard dose—that still does not mean that scientific studies have shown it to be effective.,

The industry itself is promoting a "good manufacturing practices" doctrine. Annette Dickinson, director of scientific and regulatory affairs for the Council for Responsible Nutrition, a trade organization for producers of dietary supplements, said a consortium of associations submitted a document of manufacturing standards to the Food and Drug Administration in 1997. Although such a standard would say nothing about an herb's safety or effectiveness, it would result in reliable methods that the industry would have to use to ensure the identity and quality of its products. The agency has issued a notice of proposed rules but no final ruling as yet.

Nonetheless, botanicals, as herbal products are more accurately known, are enjoying an annual retail market approaching $4 billion, up from $839 million in 1991 and growing about 18 percent a year. Hundreds of products made with virtually no government oversight are crowding shelves of health food stores, food markets and pharmacies nationwide. Supplements are also widely sold by marketers like Amway, through catalogues and on the Internet.

Now, even major pharmaceutical companies like Warner Lambert, American Home Products, Bayer and SmithKline Beecham are introducing herbal products, adding respectability to this marginalized market.

Some herbs—like echinacea, goldenseal, American ginseng and wild yam—have become so popular that their continued supply from natural sources is in danger. As the plants become scarcer and more expensive, products containing them are increasingly likely to be adulterated and may even contain none of the herb listed on the label. Peggy Brevoort, president of East Earth Herb Inc., a company in Eugene, Oregon, that produces botanicals, said that the demand for Saint-John's-wort, used for mild depression, and kava, a calmative said to reduce anxiety, now exceeds their supply, introducing the "danger of adulteration" by "unscrupulous dealers."

At the same time, two major new publications—a 1,244-page *Physicians' Desk Reference for Herbal Medicines*, produced by the same company that publishes the *Physicians' Desk Reference*, and an English-language edition of Germany's therapeutic guide to herbal medicines, *The Complete German Commission E Monographs*—have been issued to help educate physicians, pharmacists and interested consumers about the known uses, proper dosages and safety concerns of more than six hundred botanicals now sold in this country. The evaluations in both books are based on studies, most done in Germany and reviewed by teams of experts.

The National Institutes of Health now lists on the Internet international bibliographic information on dietary supplements, including herbal products. The address is www.nal.usda.gov/fnic/IBIDS/.

In addition, a few medical and pharmacology schools have introduced courses in phytomedicine, the study of botanicals. And the American Pharmaceutical Association has included a program on herbal medicine in its annual meeting. Still, most doctors remain wary of botanicals, especially when patients choose self-medication with plant extracts over established medical remedies.

The very act of Congress that has fostered this growth—the 1994 Dietary Supplement Health and Education Act—has also permitted chaos to reign in the botanical marketplace, with no mechanism to assure that products are safe or effective. Pushed heavily by Senator Orrin G. Hatch of Utah, the home base of many supplement makers, and passed over the objections of the FDA, the law created a new product class, the dietary supplement, that was not subject to regulations applied to drugs. Now any substance that can be found in foods, regardless of amount or action and including substances that act as hormones or toxins, can be produced and sold without any premarket testing or agency approval.

Marketed as neither foods nor as drugs, herbal products are not obliged to meet any established standards of effectiveness or safety for medicinal products, which require extensive laboratory and clinical trials before approval. As with other substances classified as dietary supplements, the FDA can restrict the sale of an herbal product only if it receives well-documented reports of health problems associated with it. The agency took four years, and more than one hundred reports of life-threatening symptoms and thirty-eight deaths, to act against ephedra, often sold as the Chinese herb ma huang, a stimulant that can prove disastrous to people with heart problems.

With FDA authority limited by the 1994 law, the Federal Trade Commission, which monitors advertising, has taken a more active role in monitoring supplement makers.

The FTC in 1998 took legal action against seven manufacturers that had broken rules requiring that advertising be truthful and verifiable. The companies were selling remedies or purported cure-alls for ailments like impotence, cancer and obesity.

The commission also sent E-mail warnings to 1,200 Internet sites that it said had made "incredible claims" for drugs, devices and supplements, including herbal remedies that would supposedly ward off AIDS. Also in 1998, the commission issued its first set of advertising guidelines aimed specifically at the supplement industry.

Still, the current regulations have created a quagmire of consumer confusion and set up potential health crises that even industry officials say could ultimately hurt producers as well as users of herbal products. Under the 1994 law, consumers have no assurance that an herbal product contains what the label says it does or that it is free from harmful contaminants. Independent analyses of some products, particularly those containing costly or scarce herbs, revealed that some have little or none of the purported active ingredient listed on the label.

Adding to the confusion is that botanical makers are allowed to describe products only in terms of their effects on the structure or function of the body, not their potential health benefits. Thus, a product label might say "promotes cardiac function" but it cannot say "lowers cholesterol."

Likewise, although the law does allow health warnings on the label, most manufacturers have yet to include them.

Consumers are warned, however, that federal drug safety officials are not watching the store. All botanicals must display a disclaimer on the label following the description of the product's structural or functional role: "This statement has not been evaluated by the Food and Drug Administration. This product is not intended to diagnose, treat, cure or prevent any disease." To which Dr. Tyler commented, "If that is true, why on earth would anyone use it?"

The seeds of the modern herbal market were sown in the 1960s when "green, organic and natural became buzzwords," Dr. Tyler said. But they did not mature until the '90s with the growing consumer interest in "self-care and controlling one's destiny," he said. Many turned to herbs as a gentler way to treat health problems and a potential tool for preserving mental and physical health.

The interest has spawned scores of Internet sites and hundreds of books on various herbs. But much of the literature is replete with poorly documented health claims and, with few exceptions (among them, Dr. Tyler's books), advocacy prevails over objectivity.

Because plants contain a mixture of relatively dilute chemicals, they naturally tend to have milder actions, both in their therapeutic benefits and side effects, than the concentrated, single chemicals in most drugs. Thus, botanicals generally take longer to act than regular pharmaceuticals and few have the potency of a prescription, the one possible exception being saw palmetto, which a well-designed study indicated may be as helpful for an enlarged prostate as the more expensive and riskier drug, Proscar.

The combination of chemicals in botanicals is potentially both a plus and a minus. When two or more chemicals enhance one another's activity, the therapeutic benefit could theoretically exceed that from an isolated substance formulated as a drug. Mark Blumenthal, who heads the American Botanical Council, noted that the herb Saint-John's-wort, widely used in Germany and increasingly in the United States to counter mild depression, is standardized for a substance called hypericin. But, he explained, "hypericin is not directly linked to its antidepressant activity." Rather, other substances in the herb seem to have diverse actions on brain chemicals, all of which work together to counter depression.

But, equally possible when using an herb with two or more active chemicals is that one will cancel the benefits of another or introduce a hazard. Without careful chemical tests and large, well-controlled clinical trials such actions are often hard to detect.

Consumer confidence in herbal medicine is bolstered by the common but erroneous assumption that "natural" equals "safe" and the public's failure to realize that many plants contain chemicals that are potent drugs or outright poisons. Natural laxatives like the herb *Cascara sagrada* are just as habit-forming and harmful to the colon as laxatives sold as drugs.

Indeed, one-quarter of prescription drugs and hundreds of over-the-counter products were originally isolated from plants. Ephedra, for example, contains a natural stimulant that is approved for use as a decongestant and bronchial dilator in some pharmaceutical products. However, when used in uncontrolled dosages or by people with certain underlying health problems, it can cause a dangerous rise in blood pressure and, in its herbal form, has been responsible for serious adverse reactions and dozens of deaths, mainly among people who inappropriately used it as a stimulant or diet aid.

Complicating the safety issue is the fact, shown in several surveys, that most patients fail to tell their physicians they use herbal supplements, and thus sometimes risk dangerous drug interactions or endure costly tests or treatments when an herb causes an unrecognized side effect. Experts say many patients withhold information about herbal drug use because they fear being ridiculed by their doctors.

Although all German physicians must take courses on herbal remedies, only a handful of American medical and pharmacology schools offer courses in this field.

In 1998, the President's Commission on Dietary Supplement Labels recommended that the FDA appoint a committee to evaluate the safety and effectiveness of herbal products. "This could be the most important step in the United States toward legitimizing herbal medicine," Dr. Tyler said.

However, the agency responded that it lacked the budget to support such an effort. American physicians have completed and published only a few well-designed studies of some popular botanicals. Among them were studies suggesting that saw

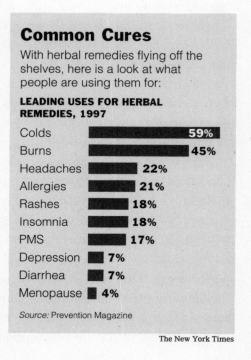

Common Cures

With herbal remedies flying off the shelves, here is a look at what people are using them for:

LEADING USES FOR HERBAL REMEDIES, 1997

Colds	59%
Burns	45%
Headaches	22%
Allergies	21%
Rashes	18%
Insomnia	18%
PMS	17%
Depression	7%
Diarrhea	7%
Menopause	4%

Source: Prevention Magazine

The New York Times

palmetto can shrink an enlarged prostate and ginkgo biloba can improve memory in patients with early Alzheimer's disease.

The Office of Dietary Supplements at the National Institutes of Health is helping to finance a three-year multicenter study of Saint-John's-wort as a treatment for clinical depression and a study of plant-based estrogens as a preventive for postmenopausal health problems.

However, thousands of studies of botanicals have been completed abroad—mainly in Germany—that strongly suggest a health-promoting role for more than 200 plant products. Germany's Commission E evaluated 380 botanicals, approving 254 as safe and reasonably effective and disapproving 126 as ineffective, unsafe or both.

The Germans use a different criterion to assess an herb's benefits—a doctrine of "reasonable certainty" that the herb has the desired effect and is safe, Mr. Blumenthal said. Whereas standard testing of a drug for approval by the United States FDA can cost as much as $500 million per product—a prohibitive amount for companies to spend on botanicals that cannot be patented—tests to establish "reasonable certainty" would cost only $1 million to $2 million, Dr. Tyler estimated.

In June 1996, Dr. Robert Temple, director of medical policy for the FDA's Center for Drug Evaluation, suggested that, rather than subjecting botanicals to the extensive tests required for drugs, the agency might consider applying less stringent criteria to assess an herb's effects, at least when a product is to be used only for a short time. He said, "A long history of safe use might provide sufficient safety information for products that are intended for short-term use."

More than four dozen botanicals or botanical formulations have been submitted to the agency as investigational new drugs. If any meet the agency's criteria for safety and effectiveness and are eventually approved as drugs, they would be allowed to make direct health claims—instead of just structure and function statements—on labels and in advertising.

Meanwhile, Dr. Joerg Gruenwald, medical director of a German phytomedicine company and primary editor of the new *Physicians' Desk Reference for Herbal Medicines*, said professionals can rely on that volume for current, documented information about botanicals. The volume, to be issued annually, updates the Commission E reports and adds several hundred other products sold in the United States, listing effects, side effects and conditions in which their use is inadvisable.

Jane E. Brody, February 1999

IN THE GARDEN OF HERBAL REMEDIES, WEEDING OUT THE BAD CHOICES

Few rigorous studies of herbal medicines have been conducted in the United States, but in Germany, a government health panel has evaluated hundreds of herbs. The table below reflects analyses by the panel and other experts on herbs.

Jane E. Brody

Herbs Thought to Be Effective . . .

HERB: **BLACK COHOSH**

WHY IT IS USED: Thought to reduce symptoms of premenstrual syndrome, painful menstruation and the hot flashes and mood disorders associated with menopause.

HOW IT WORKS: It appears to function as an estrogen substitute and a suppressor of luteinizing hormone.

CAUTIONS: Occasional stomach pain or intestinal discomfort. Since no long-term studies have been done, use of black cohosh should be limited to six months.

HERB: **CAPSICUM**

WHY IT IS USED: Best known as the hot red peppers cayenne and chili. Applied topically for chronic pain from conditions like shingles and trigeminal neuralgia. It may also be helpful for cluster headache, muscle spasms and arthritis.

HOW IT WORKS: The active ingredient, capsaicin, works as a counterirritant and decreases sensitivity to pain by depleting substance P, a neurotransmitter that facilitates the transmission of pain impulses to the spinal cord.

CAUTIONS: Overuse can result in a prolonged insensitivity to pain. More concentrated products can cause a burning sensation. Users must avoid contact with eyes, genitals and other mucous membranes.

HERB: **ECHINACEA**

WHY IT IS USED: These species of purple coneflower are thought to shorten the intensity and duration of colds and flu, help to control urinary tract infections and, when applied topically, speed the healing of wounds.

HOW IT WORKS: Though echinacea lacks direct antibiotic activity, it may help the body muster its own defenses against invading microorganisms.

CAUTIONS: Experts warn against using echinacea for more than eight weeks at a time, and against its use by people with autoimmune diseases like multiple sclerosis and rheumatoid arthritis or by those who are infected with HIV.

HERB: **FEVERFEW**

WHY IT IS USED: The dried leaves of this plant have been shown to help prevent (but not treat) migraine headaches and frequently associated symptoms of nausea and vomiting.

HOW IT WORKS: The active ingredient, parthenolide, appears to act on the blood vessels of the brain, making them less reactive to certain compounds. It may also act as a serotonin antagonist.

CAUTIONS: Most commercial preparations recommend doses that are much too high. Two hundred fifty micrograms a day of parthenolide—or 125 milligrams of the herb—is an adequate dose.

HERB: **GARLIC**

WHY IT IS USED: Active against viruses, fungi and parasites. It may also lower cholesterol and inhibit the formation of blood clots, actions that can help to prevent heart attacks.

HOW IT WORKS: When fresh garlic is crushed, enzymes convert alliin to allicin, a potent antibiotic. Garlic tablets and capsules containing alliin and the enzyme can be absorbed when dissolved in the intestines and not the stomach.

CAUTIONS: More than five cloves of garlic a day can result in heartburn, flatulence and other gastrointestinal problems. People taking anticoagulants should be cautious about taking garlic.

HERB: **GINGER**

WHY IT IS USED: A time-honored remedy for settling an upset stomach, ginger has been shown in clinical studies to prevent motion sickness and nausea following surgery.

HOW IT WORKS: Components in the aromatic oil and resin of ginger have been found to promote secretion of saliva and gastric juices.

CAUTIONS: May prolong postoperative bleeding, aggravate gallstones and cause heartburn. There is also debate about its safety when used to treat morning sickness.

HERB: **GINKGO**

WHY IT IS USED: Used medicinally in China for hundreds of years, ginkgo biloba was recently reported to improve short-term memory and concentration in people with early Alzheimer's disease.

HOW IT WORKS: It appears to work by increasing the brain's tolerance for low levels of oxygen and by enhancing blood flow to the brain and extremities.

CAUTIONS: Possible side effects include indigestion, headache and allergic skin reactions.

HERB: **KAVA**

WHY IT IS USED: This South Pacific herb, also known as kava-kava, has a growing coterie of enthusiasts who use it to reduce anxiety, stress and restlessness and to facilitate sleep without developing problems of tolerance, dependence and withdrawal.

HOW IT WORKS: The active ingredients in the root and stem act as muscle relaxants and anticonvulsants.

CAUTIONS: Should not be used with alcohol or other depressants, by people who are clinically depressed or by women who are pregnant or nursing. Kava should also not be taken for longer than three months without medical supervision.

HERB: **MILK THISTLE**

WHY IT IS USED: It is thought to protect the liver against toxins and to encourage regeneration of new liver cells.

HOW IT WORKS: The seeds contain a compound called silymarin, which may help liver cells keep out poisons and promote formation of new liver cells.

CAUTIONS: When used as capsules containing 200 milligrams of concentrated extract (140 milligrams of silymarin), no harmful effects have been reported.

HERB: **PSYLLIUM**

WHY IT IS USED: A laxative that doesn't undermine the natural action of the gut. It may reduce the risk of colorectal cancer and produce a significant reduction in blood levels of cholesterol.

HOW IT WORKS: The seeds of this herb have coatings and husks that are filled with mucilage, a soluble fiber that swells with water in the intestines to add bulk and lubrication to the stool.

CAUTIONS: Increase in flatulence in some people, especially if a lot is consumed.

HERB: **SAINT-JOHN'S-WORT**

WHY IT IS USED: Numerous reports attest to this herb's ability to relieve mild depression. It may also have sedating and antianxiety activity.

HOW IT WORKS: Though products are commonly standardized for hypericin, the chemicals responsible for the herb's antidepressant activity have not yet been certainly identified.

CAUTIONS: Based on the sun-induced toxicity of hypericin in animals, fair-skinned and photosensitive people who take Saint-John's-wort are advised to avoid exposure to bright sunlight. The herb can also diminish the effectiveness of anti-rejection drugs taken by transplant recipients, and antiviral drugs used to treat HIV, and those patients should avoid Saint-John's-wort.

HERB: **SAW PALMETTO**

WHY IT IS USED: German studies on patients with enlarged prostates have shown that extracts of the fruits of this palm tree can reduce urinary symptoms even though the gland may not shrink.

HOW IT WORKS: Nonhormonal chemicals in saw palmetto appear to work through their antiandrogen and anti-inflammatory activity.

CAUTIONS: Large doses can cause diarrhea. Some experts are concerned that those taking the herb may have inaccurate prostate specific antigen (PSA) readings, used as an early warning sign of prostate cancer.

HERB: **VALERIAN**

WHY IT IS USED: Perhaps best characterized as a mild tranquilizer.

HOW IT WORKS: The dried underground parts of this plant are thought to have antianxiety and mild hypnotic effects, making it useful in treating nervousness and insomnia.

CAUTIONS: Long-term use can sometimes cause headache, restlessness, sleeplessness and heart function disorders.

. . . And Herbs to Avoid

HERB: **ACONITE, E.G., BUSHI**

WHY IT IS USED: Pain, rheumatism, headaches

REASONS FOR CAUTION: Numerous poisonings in China.

HERB: **BELLADONNA**

WHY IT IS USED: Spasms, gastrointestinal pain

REASONS FOR CAUTION: Contains three toxic alkaloids, including atropine.

HERB: **BLUE COHOSH**

WHY IT IS USED: Menstrual ailments, worms

REASONS FOR CAUTION: Can induce labor.

HERB: **BORAGE**

WHY IT IS USED: Coughs, diuretic, mood booster

REASONS FOR CAUTION: May contain liver toxins and carcinogens.

HERB: **BROOM**

WHY IT IS USED: Intoxicant, diuretic, heart problems

REASONS FOR CAUTION: May slow heart rhythm; contains toxic alkaloids.

HERB: **CHAPARRAL**

WHY IT IS USED: Arthritis, cancer, pain, colds

REASONS FOR CAUTION: Can cause severe hepatitis, liver failure.

HERB: **COMFREY**
WHY IT IS USED: Cuts, bruises, ulcers
REASONS FOR CAUTION: Contains toxins linked to liver disease and death.

HERB: **EPHEDRA**
WHY IT IS USED: Stimulant, decongestant
REASONS FOR CAUTION: Contains cardiac toxins resulting in dozens of deaths.

HERB: **GERMANDER**
WHY IT IS USED: Digestion, fever
REASONS FOR CAUTION: Contains stimulant that can cause heart problems.

HERB: **KOMBUCHA TEA**
WHY IT IS USED: AIDS, insomnia, acne
REASONS FOR CAUTION: Can cause liver damage, intestinal problems and death.

HERB: **LOBELIA**
WHY IT IS USED: Mood booster
REASONS FOR CAUTION: Large doses can cause rapid heartbeat, coma and death.

HERB: **PENNYROYAL**
WHY IT IS USED: Stimulant, gastric distress
REASONS FOR CAUTION: Liver damage, convulsions, abortions, coma and deaths have been reported.

HERB: **POKE ROOT**
WHY IT IS USED: Emetic, rheumatism
REASONS FOR CAUTION: Extremely toxic; low blood pressure; respiratory depression; and death.

HERB: **SASSAFRAS**
WHY IT IS USED: Stimulant, sweat producer, syphilis
REASONS FOR CAUTION: Contains the carcinogen safrole. Banned from use in food.

HERB: **SKULLCAP**
WHY IT IS USED: Tranquilizer
REASONS FOR CAUTION: Can cause liver damage.

HERB: **WORMWOOD**

WHY IT IS USED: Tonic, digestion

REASONS FOR CAUTION: Can cause convulsions, loss of consciousness and hallucinations.

(*Sources: The Physicians' Desk Reference for Herbal Medicines; Tyler's Honest Herbal*, by Dr. Varro E. Tyler with Steven Foster; *Tyler's Herbs of Choice*, by Dr. Tyler, with James Robbers; *Journal of the American Dietetic Association*, October 1997; *The Mayo Clinic Health Letter*, June 1997, page F7.)

MEDICINAL HERBS: MAINSTREAM MEDICINE
SIFTS THE DATA

Chatting with the man who sat next to her on an airplane not long ago, Dr. Lenore Arab could not help noticing that his skin had a telltale orange tinge. As they talked, he revealed that he was thirty-eight and had lung cancer, and in addition to undergoing standard treatment had consulted an "herbalist," who had told him to drink three glasses of carrot juice a day, eat little else and take herbs and other supplements, including beta-carotene, a yellowish-red nutrient that is converted into vitamin A in the body.

The carrot juice alone contained enough carotene to turn his skin orange, a harmless, though certainly odd-looking, condition. But the herbalist's advice was not harmless. Indeed, Dr. Arab, a professor of epidemiology and nutrition at the University of North Carolina at Chapel Hill, found it troubling.

"It was heartrending," she said, adding that she did not want to destroy his hopes, but felt an obligation to tell him that he might be harming himself.

She warned the man, as gently as possible, that research had linked beta-carotene to an increased risk of lung cancer in men who smoked, and that the substance might not be safe for someone who already had lung cancer. In addition, she told him, cancer patients needed far more nourishment than they could get from a diet of carrot juice, herbs and vitamins.

That experience, and similar encounters with other patients taking herbal products with unknown ingredients and unknown effects, recommended by people with unknown credentials, led Dr. Arab to organize a scientific meeting on the subject.

The two-day conference in Chapel Hill, "The Efficacy and Safety of Medicinal Herbs," March 2–3, 2000, was among the first in the nation to gather mainstream researchers from respected universities and to apply rigorous scientific standards to evaluating studies of herbal products. Duke University and the National Institutes of Health were co-sponsors, along with the University of North Carolina.

But the scientific scrutiny is a bit late. "The train has left the station," Dr. Arab said, noting that Americans were already engaged in a vast, uncontrolled experiment. They spend $4 billion a year on herbal remedies, which are not regulated by the Food and Drug Administration.

"People are not turning to health professionals," Dr. Arab said. "They go to magazines for information." Many do not even tell their doctors what they are taking.

But even if people did ask their doctors about herbs, most doctors could not answer. There is little information about herbs in the nation's scientific literature, and American medical schools do not teach students about them. Speakers at the conference included several researchers from Germany, where herbal medicines have been studied more extensively than in this country and are regulated like drugs by the government, which monitors growing, harvesting and processing.

Popular herbs got mixed reviews at the conference. More than twenty controlled studies of mild depression have shown that Saint-John's-wort works as well as some prescription drugs, with fewer side effects. The herb is the best-selling antidepressant in Germany, and health insurance covers it there as well as in Switzerland and Austria. It is also widely used by Americans who want to treat their own depression, but Dr. P. Murali Doraiswamy, a psychiatrist at Duke University who spoke at the conference, had reservations about it.

He said some of the studies were too small to be reliable, that long-term data were lacking and that the herb had not been compared with the most effective prescription drugs like Prozac and Zoloft. Scientific reviewers called Saint-John's-wort promising but unproven, he said, adding that many of his own patients had tried it, but often irregularly and at incorrect doses. Because depression is a serious illness and a major cause of suicide, he said the trend to self-medicate was worrisome.

Recently, cases have been reported in which Saint-John's-wort has had dangerous interactions with other drugs, including those used to treat HIV infection and to prevent rejection in transplant patients.

Several studies of Saint-John's-wort are now in progress, one sponsored by the National Institutes of Health and one by Pfizer, Inc., the drug company. In the meantime, Dr. Doraiswamy said, the jury is still out.

The herb saw palmetto, taken by many men to relieve symptoms of prostate enlargement like frequent urination, got a more positive report. Dr. Timothy J. Wilt, of the Veterans Affairs Center for Chronic Diseases in Minneapolis, evaluated eighteen studies and found that saw palmetto worked better than a placebo and as well as a prescription drug for the condition, finasteride, also called Proscar. The herb had fewer side effects and cost $15 a month, compared with $68 for the prescription drug. But Dr. Wilt said long-term studies were needed to find out whether saw palmetto would keep working and whether it might help men avoid or delay prostate surgery.

Ginseng does appear to have antioxidant properties, according to studies by Dr. David Kitts of the University of British Columbia in Vancouver. Antioxidants are thought to prevent certain types of cell damage associated with artery disease and aging, but their usefulness has not been proved and it is not clear whether they are safe for cancer patients, Dr. Arab said.

Another herb, comfrey, was condemned by Dr. Felix Stickel, of the University of Erlangen, who said the herb had been banned in Canada and Germany because it can cause liver failure. It has not been banned in the United States, though manufacturers have voluntarily removed it from products like herbal teas because its toxicity is widely known. Previously, it had been recommended both here and overseas to treat inflammation and constipation.

Other herbs received cautiously positive reviews. Dr. Arab reported that epidemiologic studies, in which researchers survey people's diets and health, indicated that eating cooked or raw garlic—but not garlic supplements—was linked to a decreased risk of stomach and intestinal cancer.

Dr. Edzard Ernst of the University of Exeter in England analyzed a series of studies of the herb feverfew, and concluded that it could be somewhat helpful in preventing, though not treating, migraine headaches.

Ginkgo biloba appeared to slow mental decline slightly in a third of patients in a placebo-controlled study of 137 people with dementia, Dr. Pierre LeBars of New York University said. The study, the first to show any benefit, was published in 1997 in the *Journal of the American Medical Association*. But the herb did not improve memory in healthy people. Dr. LeBars said more studies were needed to find out if it would really be of use in treating dementia. The form used in the study differed from the version usually sold in this country.

Certain echinacea extracts are accepted as treatment for colds in Germany, reported Dr. Rudolf Bauer of Heinrich-Heine University in Düsseldorf, who described several controlled studies showing that the herb could shorten the duration by a few days and ease symptoms. But there are three different species of echinacea and many different processing methods, and the effectiveness of different products may vary, he said, adding there was no evidence that any form of the herb could prevent colds or other infections.

Positive findings on herbs would be great news if Americans could obtain reliable products with known doses of substances that have medicinal effects. But what is actually in many of the items sold as dietary supplements in the United States is anybody's guess: some may actually contain none of what is promised on the label.

Dr. Varro E. Tyler, a distinguished professor emeritus of pharmacognosy at Purdue University, called the status of medicinal herbs in the United States a "scandalous situation" that has left the public bewildered, scratching their heads and trying to figure out things like which of a dozen different echinacea products might work. He also warned that anybody can call himself or herself an "herbalist" and offer all sorts of advice to the public.

Dr. Tyler, who has written more than thirty books about herbs, describes them as "dilute drugs," and he said they should be regulated as drugs by the FDA so that manufacturers would be required to produce uniform batches with known ingredients.

But under the 1994 Dietary Supplement Health and Education Act, herbal medicines are classified as supplements, not drugs, which means there is no monitoring of quality control by a drug agency. The act also prevents manufacturers from saying on labels that their products can prevent or treat specific diseases or symptoms.

As a result, Dr. Tyler said, the market has been flooded with "junk products" that are a waste of money. He denounced the growing trend to add herbs like Saint-John's-wort and echinacea to iced tea, soft drinks and other foods. The herbs are drugs and should be treated with respect, he said, and do not belong in canned soup any more than Prozac does.

He faulted greedy manufacturers and the FDA. He said that to approve an herbal product as a drug, the federal agency insisted that its manufacturer provide the same proof of safety and efficacy as other new drugs. But that requirement is unrealistic, he said, because the testing process can cost hundreds of millions of dollars, and herb manufacturers do not attempt it because their products are generally not patentable and they will never recoup the costs.

Since herbs have been around for so long and the vast majority have few or no side effects, Dr. Tyler said the rules should be relaxed for them, to require strong proof of safety and "reasonable" proof of efficacy, which he said could be obtained with two well-designed, placebo-controlled trials that would cost a few million dollars, instead of hundreds of millions. He predicted that FDA-approved herbal drugs would be so popular that people would flock to them, forcing manufacturers to submit to the process to be competitive.

But a spokeswoman for the drug agency said that changing the standards for approval would take an act of Congress.

Denise Grady, March 2000

ADDING CUMIN TO THE CURRY:
A MATTER OF LIFE AND DEATH

Choose any and all correct statements: People living in hot climates eat lots of highly seasoned foods because—

1. Hot spices cool them down by making them sweat.
2. Food spoils faster in hot climates and potent seasonings disguise the taste and smell of spoiled food.
3. Spices grow profusely in the tropics and it is cheaper and easier for people to eat what is locally available.
4. Spices provide important nutrients that might otherwise be in short supply in these areas.
5. Spices make foods taste better and increase consumption of nutritious but not necessarily appealing foods.
6. Pungent spices are natural preservatives that inhibit food spoilage.

If you chose any of the first four statements, logical as they may seem, two Cornell University researchers say you would be wrong. In a forty-six-page paper published in March 1998 in the *Quarterly Review of Biology*, Jennifer Billing and Dr. Paul W. Sherman argue that "some like it hot" because spice plants contain powerful antibiotic chemicals capable of killing or suppressing the bacteria and fungi that commonly contaminate and spoil foods and can poison those who eat them.

Spices that are prominent in traditional dishes from tropical and subtropical regions are used with a much lighter hand, if at all, in countries and regions where the climate is colder, the researchers found. And many of the spices that appear most often and most abundantly in recipes from hot climates—especially garlic, onion and hot peppers—can inhibit 75 percent to 100 percent of the bacteria species against which they have been tested, according to studies by food microbiologists.

The researchers concluded that a taste for spicy foods may have evolved in hot climates and been transmitted from neighbor to neighbor and to succeeding generations as a cultural "neme," the social science equivalent of a gene. While they admit that the immediate reason for using spices "obviously is to enhance food palatability," they added that "the ultimate reason is most likely that spices help cleanse foods of pathogens and thereby contribute to the health, longevity and reproductive success of people who find their flavors enjoyable."

Dr. George Williams, editor of the journal, said that transmission of a taste for highly spiced food is both cultural and genetic and can begin in the womb. He cited studies by Sandra Gray at the University of Kansas showing that "the mother's diet during pregnancy and lactation can influence the dietary habits of her baby throughout its life."

Of course, Dr. Sherman said in an interview, people have other ways than spices of preserving food—by salting, cooking, smoking or drying it, and now by refrigerating or freezing it. But he believes the contribution of spices, all of which come from plants, previously had not been adequately explored or appreciated. He pointed out that many spice plants are rich in compounds that have antimicrobial actions. These compounds evolved in plants as protection against pathogens and predators.

Dr. Thomas Eisner, a professor of chemical ecology at Cornell who has studied how animals use plant chemicals, said: "Many plant metabolites have antimicrobial potency. The use of antibiotics from natural sources is by no means a human invention." For example, he said, an assassin bug he has studied scrapes resin from the leaves of camphor weed and spreads it on her eggs to protect them from pathogens.

Dr. Sherman, an evolutionary behaviorist and professor of neurology and behavior, and Ms. Billing, then an undergraduate at Cornell, analyzed the frequency with which various spices appear in the traditional recipes of thirty-six countries, including the northern and southern halves of the United States and China. In the analysis of 4,578 recipes containing meat, poultry or fish published in ninety-three traditional cookbooks, Ms. Billing found that the hotter the climate of the region, the more spices were called for in the recipes. Especially prominent were spices like onion and garlic that have been shown to inhibit the growth of all thirty microorganisms considered in the study. Capsicums, or hot peppers, which are widely used in hot climates, inhibit the growth of 80 percent of microorganisms considered.

For example, among 120 recipes from Indonesia, 80 percent contained garlic and onion and 77 percent contained capsicums. However, in Ireland, a considerably cooler country, onions appeared in 56 percent, garlic in 23 percent and capsicums in only 2 percent of ninety recipes analyzed, even though the plants can grow there. In India, more than 80 percent of Indian recipes were prepared with onions, ginger and capsicums and 76 percent called for garlic. But in Norway, the only prominent seasonings were black and white pepper, used in less than half the recipes. Onion appeared in only 20 percent of recipes, and capsicums were not found in any of the seventy-seven recipes analyzed.

Likewise there are differences within countries with significant regional temperature differences: the northern and southern United States and northeastern and southwestern China. Dr. Sherman suggested that antimicrobial activity may explain why a relatively bland milk-based clam chowder became popular in New England while a spicier crawfish étoufée is preferred in the Deep South.

"I consider recipes a record of the cultural co-evolutionary race between us and microbes," Dr. Sherman said. "We are trying to keep ahead of the microbes that are trying to eat the same foods we eat." He outlined a likely scenario for the evolution of highly spiced foods in countries where food-borne microbes thrive: "The first spice is added and it has a positive effect. Then a second microbe comes along and another spice is added, which has a positive effect, and so on, until a lot of spices are being used, but not so many that there are negative consequences."

He also noted that many spices that themselves have relatively weak antibiotic effects become much more potent when combined, for example, in chili powder (typically a mixture of red pepper, onion, paprika, garlic, cumin and oregano) and five-spice powder (pepper, cinnamon, anise, fennel and cloves). Lemon and lime juice, while weak inhibitors themselves, also have such synergistic effects, he said.

Dr. Paul Rozin, a psychologist who studies food and satiety at the University of Pennsylvania, suggested that a primary use of spices was to inject variety into an otherwise boring menu. He said, "When food is bland or monotonous, spices are used to trick the internal plumbing into thinking that we're eating different foods," which would help keep people from getting sick and tired of eating a lot of the same food.

Cheryl Ritenbaugh, an anthropologist who studies how food influences health at the Kaiser-Permanente Center for Health Research in Portland, Oregon, pointed out that chili peppers are a New World food that did not circulate worldwide until after the time of Columbus, so their use in many tropical countries may be too recent to support the Billing-Sherman theory. However, she said, "If the climate is hot and the food monotonous, people may not eat enough, and anything that would add flavor and kill bacteria would be very welcome."

Spicy foods may also enhance digestion. Dr. Marvin Harris, an anthropologist at the University of Florida in Gainesville, said foods made with chili peppers increase salivation, prepare the gut for receiving food, foster intestinal action and help to create a sense of fullness, which would be an evolutionary advantage in countries where food was relatively scarce.

Dr. Larry R. Beuchat, a microbiologist who studies food-borne pathogens and spoilage organisms at the University of Georgia's Center for Food Safety and Quality Enhancement in Griffin, Georgia, said that the Billing-Sherman hypothesis has merit. Even at the low levels used in recipes, plant chemicals have antimicrobial activity, he said, adding that the use of essential oils, which are oil-based extracts of plant chemicals, "is one of the oldest methods of preserving meat and was used in mummification."

Dr. Sherman pointed out that in large quantities, some of the antimicrobial chemicals found in spice plants are mutagens, carcinogens and teratogens, substances that can cause genetic damage and birth defects. This may be why women in the first trimester of pregnancy and children who are growing rapidly tend to avoid spicy foods, he said. "During rapid growth, even though there is still a danger of ingesting microbes, the risk of ingesting harmful plant compounds from spices might be worse," he suggested.

Dr. Sherman and Ms. Billing discounted competing explanations for the prevalence of spices in foods from hot climates. They wrote that because spices are consumed in tiny quantities, they provide little of nutritive value. Only hot peppers, but not most of the prominently used spices, induce sweating "and even chilies do not increase perspiration in many people."

That the use of spices evolved and spread simply because they disguise the smell or taste of spoiled foods makes little evolutionary sense because people who ate them would be more likely to get sick and die.

The researchers found no relationship between mean annual temperature and numbers of spices that grow in each country. Nor do tropical countries rely only on spices that are locally grown. "People do not use every spice that grows in their country, but they do use many spices that must be imported, and for centuries have gone to great lengths to obtain them," they wrote. Although pepper, for example, is one of the most frequently used spices in all thirty-six countries studied, it grows in only nine of them.

In further support of their argument, Dr. Sherman and Ms. Billing noted that "flavors of many widely used spices are not immediately appealing." Rather, people have to learn to like them. "The fact that parents encourage their children to eat (displeasing) spices, and that children come to prefer them by adolescence, strongly suggests that using spices is somehow beneficial," the researchers concluded.

Jane E. Brody, March 1998

CHINESE MEDICINE: PURVEYOR OF PILL AND POTION MIXES THE WEST AND THE EAST

As he navigates behind the counter at the Kamwo Herb and Tea Company, a bustling Chinese pharmacy on Grand Street in Manhattan's Chinatown, Tom Leung always weighs the freak-out factor. "Here's something that will definitely freak you out," he said as he nimbly assembled a prescription for an arthritic woman who was not well acquainted with traditional Chinese medicine. "Cicadas."

No debating that. The formula mandated a dosage of the shells of expired flylike serenading insects.

Usually, the prescription is bundled loosely for the patient to boil as tea and then strain. But Mr. Leung funneled these ingredients straight into a mammoth tea bag. "This is for a non-Chinese customer, and she might not be real happy about seeing a cicada going into her tea," he said. "My theory is you make people as comfortable as possible."

So goes his weekday world, as Mr. Leung works as a Chinese-style pharmacist sorting through drawers of dried sea horses, magnolia flowers, deer antler and licorice root, dispensing prescriptions from herbalists and acupuncturists.

Then there is the Western Tom Leung. On sporadic weekends, he fills prescriptions behind another counter. This one is at the pharmacy at either the Kmart at Pennsylvania Station or the Kmart at Astor Place, where he apportions pills into small bottles and keeps mum about the benefits of cicadas for the joints.

At a time when alternative medicine is increasingly intersecting with conventional medicine, Tom Leung's professional bifurcation is perhaps an inevitable by-product. In medicinal outlook, he is part Eastern, part Western, the ultimate hybrid pharmacist. It can make for complicated weeks. Indeed, Mr. Leung admits he sometimes finds himself mildly confused over which white coat he is wearing.

Someone will stop in at Kmart with a headache associated with dizziness and Mr. Leung points them to Tylenol or Motrin. If the same person visits Kamwo, Mr. Leung feels it his duty to recommend some chuan xiong and bai zhi, which happen to be roots. Such is pharmaceutical life when East meets West in the same body and neither yields.

"A customer came into Kmart last week and said he had trouble sleeping and relaxing," said Mr. Leung, a chipper, companionable man of twenty-eight. "Knowing the side effects of sleeping pills, I didn't want to just tell him to take Sominex or something. As a Kmart employee that day, I couldn't say, go buy these herbs. So I told the person less coffee in the afternoon and don't eat after nine at night."

Chinese medicine makes use of often disagreeable-tasting brews of herbs, grasses, bark, branches, chemicals and animal parts in a tradition that traces back thousands of years. By and large, prescriptions are boiled into a tea or soup and drunk. At Kamwo, a pharmacist wraps the herbs in a square piece of paper. They look like salad preparations, the beginnings of a bird's nest, something the cat dragged in.

Western medicine, of course, is pretty much all pills and liquids in a bottle.

Like a growing number of his customers, Mr. Leung believes in both the herb and the pill. He does not see a clash between Chinese and Western medicine, and thus he keeps a mortar and pestle in both worlds. When he has a minor ailment, he visits an acupuncturist or herbalist; for acute problems, he sees a Western doctor.

"In the past, it has been, you either believe in Chinese medicine or you believe in Western medicine," he said. "Over the last five years especially, I see more of 'I'll take the best of both worlds.' Personally, I'm right in the middle. I always tell people, if I have a headache, I'll take a Tylenol, no questions asked. But if I have a persistent sore throat, I'll take herbs. Herbs are better at treating the underlying cause. Western medicine is treating the symptom—the running nose."

Grand Street was choked with people, a cacophony of noise, and patrons, Chinese and non-Chinese alike, steadily drifted into Kamwo (the word means golden crop), a long, slender expanse crammed with jars and counters and drawers of herbal relief. Dead geckos hung on the wall (yes, they go into prescriptions too). Three employees were busily measuring out formulas.

Since Mr. Leung is by far the most fluent in English, he tackles most of the growing number of non-Chinese customers. In his two years at Kamwo, the non-Chinese business has jumped to nearly 20 percent from less than 5 percent.

A sinewy man wanted something for rheumatism. Mr. Leung said he had something for external use, but the customer did not want that. So Mr. Leung told him he needed a prescription from an acupuncturist.

"We get a lot of 'Hey, what herbs you got for a migraine?'" Mr. Leung said as he raked his hair with his fingers. "But it's not like Western medicine. You have to find out what the internal imbalance in the body is and then treat that imbalance."

Born in Hong Kong, Mr. Leung moved with his family to New York when he was six. His great-grandfather was an herbalist, as is his grandfather, as is his father, Shan Leung, who sees patients in the back of the Kamwo store.

The place has been in business since 1973 and is primarily owned by Tom Leung's uncle, Chou Leung, who is also an herbalist.

Growing up in America, Mr. Leung was uncertain whether he could make a living in Chinese medicine. It was appreciably less mainstream in the 1970s and 1980s, and so, with his parents' blessing, he pursued a pharmacy degree. He worked for three years at Walgreen's before getting restless. In 1995, he gravitated to Kamwo, where he is a manager as well as a pharmacist. Three nights a week, he takes classes to become an herbalist and acupuncturist.

Medicine—of the East and of the West—runs in the family. His sister is a pediatrician. His future brother-in-law is a Western-style internist in Chinatown. Mr. Leung's father sees him on the sly for serious ailments, for it is apostasy to some Chinese patients for their herbalist to go to a Western doctor.

Mr. Leung filled a woman's prescription "to clear dampness and break up the phlegm." Using a hand-held balance, he measured out some ban xia, a root, and pulverized it with a pestle. He added licorice, ginger, angelica—a dozen herbs in all.

In his dual world, there is the regulated Mr. Leung and the unregulated Mr. Leung. To be a Western pharmacist, a pharmacy degree and a license are required. Prescriptions must be signed by doctors.

To be an Eastern pharmacist selling herb formulas, you just need someone knowledgeable to show you how. Mr. Leung learned at a young age, mostly from his grandfather. He was putting together formulas when he was nine. There is no licensing requirement.

Prescriptions do not have to come from a doctor. The practice at Kamwo, though, is to fill only prescriptions signed by acupuncturists or herbalists. (Acupuncturists are licensed in New York; herbalists are not.)

At Kmart, he must concern himself with side effects. He must ascertain what other medications the patient is taking to be sure a new prescription does not cause a deadly mix. With herbs, he says, there is less worry.

"A formula may not work, but someone would not drop dead on the floor," he said. "There aren't really many side effects with herbs. There are some external formulas to soak your hands or feet in, and I make sure people know they're not for drinking."

Many conventional doctors complain that the efficacy and safety of herbs are unproven, but Mr. Leung feels the criticism is unfounded. "Listen, if honeysuckle were toxic, they would have found out in the last four thousand years," he said.

Last year, New York State banned ephedra, or ma huang, when sold in products aimed at achieving a drug high, for it has been linked to a number of deaths, though it is permitted in medications for asthma and other disorders. Kamwo sells it only by prescription.

There are certain herbs that do not interact well. Licorice root and hai zao, for instance, are not compatible. "You won't die," Mr. Leung said. "But it will make you pretty ill."

All told, Kamwo carries 1,500 herbs, and fills about two hundred to three hundred prescriptions a day, some of which come from around the country. Orders even arrive over the Internet. In September, an acupuncture clinic is due to open next door. Most formulas cost $4 to $5, and tend to consist of four to fifteen herbs, though Mr. Leung mixed one with thirty-four.

"Is this bad for the liver?" a man asked, holding up a box of Suan Zao Ren Tang, an over-the-counter product.

"No, that is a formula they use in China to calm your spirit," Mr. Leung said, adding, "It helps you sleep." The man took three boxes.

Someone asked about sea horses, and Mr. Leung said they strengthen the kidney and the kidney channels. Someone wondered about spotted deer antler and was advised that it gives you more qi, or energy.

A non-Asian couple stared transfixed at a row of antelope horns behind the glass counter.

Mr. Leung was amused. Out of earshot, this translator of Eastern medicine to Westerners and Western medicine to Easterners said, "Honestly, they're for show. In the past, they used them for convulsions and seizures, manifestations of internal wind. Nobody buys them now. But they create this atmosphere. People come in and say, 'Look at that!'"

N. R. Kleinfield, July 1997

A NAVIGATIONAL GUIDE TO THE
HERBAL HIGH SEAS

When the latest book on herbal remedies landed on my desk, my first reaction was to put it in the giveaway pile with all the rest of the home remedy books, especially after page 1 brought me face-to-face with cures like gin-soaked raisins for arthritis and Archway coconut macaroons for diarrhea.

But when I saw who wrote the book, *The People's Pharmacy Guide to Home and Herbal Remedies* (St. Martin's, $27.95), I decided to put aside skepticism. The authors, Joe Graedon, a pharmacologist, and Teresa Graedon, a medical anthropologist, have been writing sound and sensible books about drugs for nonscientists for more than twenty years. In their latest, the couple lay out not only the pluses but also the minuses of self-medication in language that is easy to understand. If you want a single source of good information without the usual hype, this is the book to choose.

As a skeptic of most of the claims made for herbs and dietary supplements, I had a hard time getting past the peripheral advice: garlic to get rid of fleas, cider vinegar to cure headaches and cherries to relieve gout. The Graedons do not say these home remedies necessarily work, certainly not for everyone, but they do say the remedies are harmless, so why not give them a try?

But once I moved on to the scientific information, I was more impressed. Readers should resist the temptation to jump to their favorite ailment before reading pages 7 through 22, which offer valuable precautions. The book "is not intended as a substitute for the medical advice of a physician," write the authors, who also warn that "home remedies are generally untested" and that "any symptom that persists or gets worse should be attended to by a physician."

As for interactions between herbal remedies and prescription drugs, the Graedons advise: "Please recognize that not all interactions have been discovered or reported in the literature," and "long-term side effects and interactions, in particular, have not been well explored."

Just as the Graedons' book was being released, the Food and Drug

Administration issued a warning that Saint-John's-wort causes "significant drug interaction" with the prescription drug Indinavir, used to treat HIV infection. And it was only last week that a conference sponsored in part by the National Institutes of Health called for regulation of medicinal herbs, though some speakers noted it might be too late. Americans spend an estimated $4 billion a year on herbal supplements, and the Graedons note that the industry is "virtually immune from regulation."

Despite these caveats, the authors think that "used sensibly, herbs and home remedies can be of great help in self-care" and that they "appear amazingly benign when compared with prescription medicines."

The book is divided into two parts: an alphabetical list of common ailments from asthma to warts, and a guide to herbal therapies from aloe to valerian.

A typical segment in the first section comes under the heading for insomnia. It discusses the impact of caffeine, exercise, relaxation, snacking and television, as well as the use of herbs like chamomile, valerian, hops, kava-kava and lavender. It also describes melatonin, a naturally occurring hormone that is crucial for setting the body's sleep cycle. The Graedons have some cautions about its use. That said, they fail to discuss the safety of using a hormone—any hormone—on a regular basis without medical supervision.

The section on asthma notes that the condition is so serious that "we do not believe its treatment is a do-it-yourself project." But, the authors write, adding vitamin C to the diet of someone under the care of a physician would not be risky, and some evidence suggests that vitamin C can be beneficial to lung function.

By contrast, the Graedons recommend against the Chinese herb ephedra, or ma huang, as a primary treatment for asthma, although many herbal reference books suggest it. They point out that its effects are short-lived and that it has a number of very serious side effects ranging from irregular heartbeat to death.

The second section of the book, which deals with herbal therapies, provides all the information about each herb in one place, including active ingredients, dose, special precautions, adverse effects and possible interactions. Under chamomile, for instance, readers will learn that it is used to treat digestive distress (see Peter Rabbit and chamomile tea) and as a mild sleep aid; that people who are allergic to ragweed and chrysanthemums probably shouldn't use it; and that ingesting a large amount of its dried flowers may cause vomiting.

As for gin-soaked raisins and Archway cookies, the Graedons don't pretend to know why some people find them useful, which is reason enough to recommend *The People's Pharmacy Guide to Home and Herbal Remedies* as the most sensible book of its kind.

Marian Burros, March 2000

SAINT-JOHN'S-WORT: WEED WHACKS DEPRESSION

The highly popular drug Prozac and its rival prescription medications may soon be in for competition in this country from a natural herb for the treatment of mild to moderately severe depression.

The herb, Saint-John's-wort, is already by far the favored therapy for depression in Germany, where it has been used therapeutically for centuries. In 1994, about 66 million daily doses of Saint-John's-wort were prescribed by German doctors, who turn to other drugs only when the herbal remedy fails to work.

Most of the research on the herb, which is also used to treat other common physical and emotional disorders, has been conducted in Germany. Researchers there report that it is decidedly better than placebos in medical trials and at least as good as some prescription antidepressants for treating the milder forms of depression. It is also much cheaper and appears to cause far fewer side effects than commonly prescribed antidepressants, making it a potentially preferable alternative to drugs like Prozac. While Prozac costs, on average, $80 a month, a regimen of Saint-John's-wort costs about $10 a month. And unlike Prozac, which causes distressing side effects in about one-quarter of patients, the herb has been shown in studies to cause side effects in fewer than 10 percent of patients, and, in most cases, those side effects are reported to be mild.

But before you dump your Prozac, Paxil, Zoloft or other prescribed antidepressant in favor of this increasingly popular herb, a more discriminating look at the evidence—pro and con—for the safety and effectiveness of Saint-John's-wort is in order.

Saint-John's-wort ("wort" is Old English for plant) is a weed, *Hypericum perforatum*, that grows prolifically on disturbed ground like roadsides. It was named for Saint John the Baptist, whose birthday is celebrated on June 24, when the plant usually puts forth its yellow blooms. Like other plants, it contains many different chemicals, which alone or in combination may account for its reputed therapeutic effects. Scientists do not yet know which substances in Saint-John's-wort are responsible for its apparent antidepressant activity or how they may act. Neither is it known why Saint-John's-wort has been reported to have antiviral activity, as well as the ability to relieve menstrual discomfort and winter blues and to bolster immunity.

What they do know is that there is more to Saint-John's-wort than hearsay and health food store claims. A review of twenty-three well-designed clinical trials published in 1997 in the *British Medical Journal* concluded, based on fifteen placebo-controlled trials, that extracts of Saint-John's-wort "are more effective than placebo for the treatment of mild to moderately severe depressive disorders."

The review also found evidence from eight other studies that Saint-John's-wort may work as well as some other drugs in countering mild depression, but the research team, from Munich, Germany, and San Antonio, called for more exacting studies comparing the herb with standard antidepressants like Prozac.

The researchers noted that the studies of Saint-John's-wort involved relatively small numbers of patients and that the diagnosis of depression varied from study to study and did not always adhere to the stringent criteria used in the United States. Furthermore, the preparation (liquid extracts or capsules or tablets made from ground-up plants) differed from study to study, as did the medication's potency and dosages, and none of the trials lasted longer than eight weeks. So while few short-term side effects were reported, the possible long-term hazards of Saint-John's-wort remain unknown. Although no adverse effects have been detected in long-term users in Germany, only a long-term controlled clinical study can give the herb a clean bill of health.

There is no requirement that such studies be done before the herb is sold in this country. Since it is sold as a dietary supplement, the Food and Drug Administration does not approve or disapprove it, and no documentation is required of its safety or usefulness, the kind of information required for prescription antidepressants. Because it is classified as a dietary supplement, its label may not claim that it has a specific effect in alleviating depression.

There are side effects that have been associated with Saint-John's-wort, including mild gastrointestinal discomfort (usually relieved by taking the medication with meals and a large glass of liquid), fatigue, dry mouth, dizziness, skin rashes and itching. Such side effects were reported by 2.4 percent of patients in one large study. At high doses, it may also increase sensitivity to sunlight, an effect that so far has been found only in cattle that graze heavily on it.

On the other hand, the prescription antidepressants commonly cause distressing side effects like sexual dysfunction, diarrhea, difficulty with concentration, a decrease in reaction time, drowsiness and bad reactions to alcohol.

Saint-John's-wort is not for everyone, and no one who is depressed should start taking it without first consulting a mental health practitioner who is expert in diagnosing and treating depression. That is especially important for people who are severely depressed or suicidal, because Saint-John's-wort may not be potent enough to counter severe depression. Also, even mild depression may require more than medication. Some form of psychotherapy is often needed to prevent relapses.

If you are now on a prescription antidepressant, do not add Saint-John's-wort to the regimen or abandon the prescribed drug in its favor. When combined with other serotonin-enhancing drugs, like Prozac, Saint-John's-wort may result in a serotonin overload, causing sweating, agitation, confusion and tremor. See your doctor before making any changes.

Saint-John's-wort should not be used by pregnant or nursing women or young children because of the lack of safety information.

Keep in mind that the FDA does not approve the preparations of Saint-John's-wort on the shelves of health food stores and pharmacies and that no agency checks these preparations for contents or potency. You are at the mercy of the manufacturer; the bottle may or may not contain what the label says.

As for dosages, that is also a guess. Dr. Jonathan Zuess, a doctor in Arizona who has studied herbalism and who wrote *The Natural Prozac Program* (Three Rivers Press, 1997, $10), favors the alcohol extract — about three-fourths of a teaspoon a day divided into two or three doses — that has been used in most of the German studies. If a capsule is chosen, look for brands containing 300 milligrams of the raw herb, standardized to contain 0.3 percent hypericin, one of the herb's most active ingredients. Take one capsule a day, less if you are older than sixty-five. For further guidance on products, consult *Hypericum (St. John's Wort) and Depression*, by Dr. Harold H. Bloomfield et al., from Prelude Press.

You should also keep in mind that, like prescription antidepressants, Saint-John's-wort does not work right away. It takes about four weeks to have a significant antidepressant effect, though you are likely to notice some improvement within two weeks. Since long-term safety studies are lacking, Dr. Zuess does not recommend the use of Saint-John's-wort for more than a year.

Jane E. Brody, September 1997

Later studies have found that Saint-John's-wort can interfere with the action of antirejection drugs taken by transplant recipients and antiviral drugs used to treat HIV infection; those patients should avoid the herb.

KAVA: NUMBS MOUTH, TASTES LIKE DIRT, BUT OH SO SOOTHING

A pill that calms you down without making you dull, sleepy or addicted? It may seem too good to be true, but the prospect of inner peace with no strings attached is tempting more and more Americans to try kava, an herbal product derived from the roots of a pepper plant grown on Fiji, Vanuatu and other Pacific islands.

To many people who suffer from anxiety and insomnia, kava might seem an ideal "natural" alternative to Valium and the other potentially addicting drugs prescribed to soothe ragged nerves. Kava is said to have been used for thousands of years in the Pacific to help people relax and socialize. Unlike alcohol, which can make people boisterous or belligerent, kava users report that the herb calms them without dulling the mind or causing hangovers.

There have been no scientific studies of kava in human beings in the United States. Nonetheless, Americans spent $15 million on kava in 1996, and twice that much in 1997, according to the *Nutrition Business Journal*, which projected sales of almost $50 million for 1998. Ed Smith, president of Herb Pharm, in Williams, Oregon, one of about forty American companies that sell kava, said, "Kava was virtually unknown three years ago, and now our sales are going through the roof."

The wholesale price, $14 to $20 for a kilogram of dried root (2.2 pounds), nearly doubled in the last few years, Mr. Smith said. Kava has become the subject of several popular books, and numerous Web sites sell it.

Scientific trials of kava have been conducted overseas, especially in Germany, and have found it helpful in alleviating anxiety and easing symptoms of menopause, like hot flashes, sleep disturbances and emotional problems. The active ingredients are chemicals called kavalactones, which have a mildly depressing effect on the nervous system. The German researchers found no side effects or withdrawal symptoms when people stopped taking kava.

But important questions about kava have yet to be answered. It is not known whether the products sold in the United States have the same properties as the ones tested in Germany or the traditional kava-based drinks prepared fresh in the Pacific. Researchers also do not know whether kava can be used safely for a long time or whether it can be combined with other drugs or natural products. Because it depresses the nervous system, some doctors warn patients not to take it with alcohol or drugs like Valium that have the same effect.

Kava is not totally benign. Road signs on some Pacific islands warn people not to drink kava and drive. In addition, there have been rare instances of kava abuse among Pacific islanders, resulting in problems with the skin and liver. All apparently clear up when the person gives up kava.

The original kava is a far cry from the hermetically sealed bottles now stocked in American health food stores. An eighteenth-century traveler to Polynesia wrote that kava was prepared in a "most disgustful manner." The freshly dug roots were cut up and chewed (preferably by virgins), spat into a communal bowl and mixed with coconut milk or water. The resulting fluid was then strained and passed around. People had such a good time drinking kava that Christian missionaries tried to ban it.

On some islands, kava was pounded rather than chewed. Traditionally, only men drank it. Westerners who have tried kava say it is bitter and tastes like dirt. It also numbs the mouth. In his book, *Kava: Medicine Hunting in Paradise* (Park Street Press, 1996), Chris Kilham wrote that he was glad he had worn shoes to a kava bar on Vanuatu, because the patrons did so much spitting to get the taste of kava out of their mouths that there wasn't a dry spot on the floor.

Needless to say, the kava sold in the United States is not prepared in the traditional manner. The roots are dried and ground by machines into a powder that can be sold as is, for blending into drinks; putting into pills or capsules; or making into an alcohol-based extract.

Dr. Michael J. Balick, curator of the Institute of Economic Botany at the New York Botanical Garden, said the demand for kava was leading growers in Micronesia to begin cultivating upland forests that should be preserved as watersheds. The Nature Conservancy, he said, is trying to encourage the growers to use low-lying tracts that are not so critical to the region.

Kava is sold not as a drug but as a dietary supplement and, as a result, is largely exempt from the control of the Food and Drug Administration. Supplements, unlike drugs, do not have to be proved safe and effective and are not tested or inspected by any regulatory agency. The FDA does not usually investigate a supplement unless people report problems. The agency has no evidence of health problems caused by kava, a spokeswoman said.

Under FDA rules, manufacturers may not claim that their supplements can treat or prevent disease. They can, however, make so-called structure-function claims, saying, for instance, that a product promotes strong bones or supports the immune system.

For kava, Mr. Smith of Herb Pharm said: "We can make somewhat nebulous claims. We can say it enhances well-being, but we can't say it relieves anxiety." Nonetheless, he said, people are buying it in the hope that it will ease anxiety.

If he could say anything he wanted, Mr. Smith said: "I would love to put on the label that it could be used for relieving anxiety. I know it does."

An Internet site devoted to inquiries about kava listed 660 messages in early October. The writers ranged from people seeking help with anxiety to those looking for a new way to get high. Some described the results as pleasant, but others called kava useless. One wrote: "Got nothing from the first few small hits, then I downed the remaining two-thirds of the bottle and got a very mild, slightly relaxing effect for a couple hours."

Dr. Roberta Lee, an internist in Tucson, Arizona, who became familiar with kava while practicing medicine in the Pacific, was not surprised by that story. There is no way of knowing how much active ingredient was in the product, she said, or how high the person's anxiety level might have been.

Still, Dr. Lee recommends kava to some of her patients. She said its effects were subtle, and that she urged her patients to use brands from large European manufacturers, which she declined to name. Because kava is considered a drug in Europe, she said, it is more carefully regulated there than in the United States.

"I worry about patients having access to these herbal medications without a prescription or any regulation or even general advice," she said. "People in health food stores are giving advice, and they're not pharmacists or medical people."

Dr. Lee would like to see the European studies of kava repeated in the United States. "I want to know what works on a sort of moderate anxiety level," she said. "My hunch is that it probably wouldn't be appropriate for someone with very major anxiety."

Ultimately, she said, if kava does prove useful, it will be "just one tool" in treating anxiety, along with diet, exercise, counseling and other forms of therapy.

Denise Grady, October 1998

THE HIGH PRICE OF EPHEDRA'S BUZZ

The herb is called ephedra, or ma huang, and it comes from a shrub-like plant grown widely in Asia. It can be found in more than two hundred diet supplements, in pills and powders, drinks and diet bars, for sale in health food stores and on the Internet.

Its advocates say it decreases appetite, raises metabolism, improves concentration, burns fat and even enhances sexual performance. In thousands of postings on the Internet, users praise it for raising their energy, helping them lose weight and sharpening their muscle tone.

But to its critics, ephedra is a potentially dangerous substance that urgently needs more study and regulation. They point out that its active ingredient, ephedrine, is a central nervous system stimulant similar to amphetamine, and they say reactions to it can vary widely.

Ephedrine has been widely studied over the past few years, and studies suggest that it can produce a wide array of possible side effects, including anxiety, insomnia, high blood pressure, rapid heartbeat, psychosis, kidney damage, dependency, heart attack, stroke and death. And the Food and Drug Administration says it has received hundreds of reports from physicians, health authorities and others about adverse reactions to ephedrine-based products.

Critics and proponents alike agree on one thing: ephedra is flying off the shelves. Metabolife International, Inc., a five-year-old San Diego company that sells an ephedra-based pill called Metabolife 356, said 1999 sales were expected to reach $900 million.

A critic, Dr. Jacqueline Berning, a professor of nutrition at the University of Colorado, whose clients include many professional athletes, says the use of ephedrine-based products is "rampant among athletes," even though they have been banned by the National Collegiate Athletic Association and the United States Olympic Committee.

Ephedra's active ingredient, ephedrine, has been in over-the-counter cold and asthma medications since the 1920s, and the ephedra plant has been used for thousands of years in Chinese medicine. Still, the combined effects of the herbal potpourri found in many diet supplements have not been studied. While over-the-counter drugs are subject to Food and Drug Administration regulation, herbal supplements are essentially unregulated, assumed safe unless proved otherwise.

The ephedrine debate raises questions about the efficacy and safety of a product from an unregulated industry still in its infancy. "The public has a blind spot with the herbals," said Dr. Bill Gurley, of the College of Pharmacy at the University of Arkansas. "I have a feeling over time enough serious cases of addiction will pile up and enough adverse events will be reported to change that perception."

Dr. Gurley conducted a study that suggested wide variations in product ingredients and quality. "Ephedra supplements are derived from plants that can contain any number of ephedrine-like alkaloids," he said. "These alkaloids vary not only in pharmacological activity and potency, but certain combinations may be additive or synergistic in their effect."

In testing nineteen ephedrine-based supplements, Dr. Gurley said, he found wide variations in alkaloid content. Some products contained significantly less of the active ingredients than listed on the label, some significantly more.

In 1997, in response to reports of adverse reactions, the Food and Drug Administration proposed restricting doses of ephedra to 8 milligrams at a time and 24 milligrams a day, and prohibiting the addition of caffeine to ephedrine products. (The American Herbal Products Association, a trade organization that sets standards and guidelines for the diet supplement industry, recommends that dosages not exceed 25 milligrams at a time, or 100 milligrams a day; a Metabolife pill has 12 milligrams, according to the label.)

After a lobbying effort by the diet supplement industry, a congressional subcommittee asked the General Accounting Office to investigate the research behind the FDA's proposal. In August 1999, the accounting office issued a report assailing the agency's findings as sloppy science. "The FDA needs to provide stronger evidence on the relationship between the intake of dietary supplements containing ephedrine alkaloids and the occurrence of adverse reactions," the report said.

In recent years, ephedrine-based products figured prominently in two widely publicized cases, both involving deaths.

In 1999, in British Columbia, a judge ruled that Julia Campagna, a twenty-eight-year-old woman from Kirkland, Washington, was not criminally responsible in the deaths of two teenage girls in a fiery car crash near the United States border in May 1998. Court-appointed psychiatrists testified that Ms. Campagna had been in a state of psychosis, a reaction to the ephedrine-based supplement Xenedrine, which she had taken for five days.

In 1998, Anne Marie Capati, a thirty-seven-year-old knitwear designer from Huntington, New York, died after suffering a stroke at a fitness club in Manhattan. Ms. Capati, who suffered from high blood pressure, had been taking Thermadrene, an ephedra supplement manufactured by SportPharma of Concord, California. According to her husband, who sued the manufacturer, the fitness club and his wife's personal trainer, she had been taking the recommended dose for five days, "to lose the last five pounds and firm up."

The warning label on Thermadrene (and many other brands, including Metabolife) makes clear that ephedrine-based products should not be taken by people with certain medical conditions, including high blood pressure.

In an interview, Michael Ellis, the chief executive of Metabolife and a board member of the American Herbal Products Association, strongly defended ephedrine-based supplements. "I read about the Long Island woman's death, and it's tragic," he said. "This case points out why we need consistency in the warning labels. But let's keep this in perspective."

With millions of people taking ephedrine each year, Mr. Ellis argued, a few cases of adverse effects are to be expected. "Some people die from eating peanut butter or strawberries," he said. "Everything carries risk." He has urged the FDA to appoint a working group of scientists, consumers, herbalists and industry representatives to develop new guidelines for dietary supplements containing ephedra and other herbs.

As for the purity of Metabolife, he said: "We believe we are responsible. We label correctly, and we have a nonprofit third party give us a certification of good manufacturing practices."

Mr. Ellis was at the center of an ephedra-related controversy. After being interviewed for the ABC News program *20/20*, and anticipating a hostile report about his company and product in 1999, Mr. Ellis took pre-emptive action.

In a $1.5 million advertising campaign Metabolife announced the creation of a Web site posting the unedited seventy-minute interview. Commercial spots ran on 1,500 radio stations, and there were a number of full-page newspaper advertisements (including one in the *New York Times*).

Eleven years ago, Mr. Ellis, a former police officer, was arrested in San Diego and charged with using ephedrine to produce methamphetamine, a highly addictive street drug. He pleaded guilty to using a telephone in the trafficking of drugs and was sentenced to five years' probation.

"I did something very wrong, something very much out of character, and something I am very sorry about," he said, and later added: "Metabolife has been looked at inside and out. We have a report from a DEA-approved lab that shows you can't make methamphetamine out of Metabolife. Obviously we are not breaking any laws."

Mr. Ellis said he was hopeful that the attention would help him make a point. "If this product and industry are going to have longevity, we have to come out and say, 'You can't pop supplements like they are carrots; this is another form of medicine.'"

The sentiment is shared by many mainstream physicians. "The public should be informed," said Dr. Gurley, of the University of Arkansas. "A drug is a drug whether it's from a natural source or you make it in a laboratory."

Mary Duffy, October 1999

[4]

They Are Essential, but
Not in Megadoses

Vitamins and Minerals

Diseases due to vitamin deficiency were first described centuries ago. Historical accounts tell of conditions like scurvy and beriberi, though the authors could not have known that deficiencies of vitamins C and B$_1$ or thiamine, were to blame. By the 1740s it was known that citrus fruits could somehow keep sailors from getting scurvy on long voyages, and in the late 1800s doctors realized that sailors could also avoid beriberi, which affects the nervous system, by eating meats and vegetables, or unpolished rice; it was later determined that polishing rice removes thiamine, which is contained in the bran and hull. By the 1920s, scientists had begun to identify specific vitamins. All are substances that the body must have; without them, illness will occur.

Most vitamins work with enzymes, which are proteins that help to speed up essential chemical reactions in the body. The vitamins themselves are neither protein nor enzyme; most are classified as coenzymes, molecules that attach to enzymes and enable them to do their jobs. Some minerals function in the same way.

For decades, doctors and nutritionists have insisted that people in well-nourished, affluent societies like the United States had little or no need to take extra vitamins or minerals, because a balanced diet would provide all their needs. Moreover, white flour and cereals in the United States are fortified with B vitamins, and vitamin D is added to milk. Researchers have pointed to studies showing that people who take extra vitamins do not live longer or have less risk of cancer than those who do not bother with the pills. Experts warn, too, that overdoses of some vitamins can be dangerous: too much vitamin E may contribute to bleeding, for instance, and excess vitamin A can cause headaches, liver and bone damage and a host of other problems. High doses of vitamin C or folate may interfere with drugs used to treat cancer. Supplements of beta-carotene, which is made into vitamin A in the body, have been linked to an increased risk of cancer.

But along with the warnings about excess come new findings that some people actually can benefit by taking certain vitamins, either because they do not eat a balanced diet or because conditions like pregnancy increase their requirements for certain nutrients. Folic acid taken before and in the earliest stages of pregnancy, for instance, helps to prevent devastating birth defects of the brain and spinal cord. Folic acid can also help to lower blood levels of homocysteine, a substance linked to heart disease and found at dangerous elevations in many people. Research has also found that many elderly people are deficient in vitamin D and may need supplements to avoid the bone-thinning disorder osteoporosis.

Despite the evidence that supplements can be useful for some people, most nutrition experts stand by classic advice that no supplement can take the place of a varied diet, high in fruits, vegetables and whole grains. Not only does such a diet provide substances known to be essential, but it also may supply important nutrients that have not yet been identified.

IN THE GRIP OF VITAMIN MANIA

Whatever health-conscious consumers might be looking for, there is a vitamin or mineral pill that promises it. Products for sale purport to offer cancer protection, a hardier heart, extra energy, enhanced immunity, less stress, a longer life, an antidote to pollution, stronger bones, less body fat, relief from premenstrual syndrome, athletic prowess and heightened sexual powers.

"Vitamania," as some critics call it, is sweeping the country, with sales of vitamins and minerals soaring to records.

An estimated 100 million Americans are spending $6.5 billion a year on vitamin and mineral pills and potions, up from $3 billion in 1990, according to the Council for Responsible Nutrition in Washington, a trade group for the vitamin supplement industry. Consumers are, in effect, volunteering for a vast, largely unregulated experiment with substances that may be helpful, harmful or simply ineffective.

The labels on the bewildering array of vitamin bottles in a drugstore or health food store give few clues that the products can be harmful as well as helpful. And they do not mention that because the Food and Drug Administration considers vitamins and minerals "dietary supplements," no testing for safety or usefulness—or even for whether the supplements contain what they say they do—is required before they are marketed.

Clear and consistent information about vitamins and minerals is hard to get, even from experts in nutrition, because of a lack of good long-term studies, or from the government, which has a bewildering array of standards.

"No rational person can understand this stuff," said Dr. Marion Nestle, chairman of the department of nutrition and food studies at New York University. "All the different numbers are almost guaranteed to make the situation more confusing rather than less."

The answers about how much of any vitamin a person needs often depend on the person's age, sex and stage of life. Nor is there a consensus about whether taking vitamins and minerals in addition to food is valuable for a person who is eating a relatively healthy diet.

Some facts are not in dispute. Vitamin and mineral pills can reverse or prevent deficiencies that can result in diseases like scurvy and rickets. But the questions that most Americans want answered are whether vitamin and mineral pills will fend off cancer, heart disease and osteoporosis and lead to overall well-being and longer life.

There are no easy answers. Nutrition studies are filled with hints but few conclusions. Current evidence indicates some serious shortfalls in the consumption of essential vitamins and minerals, especially by young women and the elderly. And there are tantalizing indications that there could be significant health advantages from taking supplements of some vitamins and minerals in doses larger than those needed to prevent outright deficiencies.

At the same time, however, there are risks when nutrients are taken separately from the foods that contain them and in doses far larger than the body was designed to process. For the average healthy person who consumes a variety of foods, there is scant evidence that vitamin and mineral supplements are beneficial. Even for segments of the population who may need more vitamins—smokers, people who are ill or poorly nourished, the elderly and pregnant women—the long-term benefits are unclear at best.

And national surveys by government and university scientists have shown that most of the people who take vitamins are those who are least likely to need extra nutrients: nonsmokers who do not drink heavily. They also consume more nutrients from foods, eat more fruits and vegetables, are better educated and have higher personal incomes than people who do not take vitamin and mineral pills.

Despite all those advantages, vitamin takers do not live longer or suffer fewer cancer deaths than those who do not take vitamins, according to a thirteen-year study of 10,758 Americans. A research team from the Centers for Disease Control and Prevention in Atlanta reported in 1993 that the study "found no evidence of increased longevity among vitamin and mineral supplement users in the United States." The team also failed to find any mortality benefits from supplements among people with special nutritional needs, like smokers, heavy drinkers and people with chronic diseases. And there is little, if any, evidence that taking vitamin and mineral supplements can compensate for dietary deficiencies that result from careless eating habits.

Furthermore, there are known dangers of vitamin use. High doses of vitamin E can interfere with the action of vitamin K, which promotes blood clotting. Large amounts of calcium can limit the absorption of iron and perhaps other trace elements. Zinc can reduce the level of copper in the body, impair immune responses and decrease the level of protective high-density lipoproteins in the blood, often called the "good" choles-terol. Folic acid can react badly with anticonvulsant medications and mask signs of a B_{12} deficiency. Iron supplements can be deadly to small children. In fact, the most common cause of poisoning deaths among children is not caustic cleaning agents or aspirin, but iron supplements intended for adult use.

There is unfortunately only one simple path through the vitamin and mineral maze. And it is to follow the same boring but tried-and-true advice that parents and health classes have been giving out for ages. Eat a balanced and varied diet that is low in fat and high in fruits and vegeta-bles and complex carbohydrates.

The current boom in the vitamin and mineral business got a lift in October 1994, when Congress passed the Dietary Supplement Health and Education Act, which for the most part keeps the FDA's hands off vitamin and mineral supplements unless something goes wrong.

Matthew Patsky, an analyst with the investment firm of Adams, Hark-ness & Hill in Boston, follows the broad field of dietary supplements, which includes vitamins, minerals and herbs, hormones like melatonin and hard-to-classify substances like shark cartilage. All are somehow considered "dietary," even those that would not normally be part of any-one's diet.

Mr. Patsky said in an interview that the stocks of the manufacturers of dietary supplements that he follows, which dropped in 1994, surged 70 percent in 1995, 57 percent in 1996 and 42 percent in the first half of 1997. The business "wildly outperformed the overall market and contin-ues to do so in 1997," he said.

The dietary supplement law was passed after a struggle between the FDA and the manufacturers. The agency, in reevaluating its labeling rules, had been planning to apply existing regulations for items like drugs to vitamins, minerals, herbal preparations and other supplements. Those rules would have prevented manufacturers from making health claims of any sort for any supplements without agency approval. The industry responded with intensive lobbying, aided by a letter-writing campaign by consumers who feared that government rules would limit their access to supplements of all kinds.

An end result, the 1994 law, was something of a compromise. Labels on vitamin and mineral products cannot make claims that a product cures a disease or has a specific beneficial health effect without special FDA approval. The law does, however, allow general statements on the label about a vitamin's or mineral's function in the body.

The agency agreed to allow companies to list direct health benefits for only two supplements: calcium, to prevent bone loss, and the B vitamin folic acid for pregnant women, to prevent certain birth defects involving the brain and nervous system, including spina bifida.

In contrast, the label on a bottle of vitamin A capsules may say "essential for the normal function of vision," but it cannot claim that the product will prevent or treat vision problems. Vitamin B_1 might be described as playing "a vital role in nerve function," but it cannot be called a neurological treatment.

Not that the lack of specific claims on labels has stopped people from assuming that the products offer therapeutic benefits, based on meager evidence, anecdotes and, sometimes, their doctors' recommendations, or based on extrapolations of the nutrients' normal roles in the body. Claims that products have direct benefits are made in many health magazines and newsletters, over the radio, by other media "experts" and by some employees of health food stores.

Faced with a growing need for more research, the National Institutes of Health, at the behest of Congress, established an Office of Dietary Supplements in November 1995 to promote scientific study of dietary supplements. Although there are forty known essential nutrients, almost all vitamins and minerals, "there are close to one thousand dietary supplements," said the office's director, Dr. Bernadette Marriott. "Where do we begin?"

Dr. Marriott, a specialist in nutrition and behavior who had been deputy director of the Food and Nutrition Board of the National Academy of Sciences, said she saw her role as helping to stimulate research on the role of supplements in fostering optimal health.

Meanwhile, the consumer who delves deeply into the guidelines for taking vitamins and minerals finds that different amounts of nutrients are suggested for people of different ages, weights and sexes, and that experts disagree about the amounts of vitamins needed and the amounts in various foods.

The Food and Nutrition Board, which sets recommended intakes of vitamins and minerals, in 1997 revised the Recommended Dietary Allowances, which vary for different people, and created guidelines called Dietary References Intakes to reflect, in part, the new interest in vitamins and minerals and their role in preventing disease. In addition to the quantities needed to head off nutrient deficiencies, the board created a separate listing of higher amounts for some nutrients that appear to have important roles in preventing serious diseases and promoting optimal health.

The board's Committee on the Scientific Evaluation of Dietary Reference Intakes said it would "consider how the risk of chronic disease can be related quantitatively to nutrient intakes and dietary patterns."

Calcium recommendations were adjusted upward, to higher levels that might help prevent osteoporosis rather than merely avoiding a calcium deficiency. In addition, the committee issued new recommended intakes in 1997 for phosphorus, magnesium, vitamin D and fluoride. It expected to develop the same guidelines for all nutrients and for food components like fiber and phytoestrogens, plant-derived hormones.

But the DRIs are not the numbers that most people see. The FDA requires the makers of vitamins and minerals to print the agency's Reference Daily Intakes.

That list is derived from the numbers of the Food and Nutrition Board and is loosely meant to be an amount that would stave off deficiency in a healthy adult. But these are not true recommendations, and some are, in fact, higher than the board's recommendations.

Details on any given vitamins aside, experts agree that many, and perhaps most, Americans are shortchanging themselves on one or more essential nutrients and that in the process they may compromise their chances for living long, healthy lives.

"The style of eating in this country has changed dramatically in the last decade," Dr. Marriott observed. "There's a lot more eating out, which is bound to affect nutrient intake. Americans are fatter than ever, but that doesn't necessarily mean they are well nourished."

Most people who are interested in supplements do not focus on avoiding deficiencies but rather hope to achieve more subtle and often long-term health effects, like improved stamina, protection against heart disease and cancer, and treatment of a whole host of conditions, like carpal tunnel syndrome and premenstrual tension. Some of the goals are reasonable; some are not.

The National Cancer Institute maintains that if Americans consumed at least five servings of fruits and vegetables a day, they would be most likely to take in the amounts of nutrients linked, in laboratory and population studies, to protection against several major cancers and that they would not have to worry about pills. But with the national clamoring for hamburgers, french fries and pizza, only 15 percent of Americans eat that many daily servings of nutrient-packed foods.

Such nutrients can also lower coronary risk. About a third of middle-age and elderly people have high blood levels of an amino acid, homocysteine, which studies suggest may be as important as smoking and even more important than cholesterol as a risk factor for heart disease and stroke. Homocysteine levels rise when a diet is relatively deficient in certain B vitamins, particularly folic acid, which is primarily found in dried beans and peas and dark green leafy vegetables, as well as B_6 and B_{12}.

This is one case where there is strong support for taking supplements, said Dr. Jeffrey Blumberg, a professor of nutrition at Tufts University. "These people should be doing two things," he said, "eating more foods containing B vitamins and taking a B-complex supplement. Even though we don't yet have placebo-controlled clinical trials to prove it, the data are compelling enough now to justify people doing something about it."

Dr. Blumberg is a strong advocate for bringing nutrition into the medical mainstream, and he said he hoped that researchers determined what levels of vitamins would improve overall health.

"We're seeing a paradigm shift in thinking beyond the minimum nutrient intakes to prevent deficiencies to levels that can promote health and prevent chronic diseases," he said.

The Nationwide Food Consumption Survey, conducted in 1987 and 1988 among 5,884 adults by the Department of Agriculture and analyzed by Dr. Suzanne P. Murphy, a research nutritionist at the University of California at Berkeley, revealed that 22 percent of those surveyed were eating diets that provided at least two-thirds of the recommended daily amounts of fifteen essential vitamins and minerals. There were deficiencies of nutrients like calcium, zinc, folic acid, magnesium and vitamins A, B_6, C and E. The most poorly nourished were young women nineteen to twenty-four. For women twenty and older, average intakes were below the recommended amounts for six nutrients: vitamins B_6 and E, calcium, magnesium, iron and zinc. For men, there were deficiencies in zinc and magnesium. Fewer than one-fourth of the women and fewer than half of the men consumed the recommended amounts of calcium, magnesium and zinc. The data of the 1994 Food Consumption Survey showed little or no improvement over the earlier findings, Dr. Murphy said.

Can vitamins and minerals in pills compensate for dietary deficiencies that result from careless eating habits? Most experts, even those who believe in supplementing a seemingly balanced diet, say no. They emphasize that there are many health-promoting substances in foods other than vitamins and minerals and that haphazard diets are likely to be unhealthy, even if people use vitamin and mineral supplements to bring their consumption of essential nutrients up to the recommended levels.

Though doctors, who are largely unschooled in matters of nutrition, often shy away from all megadoses, some studies by nationally recognized researchers have indicated that extra doses of some vitamins and minerals can help prevent several devastating health problems, including serious birth defects, heart disease, sight-robbing eye disorders, osteoporosis and even some cancers.

In 1970, Dr. Linus Pauling announced that megadoses of vitamin C could prevent the common cold. Although its ability to prevent colds has yet to be proved in a well-designed scientific study, vitamin C in large doses has been shown to attenuate the symptoms of many colds. But its more important role may be as an antioxidant, a substance capable of defusing highly reactive agents that can injure cell membranes or genes or transform innocuous chemicals into damaging ones. Nutrients known to be antioxidants include vitamin E, beta-carotene and selenium.

In studies at the Southwestern University Medical Center in Dallas, researchers showed that megadoses of vitamin E—amounts way beyond those to prevent a deficiency—could block the change in low-density lipoprotein cholesterol that allows it to be deposited on artery walls. Other laboratory studies have documented the anticlotting action of vitamin E. And a number of large long-term studies in men and women have correlated high intakes of vitamin E with protection against heart disease and strokes caused by blood clots.

As for selenium, a study of six hundred men found that taking a daily supplement of 200 micrograms for ten years dramatically reduced the incidence of prostate, esophagus, colon-rectum and lung cancers and cut total cancer deaths in half. Earlier studies had linked a low intake of selenium to an increased risk of developing heart attacks, strokes and other diseases related to high blood pressure.

Thus far, however, virtually all the evidence for health benefits derived from supplements of individual nutrients or groups of nutrients is considered suggestive but not conclusive. Until, and unless, long-term studies are performed on large numbers of healthy people who are randomly assigned to take supplements or placebos, the evidence remains indefinite. Given the enormous cost of studies that are years long, the definitive studies may never be conducted.

Attempts to counter illness with vitamin supplements can also backfire. Dr. Larry Norton, medical director of the Lauder Breast Cancer Center at the Memorial Sloan-Kettering Cancer Center in Manhattan, said research at his institution showed that large doses of vitamin C could blunt the beneficial effects of chemotherapy for breast cancer. The research showed that breast cancer cells had large numbers of receptors, or docking places, for vitamin C, suggesting that the vitamin acted like a growth tonic for the cancer cells.

And a recent experiment showed that free radicals, chemicals that damage cells in ways that may lead to cancer, are also necessary for some of the mechanisms that stop cancer once it gets going. So a substance like vitamin C, in large doses, could have unpredictable effects. It is also known that folic acid can negate the effects of methotrexate, a drug used to treat cancer.

"I'm not antivitamin," Dr. Norton said. "But the safest thing to do is to have a healthy lifestyle and consume vitamins in foods."

An excess of a vitamin or mineral can sometimes be just as harmful as a deficiency, whether or not a person is already ill. Nutrients known to be harmful when excess amounts are consumed include vitamins A, D and B_6; the minerals zinc and selenium, and perhaps even vitamins C and E. Too much vitamin A can cause headaches from increased brain pressure, liver and bone damage, hair loss, skin disorders, psychiatric symptoms and, when taken in early pregnancy, birth defects. Too much B_6 can damage nerves. Too much vitamin C can interfere with tests for blood in the stool. And in men and postmenopausal women, who tend to accumulate iron in their bodies, supplements containing iron could result in heart disease, cancer and serious infections.

For the majority of vitamins and minerals in tablets and capsules that are sold in pharmacies and health food stores, the numerous hints of benefits far exceed the facts. In its most recent position statement on supplements, issued in January 1996, the American Dietetic Association, the nation's largest organization of nutrition professionals, advised, "The best nutritional strategy for promoting optimal health and reducing the risk of chronic disease is to obtain adequate nutrients from a wide variety of foods."

The reason is that there are many unknown compounds in foods that can have powerful biological effects, like preventing cancer. Many dietary experts now question the wisdom of isolating single nutrients from the usual company they keep in foods.

That concern was fueled by two large long-term studies that have seriously tempered enthusiasm for a very popular supplement, beta-carotene, a nutrient in fruits and vegetables that the body converts to vitamin A. Beta-carotene is a potent antioxidant that has long been heralded as a possible preventive of common lethal cancers. Though there were undeniable shortcomings in both studies, their findings showed no benefits, instead indicating that supplements of beta-carotene might increase, rather than quell, the chances of developing cancer.

One possible explanation for the findings emerged from two studies at the University of Arizona Cancer Center. Both laboratory animals and people who were given beta-carotene supplements had low blood levels of vitamin E, which may be more important than beta-carotene in protecting health. Furthermore, growing evidence suggests that—at least for beta-carotene and the forty other carotenoids in common foods—it is the combination of food-borne nutrients and other substances in plant foods, like fiber and various plant chemicals, that may provide specific benefits. Thus, taking supplements of one or two of those substances is unlikely to have the desired effects on health.

Also worrisome, the dietetic association says, is the risk of chemical excesses or nutrient imbalances that may result from taking pills rather than eating the foods themselves. For beta-carotene and other essential nutrients, particularly the "trace" minerals needed in minute amounts, taking too much of one nutrient may increase the need for another, creating a deficiency. Or supplements may interact adversely with other drugs or worsen disorders.

"If you're taking large amounts of single nutrients," Dr. Marriott said, "that's cause for concern. Patients should be sure to tell their health-care practitioners what supplements they're taking."

Most toxic reactions to vitamins and minerals come from taking something out of a bottle, not from food. In the case of selenium, for example, the toxic dose for adults is only five times the amount recommended for daily intake.

Dr. Marriott cautioned: "Buyers need to beware. They must be very careful about choosing supplements. They should look critically at the information.

"Maybe the study had only six participants, all young men. How does this apply to me, a woman over fifty? People are so enthusiastic about nutrition, they tend to jump on every study that's published."

Jane E. Brody, October 1997

TOO MUCH OF A GOOD THING

Even though millions of Americans take vitamins C and E and other antioxidants in the hope of warding off illness and aging, a new report says there is no evidence that the large doses that have become popular can prevent chronic disease or that most Americans need to take supplements at all.

In fact, large doses of vitamins C and E and selenium can be harmful, according to the new report by the Institute of Medicine, a branch of the National Academy of Sciences. Because of concerns about toxicity, for the first time, the institute set upper limits for the nutrients and emphasized that most Americans already get enough of the nutrients from the food they eat.

There has been great interest in antioxidants in recent years because studies have hinted that they might play a role in disease prevention. Antioxidants counteract the adverse effects in the body of highly reactive forms of oxygen and nitrogen, known as free radicals, which accumulate from normal metabolism. Free radicals can damage cells, and are thought by some scientists to contribute to aging, cancer, cardiovascular disease, eye problems like cataracts and macular degeneration, Alzheimer's disease and Parkinson's disease and some complications of diabetes.

But the authors of the institute report, directed by Dr. Norman Krinsky of the department of biochemistry at Tufts University in Boston, could not find convincing evidence that taking vitamins or selenium would help prevent any of those diseases. Although many studies have shown that people who eat diets rich in fruits and vegetables have a lower risk of many types of cancer, the studies could not pinpoint particular nutrients as providing the benefit, and many researchers believe that fruits and vegetables contain other substances, as yet unidentified, that may have important effects on health.

The findings were similar for heart disease. Although one study did find a benefit from vitamin E supplements, three others found it made no difference. For cataracts, studies did show a lower risk in people who had higher blood levels of antioxidants. But the studies did not convince the panel that supplements could prevent cataracts. For macular degeneration, studies have shown a lower risk in people who eat a lot of fruits and vegetables, but cause and effect have not been proved, the study said.

Dr. Keith Ayoob, a pediatric nutritionist at Einstein Medical Center in New York and a spokesman for the American Dietetic Association, said the report "seems to suggest that there's a lot of power in food, and that we have a lot more data on food than we do on supplements."

Nonetheless, the panel recommended small increases in the recommended daily intake of vitamins C and E, which can be obtained through a diet rich in fruits and vegetables.

For vitamin C, the group recommended that women consume 75 milligrams per day, and men 90 milligrams. Smokers need 35 milligrams more than nonsmokers. Vitamin C is plentiful in citrus fruit, potatoes, strawberries, broccoli and leafy green vegetables. But for those who take supplements, no one should take more than 2,000 milligrams of vitamin C a day, the report said, because it can cause diarrhea.

For vitamin E, the recommended intake for men and women is 15 milligrams, or 22 International Units, or IU, of alpha tocopherol. Vitamin E is in nuts, seeds, liver, whole grains and leafy vegetables. The upper limit for vitamin E, which a person could achieve only by taking supplements, is 1,500 IU if the product is "d-alpha tocopherol," or 1,100 IU if the product is "dl-alpha-tocopherol," a synthetic version of the vitamin. Higher amounts could cause hemorrhaging, the report said.

For selenium, the recommended intake for both men and women is 55 micrograms per day. Selenium is found in brazil nuts, seafood, garlic, liver, meat and grains.

More than 400 micrograms a day can bring on selenosis, which causes loss of hair and fingernails.

The report also considered the antioxidants known as carotenoids, including beta-carotene, which is converted into vitamin A in the body. But the panel said there was not enough evidence to recommend a daily intake or set upper limits. The only people in need of supplements would be those with vitamin A deficiencies, which are uncommon.

Denise Grady, April 2000

THE PERILS OF HOMOCYSTEINE

What's "normal"? That's the question dozens of researchers and some physicians are now asking themselves about homocysteine, a substance in blood that may rival cholesterol as a major actor in the nation's leading killer, heart disease, and play an important role in other common health problems as well.

Recent evidence has implicated elevated blood levels of homocysteine, an unhappy by-product of normal metabolism, in conditions ranging from miscarriages and birth defects to strokes, Alzheimer's disease and other disorders that afflict older people, including osteoporosis and presbyopia, the eye changes that force the middle-aged to acquire reading glasses.

And since hostility and stress raise blood levels of homocysteine, it may explain why these emotional states are linked to heart attacks.

Though strong hints of homocysteine's ability to damage arteries date back more than thirty years, until the 1990s its importance in cardiovascular disease was completely overshadowed by cholesterol. While concerns about elevated cholesterol levels fingered dietary fat as the culprit, high levels of homocysteine are associated with a diet rich in animal protein, the source of homocysteine's parent compound, the amino acid methionine.

Furthermore, as Dr. Meir Stampfer of the Harvard School of Public Health pointed out, "There was no commercial interest in studying homocysteine," since the way to reduce it—eating less meat and taking supplements of B vitamins—is inexpensive and not patentable. For cholesterol, on the other hand, pharmaceutical companies seeking to sell cholesterol-lowering drugs paid for many studies.

In addition, homocysteine's potential role in common disorders may have been overlooked because the levels associated with an increased risk of health problems are still listed as normal by medical laboratories—8 to 20 micromoles per liter of blood plasma. However, recent studies have linked levels as low as 15 micromoles to an increased risk of heart attack, stroke, peripheral vascular disease and venous thromboembolism, potentially life-threatening blood clots in the veins.

Among the fifteen thousand doctors participating in the Physicians' Health Study, those with a homocysteine level of 15 micromoles or higher had a heart attack rate three times as high as those with lower levels over a period of just five years, Dr. Stampfer and his Harvard colleagues found. Even a level of 12 micromoles can double coronary risk.

Dr. William Castelli, former director of the Framingham Heart Study, who now heads the Framingham Cardiovascular Institute in

Massachusetts, considers levels higher than 9 micromoles to be elevated, placing people at increased risk of a heart attack or stroke. In the Framingham study, he said, about 40 percent of the people had homocysteine levels greater than 9.

"Homocysteine is an important new risk factor for cardiovascular disease," Dr. Castelli said in an interview. "There are about seventeen studies now under way to determine the benefits of lowering homocysteine levels. We're still missing crucial data. We don't yet know if lowering homocysteine will result in a lower rate of heart attacks or strokes." The studies are being financed by the National Institutes of Health.

But Dr. Castelli and others pointed out that since the way to bring down homocysteine—eating less meat and taking supplements of the B vitamins folate, B_6 and B_{12} that are required by the enzymes that process homocysteine—is harmless and inexpensive, people should not have to wait five or more years for the research results before trying to lower their own homocysteine levels.

There are several ways in which homocysteine can damage blood vessels. It injures the cells that line arteries and stimulates the growth of smooth muscle cells; both effects can result in lesions that narrow the channels through which blood flows. Homocysteine can also disrupt normal blood-clotting mechanisms, increasing the risk of clots that can bring on a heart attack or stroke.

Damage to the small blood vessels in the brain may explain the relationship that has been found between elevated homocysteine levels and the loss of cognitive function and Alzheimer's disease, say Dr. Jacob Selhub and colleagues at the United States Department of Agriculture Human Nutrition Research Center on Aging at Tufts University in Boston. Starting in 1983, they noted, several studies have linked an inadequate supply of B vitamins to a decline in cognitive function in the elderly, and some studies have shown that taking supplements of B vitamins improves cognitive performance.

For example, in the *American Journal of Clinical Nutrition*, Dr. David A. Snowdon and colleagues at the University of Kentucky College of Medicine in Lexington described a study of thirty nuns who had lived in the same convent and eaten from the same kitchen until their deaths at ages 78 to 101. Blood samples taken years earlier revealed that those who had low blood levels of folate were far more likely to have suffered atrophy of the cerebral cortex. The lower the folate levels, the more severe the brain atrophy.

As for other disorders common in the elderly, Dr. Carlos L. Krumdieck and Dr. Charles W. Prince, nutrition scientists at the University of Alabama Schools of Medicine, Dentistry and Health Related Professions in Birmingham, have described a link between moderately elevated homocysteine levels and the occurrence of senile osteoporosis and presbyopia. They pointed out that the contribution of chronically elevated homocysteine levels "to diseases of old age may have gone unrecognized because we are conditioned to accept them as inescapable consequences of growing old."

The harmful effects of homocysteine on blood vessels and blood clotting may also explain the link between elevated levels of this amino acid and various pregnancy complications, including repeated early miscarriage; pre-eclampsia, or pregnancy-related hypertension; premature birth; very low birth weight; and certain birth defects.

Researchers at the University Hospital Nijmegen St. Radboud in the Netherlands reported in the journal *Obstetrics and Gynecology* that 123 women who had experienced repeated early miscarriages had "significantly lower serum folate concentrations" and higher levels of homocysteine than a comparison group of 101 women who had not had miscarriages.

In another report, in the *American Journal of Clinical Nutrition*, researchers in Bergen, Norway, found that among 5,883 women who had a total of 14,492 pregnancies, those with the highest levels of homocysteine were significantly more likely to have experienced pregnancy complications like pre-eclampsia, premature birth and very low birth weight than women with the lowest homocysteine levels.

It has been known for some time that increasing a woman's intake of folate during the first three weeks of pregnancy can greatly decrease the risk of often lethal spinal deformities like spina bifida and anencephaly in the fetus. This prompted the Food and Drug Administration to order, as of January 1998, fortification of all flour and grain products with folate, a measure that Dr. Selhub said had reduced elevated homocysteine levels in the general population by about 10 percent. Although a practicing physician reviewing a patient's laboratory test report may understandably dismiss a homocysteine level of, say, 12 micromoles as normal, a 1995 analysis of twenty-seven studies indicated that there was no absolute safe blood level of this substance. Rather, as with cholesterol, the risk associated with homocysteine is on a continuum; an increase of only 5 micromoles in the plasma level of homocysteine can raise a person's chances of developing cardiovascular disease by as much as a 20-milligram rise in cholesterol would. Other reports have equated homocysteine's risk to the cardiovascular system with the damage done by smoking or a high blood level of cholesterol.

In fact, the emerging appreciation of the risks associated with so-called normal levels of homocysteine parallels the experience with cholesterol. As recently as two decades ago, doctors regarded cholesterol levels in blood plasma of 240 milligrams as normal, but now levels above 200 milligrams are recognized as increasing a person's risk of developing cardiovascular disease. And, as with cholesterol, homocysteine levels tend to rise with age and are generally higher in men than in women, at least until women reach menopause.

Homocysteine also appears to exacerbate the effects of other cardiovascular risks. For example, high homocysteine "substantially increases the risk associated with smoking and hypertension," Dr. Iftikhar J. Kullo and colleagues at the Mayo Clinic pointed out. And among people with diabetes, a study from the Netherlands found that for each 5-micromole rise in homocysteine, the risk of dying from any cause over a five-year period was more than triple that of nondiabetics with the same homocysteine levels.

Homocysteine is an amino acid, an intermediate product that builds up when the amino acid methionine cannot be converted to cysteine because an enzyme is lacking or is present in inadequate amounts. The B vitamins folic acid, or folate, and B_6 and B_{12} are crucial to these conversion enzymes. But it has not yet been demonstrated that taking vitamins to lower homocysteine will prevent heart disease or any other disorder linked to homocysteine.

What is known so far is that vitamin therapy can slow and even reverse clogging of the carotid arteries that feed the brain, which should reduce the risk of stroke. Dr. Daniel G. Hackam and colleagues at the Siebens-Drake/Robarts Research Institute in London, Ontario, showed a reversal of carotid artery clogging in patients with homocysteine levels both above and below 14 micromoles who took 2.5 milligrams of folic acid, 25 milligrams of B_6 and 250 micrograms of B_{12} daily for a year. They concluded that "these observations support a causal relationship between homocysteine and atherosclerosis and, taken with epidemiological evidence, suggest that in patients with vascular disease, the level to treat may be less than 9 micromoles per liter."

The homocysteine story actually began in 1969 when Dr. Kilmer S. McCully reported that children born with a genetic error of metabolism that causes their homocysteine levels to skyrocket to hundreds of micromoles died with advanced disease in their arteries at a very young age.

In the last two decades there were occasional reports of advanced clotting in arteries feeding the brains of children with homocystinuria, as the genetic condition is called. In other cases, seriously thickened walls of the carotid arteries were found in young adults born with only one of the two genes that cause homocystinuria.

But, perhaps because in most people homocysteine levels rarely exceed 30 micromoles, until recently few researchers appreciated the significance of Dr. McCully's finding or any of the subsequent observations in people with homocysteine levels in the hundreds of micromoles.

Meanwhile, Dr. McCully lost his research financing and his job at Massachusetts General Hospital and Harvard Medical School and was forced to do what little he could to pursue the homocysteine hypothesis on his own while working at the Veterans Affairs Medical Center in Providence, Rhode Island.

Dr. McCully, who is now enjoying renewed respect with the emergence of homocysteine as a cardiovascular risk factor, considers arteriosclerosis, a clogging of the arteries with fats and other substances, to be a disease of "protein intoxication." While Americans are busy focusing on fat avoidance to lower cholesterol, he believes they should be reducing their consumption of animal protein to lower homocysteine.

Indeed, a study published in *Preventive Medicine* by Dr. David J.

DeRose of the Lifestyle Center of America in Sulphur, Oklahoma, and colleagues showed that a diet devoid of animal products, caffeine and alcohol, along with exercise, stress management and spiritual support—but no B vitamin supplements—reduced homocysteine levels in forty men and women by an average of 13 percent in just one week.

"I'm thrilled that scientists all over the world are now taking up the question of homocysteine and heart disease," Dr. McCully said. "An avalanche of studies has demonstrated the validity of this approach, and I anticipate that the studies now under way will prove that controlling homocysteine is the best way to deal with heart disease."

Jane E. Brody, June 2000

TAKING ACTION AGAINST HOMOCYSTEINE BEFORE THE VERDICT IS IN

Preventive medicine often involves making a best guess based on less than complete scientific information. So it was with smoking, when people were advised to quit long before there was incontrovertible proof that it caused cancer. So it was also with cholesterol, when people were told to lower their blood levels long before research showed that doing so prevented heart attacks.

And so it is now with homocysteine, an amino acid in blood that when elevated has been linked to heart attacks and strokes as well as a host of other health problems, from miscarriage to Alzheimer's disease.

While more than a dozen studies have found that people with even moderately raised levels of homocysteine have a threefold increased risk of suffering heart attacks or strokes, it is not yet known whether reducing homocysteine levels will prevent cardiovascular problems. Nor is it known whether homocysteine itself is the culprit (although ample evidence suggests it is) or whether homocysteine is merely an indicator for something else that does the damage.

Still, most researchers studying the matter say that it would be prudent not to wait until science reaches a verdict in two to five years. Their best advice is to spend the $80 or so on a blood test to determine your homocysteine level and, if it is higher than 9 micromoles per liter of plasma, change your diet to bring it down.

Among those especially at risk of high homocysteine levels are people with chronic kidney failure, those with thyroid deficiencies, people who have received organ transplants and those living on high-protein, low-carbohydrate diets. Among those with other cardiovascular risk factors, including smoking, hypertension or high cholesterol, having even a moderately raised homocysteine level can significantly increase their risk.

In an important way, our problems with cholesterol and homocysteine begin with diets rich in animal protein. For cholesterol, it is the saturated fat that is mainly derived from animal protein foods, along with dietary cholesterol that comes only from animal products, that raises blood levels of this artery-clogging substance. For homocysteine, animal protein itself is the indirect source. Homocysteine is an intermediate product derived from the metabolism of methionine, an essential amino acid predominant in animal protein.

Three B vitamins—folic acid (also called folate), B_6 and B_{12}—are involved in processing homocysteine to keep it from building up in the blood to levels that can cause harm. Of the three, folic acid is the most important. When folic acid is present in adequate amounts, homocysteine is converted back to methionine. Folic acid is found in significant amounts in green vegetables like asparagus, broccoli, spinach, cabbage and romaine lettuce, and in orange juice, lentils and wheat germ.

But according to studies by Dr. Elias Seyoum and Dr. Jacob Selhub at the Jean Mayer Human Nutrition Research Center on Aging at Tufts University in Boston, two foods on the no-no list for cholesterol happen to be the best sources of folate that is readily available to the body: egg yolk and cow's liver. Eggs and liver are also important sources of vitamin B_{12}, which aids in converting homocysteine back to methionine. Though low in fat, these two foods are among the richest sources of dietary cholesterol and thus have been all but eliminated from the diets of many people trying to keep their blood cholesterol levels low.

Availability of folate is also influenced by how foods are prepared. Since B vitamins are soluble in water, when vegetables are cooked in water, much of the folic acid leaches out. Dr. Selhub recommends using the cooking water, for example, to prepare a soup or stew, to recapture the lost B vitamins. To better preserve B vitamins, vegetables can be steamed or cooked in a microwave oven with little or no water.

Other good sources of folate are fortified grains (products like bread and pasta made with wheat flour) and cereals. In 1998, the Food and Drug Administration mandated the addition of folate to these inexpensive and commonly consumed foods to reduce pregnant women's risk of having babies with neural tube birth defects, spina bifida and anencephaly. Folate fortification has had a side benefit of lowering homocysteine levels.

But people living on the now-popular high-protein, low-carbohydrate diets are receiving a double whammy. In addition to consuming huge amounts of methionine-rich animal protein foods, they are likely to be sorely deficient in folate and at risk of developing dangerously high blood levels of homocysteine unless they take a daily vitamin supplement that contains at least 400 micrograms of folate.

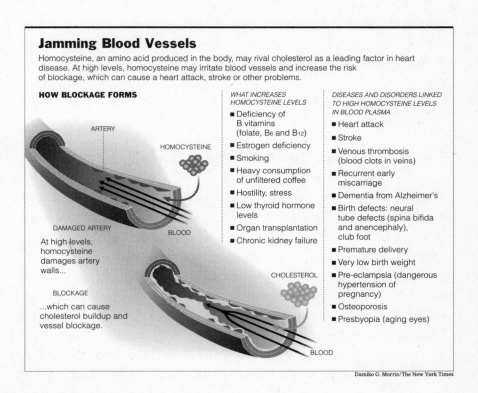

Jamming Blood Vessels

Homocysteine, an amino acid produced in the body, may rival cholesterol as a leading factor in heart disease. At high levels, homocysteine may irritate blood vessels and increase the risk of blockage, which can cause a heart attack, stroke or other problems.

HOW BLOCKAGE FORMS

ARTERY

HOMOCYSTEINE

DAMAGED ARTERY

BLOOD

At high levels, homocysteine damages artery walls...

BLOCKAGE

...which can cause cholesterol buildup and vessel blockage.

CHOLESTEROL

BLOOD

WHAT INCREASES HOMOCYSTEINE LEVELS

- Deficiency of B vitamins (folate, B_6 and B_{12})
- Estrogen deficiency
- Smoking
- Heavy consumption of unfiltered coffee
- Hostility, stress
- Low thyroid hormone levels
- Organ transplantation
- Chronic kidney failure

DISEASES AND DISORDERS LINKED TO HIGH HOMOCYSTEINE LEVELS IN BLOOD PLASMA

- Heart attack
- Stroke
- Venous thrombosis (blood clots in veins)
- Recurrent early miscarriage
- Dementia from Alzheimer's
- Birth defects: neural tube defects (spina bifida and anencephaly), club foot
- Premature delivery
- Very low birth weight
- Pre-eclampsia (dangerous hypertension of pregnancy)
- Osteoporosis
- Presbyopia (aging eyes)

Damiko G. Morris/The New York Times

But for some people, this amount of folate is insufficient to reduce homocysteine to safe levels. For example, Dr. Selhub said, people who have had kidney transplants need 2.4 milligrams of folate—six times the amount in an ordinary supplement—to lower homocysteine.

Along with folate, people with high homocysteine levels are usually advised to take supplements of vitamins B_6 and B_{12}. Foods rich in B_6 include broccoli, spinach, avocado, banana, oatmeal, wheat germ and chicken. B_{12} is found only in animal foods: liver and other meats, fish, eggs and milk.

In a study in Germany among 150 women of childbearing age, those who took a 400-microgram folic acid supplement daily for four weeks experienced an 11 percent drop in homocysteine. But those who in addition to folic acid took 400 micrograms of B_{12} had an 18 percent drop in homocysteine, according to Dr. Anja Bronstrup and colleagues at the University of Bonn's Institute of Nutritional Science.

Another way to reduce homocysteine may be to reduce stress. Even mild stress can temporarily raise homocysteine levels, a study by Dr. Catherine Stoney at Ohio State University showed. Lowering homocysteine could be one reason for the observed cardiovascular benefits of meditation.

Jane Brody, June 2000

IRON: TOO MUCH IS DANGEROUS

Generations of Americans have been exhorted to eat spinach or liver for the iron that supposedly made Popeye's muscles bulge, or to take iron-rich tonics like Geritol to revive their "tired blood." But while some iron in the diet is critical for health and life itself, the overconsumption or overabsorption of this well-known mineral is now under intense scrutiny as a possible cause or contributor to killer ailments like heart disease and cancer as well as serious infections.

The story of iron is a classic illustration of "Just because a little is good does not mean more is better." Iron is essential to the formation of the oxygen-carrying pigments hemoglobin in the blood and myoglobin in the muscles. But scientists who study iron warn that people should not take iron supplements or stuff themselves with iron-rich foods unless medical tests have demonstrated an iron deficiency. Some researchers are also concerned about the widespread use of vitamin C supplements, which can enhance the absorption of dietary iron when both are present in the gut at the same time. And questions have been raised about the wisdom of fortifying cereals and bread with iron in a country like the United States where a lot of iron-rich meat is consumed by most people.

The body has an imperfect mechanism for regulating the amount of iron people absorb and store in their tissues. Iron overload may result when the diet is overly rich in iron from, say, the consumption of lots of red meat or supplements when the body is not iron-deficient. Laboratory and clinical evidence suggests that an excess of iron in the tissues can promote coronary artery disease and foster the growth of latent cancers and infectious organisms.

Foods and supplements are not the only sources of iron. It can also be inhaled, and smokers (tobacco leaves are rich in iron) as well as workers in industries that spew particles containing iron into the air may risk lung cancer in part because their lungs are chronically exposed to excess iron.

The body has only one way to rid itself of iron, through bleeding, which is why symptoms of iron overload do not usually show up in menstruating women until after menopause. Bleeding may also contribute to the protection against heart disease and colon cancer associated with vigorous exercise and the regular use of aspirin and related drugs; both cause the repeated loss of tiny amounts of blood from the digestive tract.

For at least one and a half million Americans who have a genetic disorder called hereditary hemochromatosis, there is no question that even moderate amounts of dietary iron can lead to accumulations of "rust" in organs throughout their bodies. Unless this disorder is identified before it causes serious organ damage and treated by frequent bloodletting, it can result in such potentially fatal conditions as heart disease, cirrhosis or cancer of the liver as well as thyroid disease, diabetes, arthritis and infertility.

In the early stages of hemochromatosis, symptoms like chronic fatigue, abdominal pain, impotence and menstrual disruption mimic so many other conditions that doctors often miss the correct diagnosis until vital organs are irreparably damaged. Although many doctors now in practice were taught that this is a rare condition that occurs primarily in white males of northern European descent, it is now known to be the most common genetic abnormality, surpassing the combined cases of cystic fibrosis, phenylketonuria, or PKU, and hereditary muscular dystrophy, and occurring equally in men and women. But because most women menstruate for thirty or forty years, the problem may not show up in women until after menopause. Furthermore, it has now been shown to occur as frequently in Hispanics as in non-Hispanics in the United States. A related genetic condition has also been identified in African blacks, but its incidence has not yet been studied in African-Americans.

In 1996, researchers at Mercator Genetics, Inc., a gene discovery company in Menlo Park, California, reported identifying the gene that appears to cause hereditary hemochromatosis, a finding that could lead to a simple screening test for this disorder before it results in serious con-

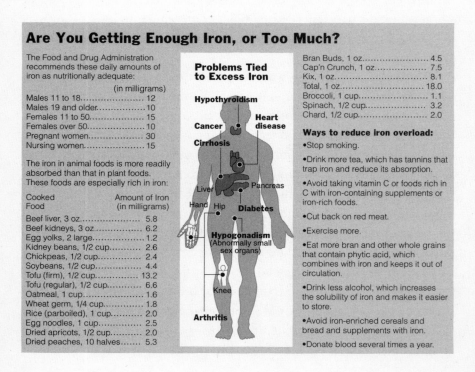

Are You Getting Enough Iron, or Too Much?

The Food and Drug Administration recommends these daily amounts of iron as nutritionally adequate:

(in milligrams)

Males 11 to 18	12
Males 19 and older	10
Females 11 to 50	15
Females over 50	10
Pregnant women	30
Nursing women	15

The iron in animal foods is more readily absorbed than that in plant foods. These foods are especially rich in iron:

Cooked Food	Amount of Iron (in milligrams)
Beef liver, 3 oz	5.8
Beef kidneys, 3 oz	6.2
Egg yolks, 2 large	1.2
Kidney beans, 1/2 cup	2.6
Chickpeas, 1/2 cup	2.4
Soybeans, 1/2 cup	4.4
Tofu (firm), 1/2 cup	13.2
Tofu (regular), 1/2 cup	6.6
Oatmeal, 1 cup	1.6
Wheat germ, 1/4 cup	1.8
Rice (parboiled), 1 cup	2.0
Egg noodles, 1 cup	2.5
Dried apricots, 1/2 cup	2.0
Dried peaches, 10 halves	5.3

Problems Tied to Excess Iron

Hypothyroidism

Cancer

Heart disease

Cirrhosis

Liver

Pancreas

Hand Hip Diabetes

Hypogonadism (Abnormally small sex organs)

Knee

Arthritis

Bran Buds, 1 oz	4.5
Cap'n Crunch, 1 oz	7.5
Kix, 1 oz	8.1
Total, 1 oz	18.0
Broccoli, 1 cup	1.1
Spinach, 1/2 cup	3.2
Chard, 1/2 cup	2.0

Ways to reduce iron overload:

• Stop smoking.

• Drink more tea, which has tannins that trap iron and reduce its absorption.

• Avoid taking vitamin C or foods rich in C with iron-containing supplements or iron-rich foods.

• Cut back on red meat.

• Exercise more.

• Eat more bran and other whole grains that contain phytic acid, which combines with iron and keeps it out of circulation.

• Drink less alcohol, which increases the solubility of iron and makes it easier to store.

• Avoid iron-enriched cereals and bread and supplements with iron.

• Donate blood several times a year.

sequences. Hemochromatosis, which is inherited as an autosomal recessive trait, like blue eyes and PKU, requires the presence of two abnormal genes, one from each parent, to cause the condition. One in ten Americans is believed to carry one abnormal gene; if two such people have children, one in four of their offspring, on average, will have hemochromatosis and half will themselves carry the gene and be able to pass it to their own children.

There is growing evidence that even people without an inherited disorder can develop problems associated with iron overload. Iron is a catalyst for the formation of free radicals, highly active chemicals that are implicated in heart disease, cancer and the aging of cells. Dr. Eugene D. Weinberg, a professor emeritus of microbiology at Indiana University in Bloomington who has studied the effects of iron for three decades, is one of a number of researchers who have warned that an overabundance of iron could be undermining the health and shortening the lives of millions of Americans.

In an interview, he pointed out that both cancer cells and infectious organisms need iron from their host to grow. Cancer cells can live in a semidormant state for a long time, he explained, but they cannot multiply without iron and oxygen from blood. He said smokers, asbestos workers and people who grind or weld steel, mine iron or paint with iron oxide powder could acquire high levels of iron in their lung tissues, increasing their risk of lung cancer.

Dr. Weinberg added: "Every pathogen needs iron, which it must get from its host. If there is excess iron in the tissue the pathogen is growing in, it will foster multiplication of the pathogen." For example, one study found that the bacteria that cause Legionnaire's disease would not survive if the level of iron in lung cells was very low.

As for heart disease, a study conducted among 1,900 middle-aged men in Finland indicated that a high iron level was second only to smoking as a cause of heart attacks. Although three American studies failed to confirm or refute this finding, the methods used in these studies were less precise. The Finnish researchers found that the greatest risk of having high iron occurred in men with high cholesterol levels. In those with low cholesterol, iron had no impact on the risk of heart attack, suggesting that iron's role in heart disease may involve the oxidation of low-density lipoprotein—LDL, the "bad" cholesterol—into the form that clogs up arteries. A person's iron status can be checked through several blood tests. The most useful is a ferritin test, which can be done as part of a routine blood test.

Jane E. Brody, March 1997

SELENIUM, A CINDERELLA NUTRIENT

Selenium, a mineral long feared for its toxicity, is on the road to becoming a Cinderella nutrient. As the last of forty nutrients to be proved essential to human health, selenium is now the subject of both human and animal studies that suggest it can help prevent the two leading killers in the Western world: heart disease and cancer. It may also lift the human spirit.

In a long-term study, selenium supplements taken for ten years failed in their primary mission, to protect against the development of skin cancers, but they were incidentally found to reduce other cancers by a third and to cut overall cancer deaths in half. This effect of a daily 200-microgram supplement was so dramatic that the researchers are convinced that it is real, not just a statistical fluke, even though the study was designed to examine a different question.

Earlier studies had linked low dietary intakes of selenium to an elevated risk of heart attacks, strokes and other diseases related to high blood pressure. People with low levels of selenium in their blood were shown to be three times as likely to die of a heart attack as those with higher selenium levels, a finding that may be related to selenium's apparent ability to raise blood levels of HDL, the "good" cholesterol, which helps protect against heart disease.

Improvements in well-being have also been noted in selenium studies. In a fifteen-week study by Dr. James G. Penland, a psychologist at the Grand Forks, North Dakota, Human Nutrition Research Center of the Agricultural Research Service, fifteen men fed a selenium-rich diet reported a significant improvement in mood, feeling more clearheaded and elated at the end of the study than at the start. A comparable group of men given a selenium-poor diet reported feeling worse. The test diet contained 240 micrograms of selenium daily, more than triple the currently recommended amount.

But researchers, though optimistic, remain very cautious about advising Americans to start gulping down selenium tablets. They point out that in industrialized countries, where foods come from many areas, it is possible to consume amounts of selenium that appear to be protective as part of a wholesome diet. And selenium in foods appears to be used better by the body than the form found in most supplements. While the promise of benefit from a daily supplement is strong, it has not been proved, and the possibility of toxicity for those who overdo it is serious indeed.

Early in this century, thousands of cattle, horses and sheep in Wyoming, Utah, Nebraska and South Dakota were felled by two seemingly unrelated conditions called "alkali disease" and "blind staggers." The cause in both cases was traced to too much selenium; the animals had eaten grasses and grains loaded with the mineral, which is unevenly deposited in the earth's crust. There are high levels in the soils of most states west of the Mississippi and low levels in the Northeast and Northwest and in some Southeast and Great Lakes states. The same uneven pattern persists worldwide.

Dr. Gerald F. Combs Jr., a professor of nutrition at Cornell University, said that in more than a dozen mountainous provinces in China where the soil is very low in selenium, many children developed a potentially fatal form of heart disease called Keshan disease or a growth-disrupting joint disorder called Kaschin-Beck disease.

But selenium's importance in the diet was not recognized until 1957, when researchers at the National Institutes of Health found that selenium could prevent liver damage in laboratory animals who were deficient in vitamin E. Subsequent studies found that small amounts of selenium could even cure some serious muscle and blood diseases in farm animals deficient in both vitamin E and selenium. Finally, in 1969, studies in rats found that otherwise well-nourished animals, when

deprived of selenium, suffered hair loss, cataracts and growth and reproductive problems.

Selenium at last joined the list of nutrients considered essential to animal health, leading ultimately to its inclusion as one of the nutrient minerals needed in the human diet in trace amounts. The Food and
Nutrition Board of the National Academy of Sciences considers a daily
intake of between 50 micrograms and 200 micrograms to be safe and adequate, and it has established recommended dietary amounts of 55 micrograms daily for adult women and 70 micrograms for adult men. For
infants and children up to age fourteen, recommended daily dietary
amounts range from 10 to 45 micrograms daily.

Still, justifiable fears of toxicity have persisted. In 1984, at least eleven
people were poisoned by selenium supplements that were accidentally
manufactured to contain 125 times as much selenium as the Food and
Nutrition Board deems to be safe and effective. Those affected suffered
loss of hair and fingernails, nausea and vomiting, and fatigue. Similar
toxic effects have been seen in people who took only 25 times the recommended amount of selenium.

Most Americans seem to consume enough selenium in their food to
satisfy the current recommendation. Surveys have indicated that the
average American consumes about 100 micrograms of selenium daily,
although in one study in Maryland, 17 percent of adults took in less than
50 micrograms. Selenium tends to be richest in foods high in protein.
Fish, for example, is an excellent source. However, the main sources of
selenium in the American diet are meats, poultry, fish, cereals and other
grains. Among vegetables, mushrooms and asparagus are good sources.
Brazil nuts, especially those sold with their shells on, are loaded with
selenium; two nuts a day can more than meet the daily need. Some
experts fear that vegetarians who refrain from eating fish as well as meat
and poultry may have difficulty consuming enough selenium.

The question now, though, is how much is enough. Selenium is an
antioxidant that can help to prevent the degradation of fats and cell
membranes and block the action of cancer-causing chemicals. More
than one hundred studies conducted in laboratory animals treated with
carcinogens have shown that selenium added to the animals' usual diet

protected them against a number of cancers, including cancers of the breast, esophagus and liver.

In 1997, a study directed by Dr. Larry C. Clark at the University of Arizona found that six hundred people who took daily supplements of 200 micrograms of selenium (in effect, tripling their normal daily intake) for ten years developed 71 percent fewer prostate cancers, 67 percent fewer esophageal cancers, 62 percent fewer colorectal cancers and 46 percent fewer lung cancers than did a comparable group of six hundred people who took a lookalike placebo tablet. No toxic effects of the selenium supplements were noted.

The tablets used in the study contained selenium-enriched yeast, prepared by growing yeast in water spiked with selenium. This organic form of selenium is the kind found in foods, whereas most selenium supplements currently sold consist of inorganic selenium, which may not have the same effect.

There is also a concern that selenium might encourage the growth of some cancers. In an earlier study conducted by Dr. Clark of cancer rates and the levels of selenium found in forage in United States counties, those counties where the forage contained moderate to high levels of selenium had lower rates of cancers of the lung, colon and rectum, bladder, esophagus, breast, ovary and pancreas. But the high-selenium areas also had higher rates of liver and stomach cancers, Hodgkin's disease and leukemia.

Dr. Charles Hennekens of the Harvard School of Public Health said the new finding "should be a message to researchers, not the general public." He added, "It is premature to start taking supplements, although it may turn out to be the right thing to do." One important need is for researchers to examine more closely the interaction of selenium with other nutrients; raising the intake of one nutrient may change the demand for another.

Dr. Donald Lisk, a professor of toxicology at Cornell and the researcher who discovered the high levels of selenium in Brazil nuts, noted that the tablets used in the new cancer study could be purchased over the counter in drugstores in dosages of 50 or 100 micrograms. Dr. Lisk said he had analyzed the tablets and found their contents to be as stated on the label. But he cautioned against giving any selenium supplements to children and warned adults against assuming that "if one tablet is good, five would be better."

Jane E. Brody, February 1997

OSTEOPOROSIS: WIDESPREAD VITAMIN D DEFICIENCY MAY BE TO BLAME

Widespread deficiencies of vitamin D may play a big role in causing the bone-wasting disease osteoporosis among older Americans, a study has found.

The researchers attributed vitamin D deficiencies to two factors of growing importance: insufficient dietary intake and inadequate exposure to sunlight. Sunlight stimulates production of vitamin D in the skin.

The study findings, published in the *New England Journal of Medicine*, suggest not only that millions of American adults lack enough vitamin D in their blood to protect their bones but also that newly upgraded recommendations for vitamin D intake may be inadequate to prevent osteoporosis in many older people. Although calcium is the main nutrient of concern for preventing osteoporosis, vitamin D also plays an important role.

Deficient levels of vitamin D were found in the blood of 37 percent of those who reported consuming the newly recommended amounts of 400 international units (IU) a day for people fifty-one to seventy years old and 600 international units for those over seventy. The previous recommendation for all adults had been 200 international units.

The study was conducted by Dr. Melissa K. Thomas and colleagues at Massachusetts General Hospital among 290 hospitalized patients, who might be expected to have lower-than-average levels of vitamin D in their blood. And indeed more than half of them did. Using a conservative measure of deficiency, Dr. Thomas said 57 percent of the patients were deficient, including 22 percent who were severely deficient in this essential nutrient.

Asked whether the findings in hospital patients could be applied to the general population, Dr. Thomas said that although the percentage of people with vitamin D deficiency might be somewhat lower in healthy people, the problem was still likely to be widespread. Dr. Thomas based this judgment on a separate analysis of vitamin D levels among forty-four patients who were younger and healthier and had none of the usual risk factors that might cause a vitamin D deficiency. Yet she found that 42 percent of them were deficient.

The results of this and other studies suggest that at least for adults living at northern latitudes where essentially no vitamin D is made in the skin all winter, a dietary supplement of 800 international units a day may be needed to stave off a chronic deficiency. In an editorial accompanying the new report, Dr. Robert D. Utiger, a specialist in endocrinology, pointed out that low vitamin D levels had been found in 46 percent of those who reported taking multivitamins, most of which contain 400 international units of vitamin D.

Vitamin D aids in the absorption of dietary calcium, but its most important role is in maintaining normal blood levels of calcium. In the patients labeled deficient, levels of vitamin D in the blood were low enough to cause calcium to be removed from their bones to supply the blood. Adults deficient in vitamin D cannot properly mineralize their bones, which gradually come to resemble a rubbery framework without cement.

A study of 3,270 healthy elderly French women showed that a dietary supplement of calcium plus 800 international units of vitamin D a day decreased the risk of hip fractures by 43 percent in just two years.

Dr. Michael Horlick, chief of endocrinology at Boston University Medical Center, said there was now enough evidence to conclude that "vitamin D deficiency is an unrecognized epidemic in our middle-aged and older population—both in patients and in healthy people throughout the year." For example, in a study he did among 160 Bostonians forty-nine through eighty-three years old who visited the hospital clinics, 40 percent were deficient in vitamin D.

Dr. Horlick's studies have shown that the American diet is an unreliable and generally poor source of vitamin D. The only major dietary source is milk that has been fortified with vitamin D, supposedly at a minimum level of 400 international units in each quart. But he said he found that "no more than twenty percent of milk samples throughout the nation contained at least 320 IU per quart and fifteen percent of skim milk samples had no detectable vitamin D at all, even though the labels said they were fortified with vitamin D."

"About ninety percent of the vitamin D in most people comes from casual exposure to sunlight," Dr. Horlick said. "But the concern about cancer risk has limited people's exposure to sunlight."

Speaking of a sun protection factor, he added, "If you religiously apply sunscreen with an SPF of eight to your exposed skin, you will make no vitamin D."

Jane E. Brody, March 1998

BAD NEWS ON BETA-CAROTENE: NO HELP FOR CANCER OR HEART DISEASE

Two large studies have found that contrary to the beliefs or hopes of the millions of Americans who take it, beta-carotene, a vigorously promoted vitamin supplement, is completely ineffective in preventing cancer or heart disease. One of the studies found that it might even be harmful to some people.

Federal health officials said they hoped that this would spell the end of the beta-carotene fad. The idea that a simple supplement capsule might fend off cancer and other diseases, they said, has simply proved too good to be true.

Dr. Richard Klausner, director of the National Cancer Institute, which financed both studies, said, "With clearly no benefit and even a hint of possible harm, I can see no reason that an individual should take beta-carotene."

Beta-carotene is a naturally occurring substance in fruits and vegetables that is converted to vitamin A in the body. The cancer institute recommends that rather than rely on supplements, people eat low-fat diets abundant in fruits and vegetables, whose hundreds of substances combined might be fostering the disease protection that has been sought in beta-carotene.

Americans spend $3.5 billion a year on vitamin and mineral supplements, said Dr. Annette Dickinson, the director of science and regulatory affairs at the Council for Responsible Nutrition, a trade association of supplement manufacturers. But the health claims for many of these supplements have not been verified by rigorous scientific investigation, and the Food and Drug Administration is not empowered to regulate claims that vitamin manufacturers make in advertising and promotional brochures except for those that accompany the supplements themselves on retailers' shelves.

One of the beta-carotene studies, the Physicians' Health Study, involved 22,071 doctors who were randomly assigned to take 50 milligrams of beta-carotene or a dummy pill every other day. The study ended on December 31, 1995, after twelve years, with the conclusion that beta-carotene supplements did not protect against cancer or heart disease.

The other study, the Beta-Carotene and Retinol Efficacy Trial, or Caret, tested both beta-carotene, in a dose of 30 milligrams a day, and vitamin A, in a daily dose of 25,000 international units. The 18,314 participants in this study took beta-carotene, vitamin A, both, or a placebo. Preliminary studies had hinted that beta-carotene might be especially effective in preventing lung cancer, and all the subjects in the Caret study were at high risk for lung cancer because they smoked or had worked with asbestos.

The study was halted on January 10, 1996 — twenty-one months ahead of schedule — when investigators concluded not only that the vitamins were not helpful but also that they might be harmful: the rate of death from lung cancer was 28 percent higher among the participants who had taken the supplements than among those who had taken the placebo, and the rate of death from heart disease was 17 percent higher. The reason for these increases is unclear, and they were too small to be considered statistically significant. But they were nonetheless worrisome.

These two studies were preceded by a Finnish study of 29,133 men who were smokers. That study, published in 1994, found a slight increase in the death rate among those who had taken beta-carotene. But some critics of the research said the beta-carotene dose, 20 milligrams a day, had been too low to find the benefit that they had expected. Others said the men had been studied for too short a time, five to eight years. And still others said that even if beta-carotene did not help smokers, it would help healthy people.

To underscore the importance of the newer findings, Dr. Klausner announced them at a news conference yesterday at the National Cancer Institute in Bethesda, Maryland, without waiting for the usual publication in a medical journal.

Dr. Klausner said that as a consequence of the results, researchers would immediately remove beta-carotene from another study, involving 40,000 female health professionals who have been taking beta-carotene, vitamin E and aspirin.

The Caret study's director, Dr. Gilbert S. Omenn, dean of public health at the University of Washington in Seattle, said its results were not definite proof that beta-carotene is harmful. But the reason it was halted, he said, is that its findings were reminiscent of those in the Finnish study.

"These vitamins were providing no benefit," Dr. Omenn said, "and may—with the emphasis on *may*—have adverse effects."

But Dr. Dickinson, of the supplement manufacturers' trade association, said the new results were not enough to indicate that Americans should stop taking beta-carotene, especially in lower doses or in multivitamins. Although she acknowledged that heavy smokers "ought to be aware of the Caret trial and take it into consideration," she said that "there is still a strong suggestion" that beta-carotene might be beneficial among the population as a whole.

The study researchers disagree. "There is absolutely no benefit" in beta-carotene supplements, said Dr. Charles Hennekens of the Brigham and Women's Hospital in Boston, who was the director of the Physicians' Health Study. And that finding, Dr. Hennekens added, is "the biggest disappointment of my career."

The two studies began in the early 1980s, when researchers had high hopes that beta-carotene or vitamin A might protect against cancer and heart disease. The hypothesis was that these substances served as antioxidants, mopping up dangerous chemicals known as free radicals, which, although a normal product of body function, can damage DNA, leading to cancer, and can convert cholesterol, normally inert, into a substance that can lead to heart disease.

In support of the hypothesis were epidemiological studies showing that people whose diets were rich in fruits and vegetables, the sources of beta-carotene, had less cancer and heart disease than people whose diets were not. And studies found that the more beta-carotene in a person's serum, the lower their risk of cancer.

Some scientists urged caution at the time, saying that beta-carotene in the serum might simply be a marker for fruit and vegetable consumption and that the complex mixture of chemicals involved in this consumption might be what promotes health. Or it might be that people who ate fruits and vegetables were healthier to begin with: more likely to exercise, less likely to smoke and leaner than those whose idea of a vegetable is a dollop of ketchup.

One of those cautious experts, Dr. Victor Herbert, a professor of medicine at the Mount Sinai School of Medicine in New York, warned that the vitamin supplements could actually be harmful, because beta-carotene acts as a pro-oxidant in some circumstances.

But the antioxidant craze took on a life of its own. "The enthusiasm ran ahead of the evidence," said Dr. Daniel Steinberg, a professor of medicine at the University of California at San Diego, who studies antioxidants and heart disease.

Now, given the new studies' finding that beta-carotene supplements are useless or worse, some experts are saying that at least the scientific process was brought to fruition. "The reality is that science has worked here," said Dr. Hennekens, the director of the Physicians' Health Study. Despite people's willingness to accept less-than-definitive evidence, he said, scientists pushed ahead with carefully designed clinical trials.

"The major message," Dr. Klausner said, "is that no matter how compelling and exciting a hypothesis is, we don't know whether it works without clinical trials."

Others criticize the dietary supplement industry for promoting beta-carotene so vigorously without an adequate scientific basis. "The health food industry is selling America a bill of goods," said Dr. Herbert, who added that he had long been "a leading voice against this quackery."

Dr. Peter Greenwald, director of the division of cancer prevention and control at the cancer institute, said: "We ought to give this some real thought. Someone's promoting supplements. Where does the responsibility lie to show efficacy?"

Gina Kolata, January 1996

VITAMIN E MAY BOOST IMMUNITY

A new study suggests that the near-universal decline in the health of the immune system that accompanies aging may be slowed by supplements of vitamin E.

According to findings being published in the *Journal of the American Medical Association*, various immune functions were given a significant lift by daily supplements of vitamin E for 235 days, with the best results occurring with a supplement of 200 milligrams a day. (One milligram is roughly equal to one international unit of vitamin E.)

Vitamin E is a powerful antioxidant that has received much scientific and popular attention in recent years for its purported ability to delay the ravages of age. The new study, directed by Dr. Simin Nikbin Meydani of Tufts University in Boston, involved eighty-eight healthy men and women sixty-five and older who were randomly assigned to receive one of three levels of vitamin E—60, 200 or 800 milligrams a day—or a look-alike placebo. The lowest dose tested represented twice the current daily recommended intake of vitamin E. The study measured such immune functions as the amount of antibody produced in response to a vaccine.

Since vitamin E is found primarily in vegetable oils and margarine, wheat germ, nuts and seeds, it is nearly impossible to consume amounts significantly higher than the recommended intake through a normal, wholesome diet, particularly a diet that is low in fat. Because of budgetary and health constraints, the elderly are especially likely to consume too little of this essential nutrient. Furthermore, some medications interfere with vitamin E, and chronic diseases common among the elderly may impair their ability to absorb foods rich in vitamin E.

Vitamin E in amounts of 100 to 400 international units a day have previously been linked to a reduced risk of developing heart disease and some cancers. But higher doses of vitamin E can interfere with blood clotting and may increase the risk of bleeding disorders and hemorrhagic stroke. High doses also may weaken bones and reduce the body's stores of vitamin A.

Jane E. Brody, May 1997

THE DANGERS OF TOO MUCH VITAMIN C

Those who think that if a little vitamin C is good, more must be better should think again, says a team of British researchers, who found that a supplement of 500 milligrams a day could damage people's genes.

Many Americans take that much or more, in hopes of preventing colds and reaping the widely celebrated antioxidant benefits of vitamin C. Antioxidants, which block cellular and molecular damage caused by the highly reactive molecules called free radicals, are believed to protect against heart disease, cancer, eye disorders like cataracts and macular degeneration, and other chronic health problems.

But the British researchers, chemical pathologists at the University of Leicester, found in a six-week study of thirty healthy men and women that a daily 500-milligram supplement of vitamin C had pro-oxidant as well as antioxidant effects on the genetic material DNA. The researchers found that at the 500-milligram level, vitamin C promoted genetic damage by free radicals to a part of the DNA, the adenine bases, that had not previously been measured in studies of the vitamin's oxidative properties.

The finding, published in the British journal *Nature*, corroborates warnings that have been issued for decades by American physician Dr. Victor Herbert, professor of medicine at the Mount Sinai School of

Medicine in New York. Dr. Herbert has shown, primarily through laboratory studies, that vitamin C supplements promote the generation of free radicals from iron in the body.

"The vitamin C in supplements mobilizes harmless ferric iron stored in the body and converts it to harmful ferrous iron, which induces damage to the heart and other organs," Dr. Herbert said in an interview. "Unlike the vitamin C naturally present in foods like orange juice, vitamin C as a supplement is not an antioxidant. It's a redox agent—an antioxidant in some circumstances and a pro-oxidant in others."

In contrast, vitamin C naturally present in food, he said, has no oxidizing effects. Vitamin C supplements in large doses have been linked to genetic damage as far back as the mid-1970s. In a study then, Canadian researchers found that use of the vitamin in doses larger than in the British study, but not much larger than the amounts some people take to ward off colds and the flu, damaged genetic material in three systems: bacterial cells, human cells grown in test tubes and live mice.

The lead author of the new study, Dr. Ian Podmore, said that at 500 milligrams, vitamin C did act as an antioxidant on one part of the DNA, the guanine bases. Oxidation of guanine to oxoguanine is what is usually measured to determine the degree of DNA damage through oxidation. As expected, when the volunteers took a daily 500-milligram dose of vitamin C for six weeks, oxoguanine levels indeed declined, "which is why vitamin C is generally thought to be an antioxidant," Dr. Podmore said.

But when they measured a second indicator of DNA oxidation, oxoadenine, the researchers found that it had risen rather than declined, "indicating genetic damage to this DNA base," Dr. Podmore said.

A colleague, Dr. Joseph Lunec, said that at the 500-milligram level, vitamin C's "protective effect dominated, but there was also a damaging effect."

"There should be caution about taking too much vitamin C," Dr. Lunec said. "The normal healthy individual would not need to take supplements of vitamin C."

In the United States and Britain alike, the recommended daily intake of vitamin C for healthy adults is 60 milligrams, which can be easily obtained from foods—by drinking about six ounces of orange juice, for example. Larger amounts are recommended for smokers and for pregnant and lactating women, but even these amounts can be readily obtained from foods.

Dr. Lunec took issue with the late Dr. Linus C. Pauling, the Nobel laureate chemist who took 12,000 milligrams of vitamin C daily and suggested that people could take as much of it as they wanted with no ill effect.

"We think that's not the case, to say the least," Dr. Lunec said. "You can have too much of a good thing."

The research team is now studying the effects of lower doses of vitamin C, "to see if we can maximize the protective effect and minimize the damage," Dr. Lunec said. Given the new finding, he said, "it would be unethical to test higher levels."

Jane E. Brody, April 1998

[5]

A Pill for Every Purpose

Other Supplements, from Andro to Zinc

Hormones, minerals, amino acids: the shelves of health food stores and pharmacies are jammed with products that are promoted as energy enhancers, muscle builders, remedies for insomnia, weight-loss aids, boosters of the immune system and foes of free radicals, molecules that are widely blamed for aging, cancer and other diseases.

Some have legitimate uses. Melatonin, for instance, can help people with winter depression, and it has been used successfully to treat sleep problems in blind people. Creatine may help athletes who work out a lot—but not sedentary people—to increase their strength and muscle mass. Studies have found that glucosamine and chondroitin sulfate can help to treat pain and stiffness in arthritic knees.

But claims for other supplements have been questioned or discredited. Studies are divided as to whether zinc can relieve cold symptoms, with the majority of the data indicating that it cannot. Chromium picolinate does not help people lose weight, researchers say. Shark cartilage did not help patients with advanced cancers of the brain, lung, colon, breast, bladder, prostate or lymphatic system, a 1998 study found. But as many as fifty thousand American cancer patients may have taken the cartilage pills. The substance had been advanced as a treatment because of the belief that sharks do not get cancer. Because sharks' bodies are made mostly of cartilage, it was assumed that something in cartilage must inhibit the growth of cancer. Not only has the theory not proved true in people, but another study has shown that sharks actually do get cancer. Researchers from Johns Hopkins University and George Washington University presented evidence of malignant tumors in sharks and related fishes like skates and rays at a cancer conference in April 2000, and accused promoters of the cartilage pills of "giving desperate patients false hope" and encouraging the needless slaughter of sharks and disruption of marine ecosystems.

Most Americans assume that anything in pill form must be regulated by the Food and Drug Administration, and therefore must be safe and effective, or it would never have been allowed on the market. But that is not the case with supplements; the FDA cannot act against them unless there is evidence that someone has been harmed. And unwary consumers run the risk of being the ones to provide that evidence.

A NEWSLETTER EXPLAINS IT ALL FOR YOU

After years of double-digit growth, sales of herbal supplements have slowed down. Maybe it's because there has been so much negative publicity about their safety and effectiveness. Maybe it's because, despite all the promises from the manufacturers, the supplements don't provide a quick fix. Or maybe it's because there are so many of them that most people are completely bewildered.

The confusion can be traced to the 1994 Dietary Supplement Health and Education Act, which gives manufacturers almost carte blanche to sell products with virtually no government oversight.

The leveling off of sales could also be a protest against the idea that companies can manufacture products without any quality control and make false promises. Now, a new quarterly publication, the *Dietary Supplement*, could prove to be of help to the bewildered consumer as well as to health professionals looking for an unbiased overview of what is available.

Those who want unequivocal answers will be disappointed, though. The newsletter expects readers to balance the information themselves and make informed decisions instead of relying on what manufacturers promise. Describing itself as an "independent source for the sensible, informed use of vitamins, minerals, botanicals and related products," the newsletter in its first three issues seems to be living up to the description. What it has to say about vitamin E, echinacea, glucosamine and chondroitin is both thorough and sensible.

The newsletter is the brainchild of Paul R. Thomas, who has a bachelor's degree in biology and a doctorate in nutrition education and has worked for the Food and Nutrition Board of the National Academy of Sciences. He says he takes no money from the supplement industry, and the newsletter accepts no advertising. The sixteen-page quarterly provides an in-depth discussion of a different supplement in each issue along with other information about the industry.

Each discussion asks two questions: What are the scientific evidence and expert opinion for and against the use of the supplement? What is the best advice on how to choose a supplement to gain the benefits and minimize the risks?

About vitamin E the newsletter says: "Heart disease is best prevented by eating right, getting regular exercise"—the usual advice. But it goes on to say, "It is not clear whether supplements of vitamin E add much to a heart-protective lifestyle, but for those who believe extra vitamin E may be of benefit to the heart, 200 to 400 International Units (IU) a day divided into two doses appears reasonable."

And it adds that for those who want to take vitamin E, the natural form is better than synthetic, even though it is more expensive, because it stays in the body longer. Synthetic vitamin E is labeled dl-alpha tocopherol; natural is labeled d-alpha tocopherol.

The newsletter advises using products with an expiration date, as well as some evidence of quality assurance, like a statement on the label that it meets quality and purity standards set by United States Pharmacopeia, a professional organization.

Echinacea, also reviewed by the newsletter, is the best-selling herbal remedy in this country, marketed to prevent or alleviate the symptoms of colds. The newsletter says it appears to be safe "when used by basically healthy people on an occasional, short-term basis." But it goes on to say that it is difficult to know whether echinacea works, because the clinical trials, many of which were financed by the industry, had deficiencies, and because each echinacea product contains different properties, making it impossible to recommend one brand over another.

"If you're going to try an echinacea supplement, and it's not at all clear that you should, simply pick one the next time you're coming down with a cold or flu," the newsletter advises. "If it doesn't work and you're determined to give echinacea another try with your next respiratory infection, choose a different brand."

The newsletter costs $28 a year from 11905 Bristol Manor Court, Rockville, MD 20852, (301) 881-7008, or www.thedietarysupplement.com.

Besides United States Pharmacopeia, other professional organizations are trying to improve the reliability of dietary supplements. Consumer-Lab.com is a commercial testing company that has begun to assess the quality of dietary supplements; its evaluations are posted on its Web site, www.consumerlab.com. The National Nutritional Foods Association, a trade organization for manufacturers and retailers of herbal remedies, requires members to be part of its certification program, which provides "reasonable assurance" that the products meet certain quality standards.

At the University of the Sciences in Philadelphia, a group of pharmacists is undertaking clinical evaluations of herbal supplements. *Good Housekeeping* magazine has announced that advertisers will be required to provide evidence that the ingredients claimed on the label are actually in the product in the amounts specified. And the National Center for Complementary and Alternative Medicine at the National Institutes of Health is providing $6 million to develop standardized versions of the pills of four botanicals, including echinacea, for use in future clinical trials.

In the meantime, the *Dietary Supplement* may be your best bet.

Marian Burros, October 2000

THE SEARCH FOR MUSCLE IN A BOTTLE

"Thirteen. Keep pushing. Fourteen. One more." Stretched out on a weight-lifting bench, a dumbbell in each fist, Ryan Renicker, twenty-five, grimaces. His friend and occasional personal trainer, Joshua Tomey, quietly eggs Mr. Renicker on as he hoists the weights one last time, over his chest in a butterfly motion, before easing them to the mat with a deep sigh.

Mr. Renicker works out most nights at City Gym, in Boston's Kenmore Square, before heading home from his job as a financial analyst. On this midwinter evening, he moves among exercise stations in a fury of flexed muscles. And what muscles they are. At 6 feet 2 inches and 210 pounds, Mr. Renicker has a broad chest, rocky abdominals and biceps like footballs.

But he has had help. For the last two years, Mr. Renicker has been taking a daily 5-gram dose of the dietary supplement creatine monohydrate. He spends about $30 a month on the white powder, which he buys in 2-pound tubs.

"You can feel it during a workout," Mr. Renicker said. "It gives you more energy. You don't fatigue as quickly. When I started using it, my strength went up incredibly."

Thousands of body-conscious Americans seem to agree. By one estimate, last year consumers bought $200 million worth of creatine products (which range from powdered beverages to creatine candy), making it the best-selling strength or energy supplement in the United States.

Although this amino acid compound has been gaining popularity since its introduction in 1993, creatine monohydrate and another supplement, androstenedione, garnered a glaring spotlight in the summer of 1998. In the midst of pursuing Roger Maris's single-season home run record, Mark McGwire acknowledged that he used both supplements to add oomph to his swing.

Nationwide, in taverns and on the Internet, a debate ensued over the ethics of using muscle boosters to enhance athletic performance. But men who simply want to fill out their T-shirts with firmer flesh were left wondering: Do creatine, "andro" and other legal muscle-making supplements really work? And are they safe?

There is no question that some muscle-makers are very effective—like the ones banned by most sports. A 1996 study in the *New England Journal of Medicine* demonstrated that men injected with 600 milligrams of pharmaceutical testosterone every day for ten weeks gained considerably more muscle strength and size than men who took placebo pills. (A man normally produces about 7 milligrams of testosterone a day.)

However, testosterone and other anabolic steroids (drugs that promote muscle growth by mimicking male hormones) are approved by the federal government only for the treatment of hormone deficiencies and a few other medical conditions. All major athletic organizations in the United States forbid their use. Anabolic agents that have not been federally approved are smuggled into the United States and sold on the black market. But the threat of potential side effects—including shrunken testicles, baldness, liver failure and overly aggressive behavior known as "'roid rage"—makes them attractive only to hard-core bodybuilders.

Muscle seekers wary of the law and of the health risks have long used over-the-counter pills and powders, but exercise physiologists insisted that they were wasting their money—until now. "Creatine is one of the most effective products on the market," said Dr. Melvin H. Williams, professor emeritus of exercise science at Old Dominion University in Norfolk, Virginia. Dr. Williams is the author of *The Ergogenics Edge: Pushing the Limits of Sports Performance* (Human Kinetics, 1998), in which he questions the effectiveness of many commonly used sports supplements. But Dr. Williams said there is a growing stack of scientific studies proving that creatine works, unlike most other products hyped in muscle magazines.

In an experiment conducted in 1995 at the University of Texas Southwestern Medical Center, eight highly trained men who took 20 grams of creatine every day for twenty-eight days increased their bench press by an average of 18 pounds, an astonishing leap for experienced weight lifters. Unlike anabolic steroids, creatine supplements do not work their magic by boosting hormone levels. (The few studies involving women suggest that creatine works only half as well.)

Men and women alike manufacture tiny amounts of creatine, and a small amount is found in meat and fish. Creatine provides muscle fuel during short bursts of explosive power—lifting heavy weights or sprinting, for example. The body's own stock of creatine is exhausted quickly. In theory, overloading muscles with creatine supplements allows people to lift a heavy weight more times before tiring. More repetitions lead to bigger muscles.

The reality of how creatine builds muscles is a bit more complex. Scientists know, for instance, that creatine causes muscle cells to retain water. In the simplest sense, bloated muscle cells will produce bulkier muscles. But Dr. Tim Ziegenfuss, a physiologist at Eastern Michigan University in Ypsilanti, says that when a muscle cell expands, it triggers the production of more protein, which makes muscle fibers bigger.

One thing is certain: regular creatine users gain weight. "I've seen guys put on ten to fifteen pounds of solid muscle," said Mr. Tomey, the trainer at City Gym. According to Dr. Williams, however, much of the weight gain, at least initially, is caused by retained water. Anecdotal reports suggest that creatine supplements don't work at all for 20 percent to 30 percent of people who take them, probably because they already have naturally high levels in their muscles.

There are scattered reports that creatine can cause muscle cramps and dehydration. (Dr. Ziegenfuss encourages creatine users to drink plenty of water.) And the Food and Drug Administration has on file thirty-two cases of "adverse events" involving people who used it, including one death.

Other supplements are far more problematical, like androstenedione. In the 1970s, East German female athletes are said to have been the first competitors to use synthetic andro, in the form of nasal spray. Now sold as pills, several brands of androstenedione are available in vitamin stores throughout the United States. But the nation's leading nutrition-supply retailer, General Nutrition Centers, ordered its franchisees to stop selling androstenedione in 1998. Olympic and college athletes are prohibited from using the supplement, as are players in the National Football League.

The uneasiness about andro stems from its similarity to testosterone-boosting anabolic steroids. A naturally occurring hormone produced by the adrenal gland, androstenedione is converted by enzymes into testosterone. The average man produces about 3 milligrams of androstenedione each day. Strength athletes and bodybuilders take 100 milligrams or more of andro a day in hopes of elevating their testosterone levels to promote greater muscle growth.

According to Dr. Ziegenfuss, they may be wasting their money. In laboratory tests, he has given 200-milligram doses of androstenedione to young men and found that their testosterone levels barely changed. Dr. Ziegenfuss said he has taken the supplement on and off for the last nine months. "I really haven't noticed a whole lot yet, to be honest," he said.

While taking andro for a few weeks does not seem to produce serious side effects, some scientists worry that long-term use could wreak metabolic mayhem.

"We're talking about a sex hormone," said Dr. Jerrold Leikin, a physician and the director of emergency services at Rush-Presbyterian-St. Luke's Medical Center in Chicago. Dr. Leikin, the author of *Poisoning and Toxicology Compendium* (Lexi-Comp, 1998), believes that athletes who gobble andro run the same risks as people who use anabolic steroids, including liver damage and rising cholesterol levels. "There is no reason to think they will be any different," he said.

The usual caveats apply to purchasing over-the-counter muscle pills and powders. Since the Food and Drug Administration does not regulate the content and purity of dietary supplements, there is no guarantee that the bottles bought at the local vitamin store contain what the label says. It is also a good idea to discuss the use of any supplement—and its potential side effects—with your doctor.

Creatine and androstenedione are not the only dietary supplements that bodybuilders use in hopes of bulking up. Here are other popular ones. (Experts recommend that anyone interested in taking a nutritional supplement consult a doctor beforehand.)

- Protein supplements. People who lift weights for at least an hour or two every day require up to twice as much dietary protein as those who don't. But protein bars and shakes offer little beyond convenience. Foods like skim milk and turkey breast are excellent sources of protein and cost a fraction of the price.
- DHEA. The adrenal gland produces dehydroepiandrosterone, a hormone that may convert to testosterone or other hormones. Levels begin to

drop after age thirty. Some research shows that DHEA
helps sedentary adults over fifty to lose fat and gain
muscle, but there is little proof that the hormone
makes anyone else bulk up. Many medical authorities
have condemned the use of DHEA supplements,
citing several potential side effects including liver
damage, cholesterol problems and an elevated risk of
breast and prostate cancer.

Timothy Gower, February 1999

*In the summer of 1999, Mark McGwire said he had quit using andro
and never wanted to take it again. That autumn, the Federal Trade Commission ordered two companies that marketed andro to stop claiming that
it was free of side effects. The commission said there was no scientific proof
for the claims. The companies agreed to disclose potential risks in their
advertising, labeling and promotional materials. And in November 2000,
researchers at East Tennessee State University published a study in the*
Archives of Internal Medicine *showing that andro did not help men who
were working out in a high-intensity resistance training program, but did
cause worrisome hormonal changes as well as changes in blood lipids that
increased the risk of heart disease.*

CREATINE: THE MUSCLE-BUILDING SECRET IS OUT

In 1998, as baseball fans cheered on Mark McGwire's effort to capture
the seasonal home run record set by Roger Maris in 1961, manufacturers
of a dietary supplement called creatine were cheering wildly, too. The
Cardinals' first baseman said he had been aided in his quest by the muscles and strength he acquired through creatine-supplemented workouts.

Inspired by Mr. McGwire, as well as the Orioles' outfielder Brady
Anderson, another creatine user, who was transformed from a virtual
ninety-seven-pound weakling into a hulk, and the many other professional athletes who swear by it, countless prospective athletes and
scrawny teenage boys were spending upwards of $200 million a year on

creatine. By taking this perfectly legal but minimally tested and unregulated substance, they hoped to improve their scores and/or physiques. As a result, creatine became one of the hottest-selling supplements.

There is good reason for creatine's popularity. Unlike the anabolic steroids that mimic the effects of the male sex hormone testosterone, creatine does not cause hair loss or make the testicles shrink. Although virtually nothing is known about possible long-term hazards, no obvious adverse effects have been linked to creatine use. Although sales fell significantly in 1997 after the deaths of three wrestlers taking creatine, the supplement was subsequently cleared of responsibility.

And since creatine is a substance naturally present in common foods and manufactured by the body, it has not been—nor is it likely to be—banned from use in athletic competitions. Another over-the-counter supplement used by Mr. McGwire and others, androstenedione, is converted to the steroid hormone testosterone in the body and has been banned by several leading athletic associations. Athletes who test positive for steroid use can be stripped of medals or forbidden to compete, but it would not be possible to tell whether an athlete got creatine from a steak or a bottle.

Creatine may also prove helpful beyond the playing field to counter the muscle wasting that occurs, for example, in AIDS patients, the elderly and people with cancer or chronic heart failure. Creatine is an amino acid made in the liver and kidneys and acquired in the diet from animal protein foods, especially meats, milk and some fish. The muscles of a 154-pound person need about 2 grams of creatine a day (more or less depending on muscle mass). Meat eaters get about half that from their diets (a half pound of meat has about 1 gram); the rest is made in the body. As might be expected, creatine levels are lower in vegetarians.

Creatine is stored in muscle cells as the compound phosphocreatine, which the body uses to enhance the action of the muscles. It also increases the water content of muscle cells, which adds to their size and probably their ability to function as well. The typical user of creatine supplements gains weight from an increase in lean body mass, not body fat. Users also are likely to experience a rise in blood levels of the heart-protective HDL cholesterol. Studies of the effects of the supplement on athletic performance have clearly shown its benefits are limited to anaerobic activities that involve short intense bursts of energy, like weight lifting, sprinting and slamming a baseball over the outfield fence.

Unlike endurance pursuits like running and cycling, anaerobic activities do not require a steady supply of oxygen. Researchers say that creatine is of no particular benefit to endurance athletes, who may be slowed down by the supplements because of the weight gain they cause.

Creatine's benefits are likely the result of an increased ability to train intensely and gain strength and improve body composition as a result of such training. Creatine offers no particular benefit to a sedentary person—you have to work out regularly when taking it to reap its rewards. Nor is it likely to be helpful to weekend athletes.

It is generally a good idea to have a thorough medical checkup before starting creatine supplementation and, since there are no long-term safety studies, to have periodic kidney and liver function tests and cardiac examinations. People with kidney disorders are advised not to take creatine at all.

Exercise experts who have studied creatine offer the following dosage recommendations to those who decide to take it: start with 20 to 25 grams a day for five or six days, which loads muscle cells with the most creatine they can hold. Absorption is enhanced when creatine—which can be taken in capsule, powder or other forms—is taken with a high-carbohydrate drink, although the common advice to take it with fruit juice has been nixed by some experts. After the loading dose, take a maintenance dose of 2 to 5 grams a day. As long as the maintenance dose is continued, the cells will remain saturated with creatine, these experts say.

Can you safely take it indefinitely? The answer remains unclear. What is known, however, is that taking more than the recommended amount of creatine is a waste and may increase the likelihood of an adverse reaction. Side effects reported anecdotally include gastrointestinal distress, nausea and muscle cramping, although these effects have not been noted in the course of scientific studies of the supplement.

Creatine supplements also increase the likelihood of dehydration and should not be used when dehydration is a risk, for example, when exercising in extreme heat or trying to make weight in wrestling.

A word to wise young athletes and their parents: no studies have been done on the effects of creatine supplements on the growth, development or health of children and adolescents, said Dr. William O. Roberts of MinnHealth SportsCare in White Bear Lake, Minnesota, a family physician and consultant to the magazine *The Physician and Sportsmedicine.*

Keep in mind, too, that because creatine is sold as a dietary supplement and not as a drug, it is not required to meet the standards of the Food and Drug Administration for purity or safety. Quality assurance is up to the manufacturer, and not all producers are equally careful or honorable. Be sure to choose a reputable brand; a bargain may be no bargain.

Jane E. Brody, September 1998

DHEA: BEHIND THE HOOPLA OVER A HORMONE

In a culture that worships youth, baby boomers and older people alike are ever in search of a fountain of youth. And if you believe the claims being widely disseminated in books, magazines and newsletters and on radio, television and the Internet, that Holy Grail is now available in dihydroepiandrosterone, or DHEA, a hormone, classified as a dietary supplement, that is selling briskly.

The claims for DHEA make it sound like a miracle drug that can stop and even reverse the aging process and the debilitating diseases that often accompany it. Some enthusiasts say that a daily dose of the substance has taken twenty years off their chronological ages. Commercial proponents, true believers and a few less-than-cautious researchers say it can strengthen immunity; recharge a flagging libido; melt body fat and build new muscle; prevent cancer, heart disease, diabetes and osteoporosis; enhance energy; improve mood; relieve symptoms of lupus; treat Alzheimer's disease; and increase longevity.

If even half these claims were established facts, DHEA might truly be a wonder drug. But before you rush out to buy a bottle, consider what is and is not known about its real and potential benefits and risks.

DHEA is a hormone, a weak androgen produced by the adrenal glands that can be converted in the body to testosterone and estrogen in both men and women. Its release into the blood peaks at various times: just before birth (slackening in childhood) and before puberty (slackening after age twenty-five or thirty). Blood levels of the hormone in a seventy-year-old are only about 25 percent of those in a thirty-year-old, prompting some to suggest that aging may be a DHEA-deficiency disease. But it could also mean that the hormone is not needed in large amounts by older people.

DHEA is a nonpatentable steroid that can be synthesized from pharmaceutical ingredients or extracted from wild yams. Although DHEA had been available over the counter for decades, the Food and Drug Administration deemed it in 1985 to be a drug for which unsubstantiated claims were being made, and banned its sale. Then in 1994, the hormone, along with many other potent "natural" chemicals, reemerged as a nonprescription supplement under the Dietary Supplement and Education Act, which blocks FDA regulatory action unless a label makes unproved claims or the product is proved dangerous.

Warning No. 1: The DHEA you can buy in health food stores and elsewhere has not been scrutinized by any official organization for quality or content. You may or may not be getting what you pay for.

Warning No. 2: There are no long-term studies of either the benefits or risks of the hormone. Nearly all the relatively few studies completed in people have been small and short-term. Most of the claims made for it are based on studies in mice and rats, which, unlike people, do not produce significant quantities of the hormone at any time in their lives. Therefore, its effects in these animals may be quite different from those in people. Furthermore, careful researchers say promoters have drawn unwarranted conclusions about the benefits of DHEA from their studies and have made claims based on small studies that have not been confirmed by others.

Warning No. 3: The overwhelming majority of researchers who are conducting well-designed studies of the hormone caution consumers against taking it without medical supervision. Given the many unknowns about how the hormone can be administered safely and what benefits it may bestow, the researchers say it should be used only by participants in an approved research study, in which they receive pharmaceutical-grade

DHEA and are closely monitored for ill effects. The researchers also caution against doses higher than 50 milligrams a day.

Despite its over-the-counter availability, the hormone may indeed have risks. As indicated by studies in animals and people, the possible hazards include stimulating the growth of prostate and breast cancer, damaging the liver, masculinizing women and increasing women's cardiac risk.

That said, once researchers have sorted things out, DHEA or a metabolite (a breakdown product) may indeed have a bright future as a hormone supplement in midlife to late life. At the University of California at San Francisco, Dr. Owen M. Wolkowitz and Dr. Louann Brizendine are evaluating the hormone's ability to improve memory and quality of life in patients with mild Alzheimer's disease, based on animal studies in which aged mice given DHEA performed as well on memory tests as young mice, and on the finding that elderly people with lower blood levels of the hormone did not function as well as those with higher levels. In another study of men and women with major depression, Dr. Wolkowitz said, the hormone produced significant improvement when compared with a placebo.

The hormone's ability to enhance normal immune responses has been suggested in studies of older men and women, who while taking DHEA produced higher levels of infection-fighting natural killer cells and less of a damaging immune substance, interleukin-6. Elderly patients on the hormone showed an improved response to influenza vaccine. And in patients with the autoimmune disease lupus, DHEA reduced the severity of symptoms and the amount of medication they required.

As for other claims, however, higher blood levels of the hormone were linked to only a modest decrease in cardiac risk for men and no decrease in risk for women in a ten-year study of nearly two thousand people in Rancho Bernardo, California, conducted by Dr. Elizabeth Barrett-Connor of the University of California at San Diego. Nor did she find an association between DHEA levels and bone density. Initial claims that the hormone might lower breast cancer risk have not been borne out by three studies. And two studies found higher levels of the hormone in women who developed cancers of the breast or ovary.

Anecdotal reports of a revival of sexual desire and prowess stimulated by DHEA remain just that: anecdotes, which carry no scientific weight whatsoever. *Nutrition Action* newsletter reported in March 1997 that volunteers in one study experienced no change in sexual desire while taking 50 milligrams of the substance daily for three months, and no study has yet examined the hormone's effects on sexual activity.

Likewise with studies of the hormone's effects on energy and mood. A small three-month study described "improved physical and psychological well-being" in people given 50 milligrams of DHEA a day, but a second study of a 100-milligram dose taken for six months did not produce such reports.

And Dr. Arthur Schwartz of the Temple University School of Medicine in Philadelphia said that contrary to claims on the Internet, his studies had not shown that the hormone aids in weight loss. Six other studies found no benefit from the hormone on levels of body fat in men and women.

Jane E. Brody, February 1998

GLUCOSAMINE AND CHONDROITIN SULFATE: THE ARTHRITIS IS AT BAY, THANK YOU

The two questions I was asked most often in 1997 were "Is that dietary supplement still helping your arthritic knees?" and "Are there results yet from the studies being done on this side of the Atlantic?"

In late 1996, following my arthritic spaniel's dramatic improvement upon taking a supplement containing two substances that play a role in the formation of cartilage, glucosamine and chondroitin sulfate, I decided to try the stuff myself. Two months later, ignoring bemused queries like "Are you barking yet?" I reported about a 30 percent improvement—not an absence of pain and stiffness, but less of them and little or no swelling after activities like tennis and ice skating that gave my knees a workout.

Now a year later my dog and I are still taking the supplement, though at lower daily doses. My dog, who will be thirteen in June, is free of pain and stiffness. He walks two hours a day, goes up and down stairs easily and regularly climbs a mountain road with me. I continue to play singles tennis two to four times a week and skate four or five times a week, and I have added a daily three-and-a-half-mile brisk walk to my activities.

Despite recent X rays showing advanced arthritis in one knee and moderately advanced arthritis in the other, my knees do not swell anymore and are no longer stiff after prolonged sitting. I do not have pain-free knees, but I no longer have disabling discomfort, a chronic limp or difficulty going down stairs, and I have greatly reduced my use of ibuprofen, which while relieving pain and swelling may contribute to joint deterioration.

My dog and I are not alone. My mailbox has been stuffed with testimonials from others who have ventured into this form of alternative medicine to cope with their arthritis. One elderly Brooklyn man said that after three years of crippling pain, he has thrown away his cane and now walks a mile a day. An Arizona woman in her seventies who could hardly walk now walks a mile and a half every morning with her once equally crippled thirteen-year-old dog. A sixty-seven-year-old man in North Carolina reports that after being sidelined by arthritis, he has resumed square dancing.

An orthopedic surgeon in Rochester, New York, told of one patient who canceled knee-replacement surgery after improving on the supplements.

And the Arizona doctor who turned glucosamine and chondroitin into a national craze, Dr. Jason Theodosakis, author with Brenda Adderly and Barry Fox of *The Arthritis Cure* (St. Martin's Press, $22.95 hardcover and $6.50 paperback), said he was among thousands of patients helped by one or both substances, neither of which is covered by medical insurance because they are sold as dietary supplements, not drugs.

In a follow-up work, *Maximizing the Arthritis Cure* (St. Martin's Press, $22.95), Dr. Theodosakis includes additional testimonials, among them ones from a seventy-year-old man who said he was able to dance for the first time in ten years and a priest who was no longer stiff getting off his knees in church.

No dietary supplement alone can be expected to cure osteoarthritis, the wear-and-tear degeneration of the cartilage that cushions the ends of bones in each body joint. Dr. Theodosakis devotes the bulk of his new book to exercises that foster aerobic conditioning, muscular strength and flexibility and a diet that counters overweight. I can testify to the value of both. My knees hurt when I carry just ten extra pounds in my arms for any distance. If those pounds were on my frame, they would be carried by my knees as well.

Furthermore, not everyone improves on the supplements. If cartilage has completely worn away, it cannot be rebuilt. On average, about half of those who try the supplements report reduced pain and stiffness.

But anecdotes do not establish facts. Well-designed studies are needed to prove, or disprove, the value of a remedy. Patients must be randomly assigned to take either the substance in question or a look-alike inactive or comparison remedy, and neither patients nor evaluating physicians can know who is on what until the study is completed. A Canadian physician who has been studying glucosamine alone, Dr. Joseph B. Houpt, a rheumatologist at the University of Toronto, maintains that there is little point in testing the combination regimen before defining the benefits of the individual components. Other researchers, pointing to extensive studies in Europe of glucosamine alone and a few studies of chondroitin, believe the combination is synergistic, that is, the two together produce greater benefits than would be expected simply from adding together their individual effects.

Dr. Houpt also explained that "these are difficult studies to do." Each patient must be thoroughly evaluated to document the extent of arthritic changes within the joints, pain, stiffness, swelling and functional disabilities like trouble climbing up and down stairs, walking or getting up after prolonged sitting.

Dr. Amal K. Das Jr., an orthopedic surgeon in Hendersonville, North Carolina, has completed a study of nearly one hundred patients treated for six months with both glucosamine and chondroitin sulfate. He said, "We found the combination of one thousand five hundred milligrams glucosamine and one thousand two hundred milligrams of chondroitin daily to be effective for treating the pain of mild to moderate arthritis confirmed by X ray." Patients were evaluated using numerous measures of pain, including their discomfort when walking and climbing stairs. Dr. Das said, as have others, that the supplements had caused no adverse reactions.

Another study, of thirty-four Navy Seals and divers by Dr. Alan Philippi and Dr. Christopher Leffler at the Portsmouth Naval Medical Center in Virginia, found significant relief of knee pain but no improvement in function after eight weeks on the supplements.

Several university-based studies of arthritic horses and dogs as well as basic laboratory studies continue to point to functional benefits and healthy changes in joint cartilage associated with the supplements. For example, Dr. Louis Lippiello, a biochemist at Medical Professional Associates of Arizona, found in cell cultures and in dogs that each substance independently increased synthesis of cartilage components and that the two together did even better.

Jane E. Brody, January 1998

As of February 2001, Jane Brody was still taking the supplement.

CHROMIUM PICOLINATE: FALSE CLAIMS, FABULOUS SALES

Chromium picolinate is one of the hottest dietary supplements on the market. The Federal Trade Commission says that at least nine million consumers spend $100 million a year on various forms of it.

And no wonder. If half the claims made for it were true, it would probably be as important a discovery as aspirin or penicillin. Or sliced bread. But for now, the commission contends that none of the claims made for chromium picolinate have been substantiated; one claim, the commission says, is in fact false.

That conclusion led the commission to push for a consent agreement with Nutrition 21, the San Diego company that has exclusive rights to market chromium picolinate in the United States, and with two of the many companies that sell it—Body Gold of La Jolla, California, and Universal Merchants, Inc., of Los Angeles. Under the consent agreement, which is not an admission of guilt, the companies promised to stop making unsubstantiated claims for their products.

The scientific background of the substance is this: chromium is an essential trace mineral that is required for normal insulin function, and chromium picolinate is one form of it.

Dr. Victor Moreno, the president of Nutrition 21, said that until there is scientific evidence that the commission will accept, the company will probably make only one claim: that chromium picolinate may help moderately obese people improve body composition. Dr. Moreno acknowledged that such a claim is "a far cry from what was said before."

Improving body composition means only that the body loses fat and gains muscle mass, not that there is any weight loss. Until it signed the consent agreement, however, Nutrition 21 had made the following claims, and the other two companies had followed suit with at least some of them, according to FTC documents: that chromium picolinate reduces body fat, causes weight loss without dieting or exercise, builds muscles, increases metabolism, controls appetite, reduces cholesterol, lowers elevated blood sugar levels, can treat and prevent diabetes and can improve normal insulin function.

In the settlement, the commission said that all these claims were unsubstantiated and deceptive. And the companies' contention that the claims were scientifically proven was "outright false," said Joel Winston, the assistant director of the division of advertising practice at the commission.

One piece of marketing literature from Nutrition 21 was headed: "Weight loss, fat loss and muscle loss or how to break the string of yo-yo diets." Ads for Body Gold called the product "a powerful weight loss combination." An ad for Universal Merchants' Chromatrim 100, which the ad called "a sugar-free fat-reducing chewing gum," said that the gum would "decrease appetite (especially sugar cravings)."

Mr. Winston said it was important to keep in mind that there is a difference between fat loss and weight loss: "What the ads said is weight loss, and the studies don't show much for weight loss."

In fact, if chromium picolinate does what Dr. Moreno says it does—increase muscle mass and decrease body fat—that does not necessarily add up to weight loss. In a study to measure the effects of chromium picolinate on body weight and mass, Gilbert R. Kaats of the Health and Medical Research Foundation in San Antonio found that 69 of 219 men and women, or 31.5 percent, dropped out.

The principal reason was the "relatively slow scale weight loss that occurred with many subjects in this seventy-two-day study," Dr. Kaats wrote in *Current Therapeutic Research* in October 1996. And one reason for this is that while there was a loss of body fat, there was also a gain in muscle mass.

"We're not saying that in the future there may not be evidence to support the claims," Mr. Winston said. "We are not suggesting that chromium picolinate is worthless," just that there is not enough scientific evidence yet to back up claims made for it.

In the settlement with Nutrition 21, the company was required to send certified letters to all its customers spelling out the details of the consent order.

Mr. Winston said that there are many other companies making the same unsubstantiated claims for chromium picolinate but that the commission could not prosecute them because it did not have the time or the money to do so. But by making an example of these three companies, he added, "we hope this will send a message to the industry as well as the public."

Marian Burros, January 1997

MELATONIN: NEW PROMISE FOR
WINTER DEPRESSION

A few tiny doses of the hormone melatonin each afternoon may help tame the dark demons of winter depression, studies suggest.

In two preliminary studies, Dr. Alfred J. Lewy and his colleagues at Oregon Health Sciences University in Portland showed that properly timed doses of melatonin in amounts much smaller than are being sold could reset people's body clocks and lift their spirits. Dr. Lewy maintains that the findings strongly support the theory that winter depression is a form of jet lag in which people's daily rhythms increasingly fall out of line with clock time when dawn is delayed. By midwinter, people with winter depression feel as if they are being forced to wake up hours before their bodies are ready—as if they had just flown from California to New York.

In an interview, Dr. Lewy said the effectiveness of melatonin indicated that people with winter depression suffered more as winter darkness deepened. Their internal rhythms become adapted to darkness in the morning and do not mesh with the requirements of their lives, which force them to arise and function effectively when their body clocks say it is night. Not until spring approaches does their depression begin to lift.

Dr. Lewy, a psychiatrist and an expert on circadian rhythms, said the preliminary findings suggested that taking melatonin in the afternoon might be nearly as effective as intense morning light in relieving winter depression. He predicted that a similar regimen could be used to help people recover faster from jet lag, adapt better to changing work shifts and adjust more quickly to daylight saving time.

Winter depression, also known as seasonal affective disorder, afflicts as much as 20 percent of the population. The disorder causes many people in northern latitudes to spend the winter beset by blues and lethargy. They tend to sleep more, eat more, crave carbohydrates, gain weight, think more slowly, concentrate poorly and feel fatigued, irritable and unhappy.

If the melatonin remedy holds up in larger studies, it could become the treatment of choice. Simply taking a few pills each day would greatly simplify the treatment of winter depression, which most commonly requires patients to sit in front of a light box that simulates sunlight for about an hour upon awakening every morning. For some people with winter depression, Dr. Lewy said, his studies suggest that melatonin alone might work; for others, the needed lift may come from combining the hormone and light treatment.

At the least, Dr. Lewy and others believe, melatonin might be a useful adjunct to light therapy, enabling patients to spend less time in front of a light box or enhancing the lift provided by light therapy.

Another expert on winter depression, Dr. Michael Terman, a research psychologist at New York State Psychiatric Institute, has given melatonin to a few patients who had incomplete responses to light therapy and found that the combination worked better than light alone. But Dr. Terman said the approach must be tested in large controlled studies.

Melatonin is a hormone produced only at night by the pineal gland in the brain. With sunlight, the body's primary timekeeper, melatonin helps to set the brain's biological clock, which determines all of the body's circadian rhythms, including the sleep-wake cycle, digestive functions and hormone releases.

By giving doses of melatonin equal to levels normally produced by the body in the afternoon, the Oregon researchers were able to readjust the circadian rhythms of the study subjects, convincing their bodies that night was beginning to fall in midafternoon, which meant that physiological dawn would come earlier.

Dr. Lewy and his colleagues are not sure why a disrupted circadian rhythm results in depressive symptoms in so many people. But they found that when melatonin was used to synchronize the internal timing mechanism with the need to get up when it was still dark outside, symptoms of depression were alleviated in most of the patients studied.

The researchers published the results of a pilot study of ten patients in January 1998 in the journal *Psychiatry Research*. During the winter that began in 1996, half the patients were given 0.125 milligrams of melatonin at 2 P.M. and 6 P.M. and the other half got a look-alike dummy medication. In three patients taking melatonin but only one on the placebo, the symptoms of depression were reversed, Dr. Lewy said. He added that he and his colleagues had also completed a second melatonin study this winter of twenty-six patients to determine whether the hormone, properly timed, advanced their body clocks. Nine patients took melatonin in the morning, nine took it in the afternoon and eight took a placebo.

Dr. Lewy said that the placebo and the morning melatonin, which in effect prolonged night for the patients, had virtually no antidepressant effect, but symptoms improved significantly in a substantial number of patients who took melatonin in the afternoon—this time in three doses of 0.1 milligram at 2 P.M., 4 P.M. and 6 P.M., which Dr. Lewy said better imitated the way melatonin was naturally released beginning at dusk.

Dr. Lewy and Dr. Terman emphasized the preliminary nature of these findings and cautioned against self-treatment by depressed people. There are three potential problems: possible interaction with other medications, achieving a proper dose (melatonin is sold as a "dietary supplement" without a prescription in doses no smaller than 0.3 milligrams, which is three times the amount Dr. Lewy used) and the soporific effects of melatonin. Dr. Lewy warned that some people with winter depression may become sleepy even on the very low dose he used.

ADJUSTING TO DAYLIGHT SAVING TIME

Although the yearly "spring ahead" to daylight saving time involves only a one-hour shift forward, it takes many people a week to adjust. This is because the increase in daylight at the end of the day works against the body's ability to advance its biological clock so that it meshes with the new clock time.

Dr. Alfred Lewy at Oregon Health Sciences University in Portland suggests that small well-timed doses of melatonin can ease the adaptation. Start with tablets containing 0.3 milligram of melatonin. Cut each tablet into three parts. Starting on the last Thursday before the clock change, take one-third of the tablet eight hours after your usual wake-up time, another one-third two hours later, and the final third two hours after that. (Dr. Lewy cautioned that even these doses make some people sleepy. If this occurs, cut out one or two doses.) Get out in the morning light without sunglasses, but wear dark glasses in the late afternoon until dusk. Continue this regimen for a few days.

Jane E. Brody, March 1998

MELATONIN: BRINGING SLEEP TO THE BLIND

In the early 1970s, Dr. James Stevenson, then a graduate student in psychology at Stanford University, developed a theory about why he had so much trouble sleeping.

Dr. Stevenson, who had been blind from birth, suffered insomnia at night, and in the daytime experienced "sleep attacks," which arrived one hour later each day, playing havoc with his efforts to get to classes on time. He had read that in blinded animals, the body's clock, normally harnessed to the twenty-four-hour cycle of daylight and darkness, often goes into free run, shifting sleep patterns. His own sleeping difficulties, Dr. Stevenson suspected, might have a similar origin.

A sleep researcher, Dr. Laughton Miles, later confirmed what Dr. Stevenson had concluded: in the absence of light, his body had taken up a free-running, 24.9-hour circadian rhythm of sleep and wakefulness, a schedule that shifted his natural sleeping time back by nearly an hour each day.

But Dr. Miles, who in 1977 published a scientific report on Dr. Stevenson's case, could find no way to fix the problem, nor could other researchers, who have spent two decades seeking effective treatments for the sleep problems caused by free-running circadian rhythms, which affect about half the 200,000 Americans who are totally blind.

But a study presented in 1999 at the annual meeting of the Associated Professional Sleep Societies in Orlando, Florida, suggested that the search may finally be over.

Dr. Robert L. Sack, Dr. Alfred J. Lewy and Richard L. Brandes of the Sleep and Mood Disorders Laboratory at Oregon Health Sciences University found that a daily 10-milligram dose of the hormone melatonin successfully "entrained" the free-running rhythms of six out of seven totally blind subjects, returning them to a normal twenty-four-hour sleep pattern.

"Even entraining one blind person with melatonin is important," said Dr. Charmane Eastman, director of the Biological Rhythms Research Laboratory at Rush-Presbyterian-St. Luke's Medical Center in Chicago. The study, she said, had implications not only for the blind, who often list sleep problems as one of the most difficult aspects of their disability, but also for sighted people, whose circadian rhythms can be altered by jet lag or shift work.

Dr. Lewy, director of the sleep lab at Oregon, said, "Totally blind people offer a natural way to study the human body clock, without the interference of light cues."

In an earlier study, the researchers tried using a 5-milligram dose of melatonin without success. "We got some shifting of rhythms, but we weren't able to establish a clear twenty-four-hour cycle," Dr. Sack said.

A few other investigators have reported single cases in which melatonin corrected free-running sleep-wake cycles in blind people. And Dr. Stevenson, now a research psychologist at NASA Ames Research Center in Mountainview, California, said he began taking melatonin before bedtime in 1987, and now sleeps normally. But the newer study compared melatonin with placebo pills in a group of subjects.

Melatonin is secreted by the pineal gland—a tiny structure deep in the brain—and helps regulate the body's biological clock. In sighted people, melatonin secretion is synchronized with the twenty-four-hour cycle of daylight and darkness, turning on at nightfall, and continuing for about twelve hours. But in the absence of light, most people's body clocks run on a cycle slightly longer than twenty-four hours, Dr. Sack said.

The hormone is also sold over the counter as a nutritional supplement, usually in 3-milligram tablets. Taken in the afternoon, it shifts the body's clock earlier, tricking it into thinking dusk has already fallen. Taken in the morning, however, it delays the clock, as if dawn had not yet arrived.

Scientists still know little about the effects of melatonin at different dosages: in sleep studies, researchers have used doses as small as 0.3 milligrams and as large as 75 milligrams or higher. Dr. Sack said that for some blind people, 10 milligrams may be more than is needed. He and his colleagues are conducting further research to see if dosages between 5 and 10 milligrams are equally effective.

In the study, the subjects, who did not know which treatment they were receiving, took melatonin an hour before bedtime for a period of weeks, then were switched to a dummy pill, or vice versa. The length of time it took for the melatonin to shift rhythms back to normal varied from person to person. "Without knowledge of a person's circadian phase," Dr. Sack and his colleagues wrote, "it may be difficult to know the best day for initiating melatonin treatment; thus entrainment may not occur for weeks or months."

Clifton Zang, a forty-seven-year-old man from Portland who has been totally blind since being hit in the head by a stray bullet while sitting in his pickup truck sixteen years ago, said the benefits of melatonin became apparent not long after he started taking the supplement.

"Before the study, I had no control of my sleep," Mr. Zang said. "I'd sleep any time of the day or night. I'd be awake at two in the morning and fall asleep at noon. But since I've been on the melatonin I go to sleep at eleven o'clock and wake up at five, six or seven."

Erica Goode, June 1999

REMEDY RESEARCH: SOME HINTS, FEW ANSWERS

Eager to relieve the agonizing symptoms of winter viruses, sufferers are widening the search for remedies well beyond the conventional treatments. But even as Americans gobble $12 million worth of vitamins, herbs and supplements annually, scientists and others say there is not enough solid research to evaluate their effectiveness.

That, however, is beginning to change. In the fall of 1998, alternative medicine drew attention when the *Journal of the American Medical Association* published its first issue devoted to alternative medicine. Other journals are also reporting on such therapies. Here are some of the findings about the effectiveness of several popular alternative treatments.

Echinacea

Called the most popular herb in the United States, echinacea is generating more than $300 million in sales annually. Although a 1992 study of the use of echinacea demonstrated a significant decrease in symptoms and duration of flulike illness, a review of twelve commonly used medicinal herbs published in the *Archives of Family Medicine* in November 1998 noted that of twenty-six published controlled trials evaluating the plant, none was conclusive.

The review, with lead authors from the University of Washington, concluded: "Available evidence on echinacea's therapeutic potential is incomplete, but does suggest a possible supportive role in treating infections and wounds. However, well-designed clinical trials are needed to substantiate echinacea's efficacy, clarify appropriate dosages and confirm safety." For boosting immune systems, dosages have not been standardized, but the 1992 study suggested a link between benefits and dosage.

In the same issue, Dr. Dieter Melchart of the Center for Complementary Medicine Research in Munich, Germany, reported the results of a clinical trial in which 302 volunteers received either one or two echinacea extracts or a placebo. The twelve-week study found echinacea no more effective than a placebo in preventing colds.

Garlic

Garlic is one of the most extensively studied herbs. Louis Pasteur determined that it had antiseptic properties in 1858. Results from recent clinical trials attempting to confirm medicinal uses have been mixed, according to the *Archives of Family Medicine* herbal review. In late 1997, *Antimicrobial Agents and Chemotherapy*, the journal of the American Society for Microbiology, reported the discovery of a molecular mechanism that might explain some of garlic's antiseptic power. Scientists at the Weizmann Institute in Israel contend that allicin, the main biologically active component of garlic, blocks certain enzymes associated with bacterial, fungal and viral infections.

Vitamin C

Linus Pauling, who won the Nobel Peace Prize and the Nobel Prize in Chemistry, launched a controversy still being played out in laboratories around the world when he published a book, *Vitamin C and the Common Cold*, in 1970, asserting that vitamin C could prevent colds. He later expanded his theories to include flu and cancer. He advocated taking at least 1,000 milligrams of vitamin C daily and took 12,000 milligrams a day himself, although the recommended daily allowance is 60.

No conclusive data have shown that such large doses significantly protect against the common cold, but many people remain convinced. Meanwhile, vitamin C turns up in various over-the-counter remedies and foods, and the Japanese have even added it to cola.

Zinc Lozenges

Zinc lozenges as a cold remedy surfaced with George Eby, a Texas math major who became a city planner, then fell into biomedical research in 1979 when his young daughter, suffering from leukemia, had a severe cold. The cold appeared cured after a crushed zinc gluconate tablet dissolved in her mouth. By 1984, Mr. Eby was reporting tests in which the lozenges significantly reduced how long cold symptoms lasted. In 1996 a Cleveland Clinic study found that sucking on zinc gluconate lozenges reduced the duration of cold symptoms although the lozenges tasted bad and 20 percent of the people who took them reported nausea. A later trial at the same clinic showed no benefits from zinc. Mayo Clinic specialists suggest caution for children, pregnant women and people with chronic kidney or liver disease.

Nancy Beth Jackson, January 1999

Later studies showed that although garlic can lower cholesterol, the effect is so slight, only about 4 percent, that doctors do not consider it useful. Statin drugs, by comparison, can lower cholesterol by 17 percent.

As for zinc, in November 1999, the Federal Trade Commission announced that the manufacturer of zinc lozenges had agreed to stop making claims that the product could prevent colds and relieve allergy symptoms.

[6]

Accupuncture, Magnets, Massage and Exercise

Alternative Therapies

By the time a panel of experts in the United States declared in 1997 that acupuncture was an effective therapy for some medical problems, an estimated one million Americans were already using it. In China, of course, it had been in use for 2,500 years. Its long history in Asia is undoubtedly part of its appeal to Westerners: many people reason that if a practice has lasted that long, it must have something going for it.

Although its originators believed acupuncture acted on mystical forces in the body, modern research has revealed that it makes biological sense: the needles apparently stimulate the release of natural pain-releasing substances in the body, as well as other nervous system messenger chemicals and hormones. Acupuncture may even alter immune-system functions. Its proponents say its greatest promise lies in treating conditions like nausea and chronic pain from muscle and skeletal problems. A study in 2000 showed that it could help some people overcome cocaine addiction. Acupuncture is quite safe, researchers say, with few side effects.

Expert panel or not, the medical profession has not unanimously accepted acupuncture: some doctors claim that the studies showing efficacy were hopelessly flawed and that gullible patients are being taken in and bilked by "quackupuncture." But in the meantime, people flock to acupuncturists, seeking help for everything from tennis elbow to quitting smoking.

Even older than acupuncture is t'ai chi, with its graceful, dancelike motions; it is often described as a form of meditation as well as exercise, and an aid to relaxation. Studies have shown that it can also improve balance and strength in older people, and reduce their likelihood of falls.

Some scientists see the growing popularity of these techniques, as well as massage and other medical and exercise regimens from the East, as evidence of a collective softening of the brain. But others reason that there is something to be gained from essentially harmless practices that ease pain and stress, increase strength and impart a sense of well-being.

ACUPUNCTURE IMPRESSES SOME, INFURIATES OTHERS

An independent panel of experts concluded that the ancient practice of acupuncture was an effective therapy for certain medical conditions, especially those involving nausea and pain, and should be integrated into standard medical practice for these problems.

The panel emphasized that acupuncture was remarkably safe, with fewer side effects than many well-established therapies. More than one million Americans are believed to be relying on acupuncture to treat a wide range of ailments, from headache and bowel disorders to arthritis and stroke.

The panel's findings, summarized in a sixteen-page consensus report of the National Institutes of Health, are expected to encourage more patients and physicians to consider acupuncture as an alternative or complementary treatment for some common health problems, including nausea associated with pregnancy and cancer chemotherapy, and pain following dental surgery. The report may also foster the use of acupuncture to treat chronic problems, like low back pain and asthma, for which standard medical treatments are inadequate or costly or may entail serious side effects.

The panel said its report should prompt medical insurers, including

Medicare and Medicaid, to consider covering the costs of acupuncture, at least for conditions where there is clear evidence of its benefits.

Acupuncture, which originated in China more than 2,500 years ago, involves stimulation of certain points on or under the skin, mostly with ultrafine needles that are manipulated manually or electrically. Other acupuncture methods, used less often or still considered by acupuncturists to be experimental, involve the use of herbs and heat, or low-frequency laser beams, at the various acupuncture points. Although acupuncture originally involved only 361 such points, there are now upward of 2,000 recognized by licensed acupuncturists.

Acupuncture has been slow to gain acceptance by the Western medical establishment, largely because traditional Chinese explanations for its observed effects were based on theoretical concepts of opposing forces called yin and yang, which, when out of balance, disrupt the natural flow of qi (pronounced chee) in the body.

But the panel cited growing evidence of acupuncture-induced biological effects that could at least partly explain the benefits observed in scores of studies and in clinical practice. For example, the report said, there is considerable evidence that acupuncture causes a release of natural pain-relieving substances like endorphins, as well as messenger chemicals and hormones in the nervous system. Further, it said, acupuncture appears able to alter immune functions.

"There is sufficient evidence of acupuncture's value to expand its use into conventional medicine and to encourage further studies of its physiology and clinical value," the panel concluded after spending a day and a half hearing and reviewing presentations on acupuncture research.

The panel evaluated seventeen scientific presentations summarizing hundreds of studies conducted in recent years, primarily in Western countries. But critics of acupuncture, some of whom call it "quack-upuncture," said the presentations could not have resulted in a reasoned consensus, because no naysayers had been invited to give their views.

"I fail to see how they can arrive at a consensus when only one view is presented," said Dr. Wallace Sampson, a member of the National Council Against Health Fraud who prepared the council's position paper on acupuncture, published in 1991.

Dr. Sampson pointed out that for the most part, the best-designed studies of acupuncture showed the poorest results for it, a fact also mentioned by several experts who made presentations to the panel.

The twelve-member panel, headed by Dr. David J. Ramsay, a physiologist who is president of the University of Maryland at Baltimore, represented a wide range of scientific disciplines and included some physicians who perform acupuncture or have been treated by it.

The members were charged with determining the quality of evidence for the benefits of acupuncture, the conditions for which it might be effective and what studies were needed to further define its value. The panel, which based its conclusions almost entirely on studies that meet criteria for well-designed research, was convened by various agencies of the National Institutes of Health, including the Office of Alternative Medicine.

The panel did not issue a ringing endorsement of acupuncture. But it did find the procedure to be especially useful for treating painful disorders of the muscle and skeletal systems, like fibromyalgia and tennis elbow, and possibly safer than currently accepted remedies for those disorders. As for other pain problems, including postoperative pain and low back pain, the panel said, available data suggest that acupuncture may be a reasonable option.

Among further areas cited as possibly amenable to treatment by acupuncture, usually together with standard remedies, were drug addiction, stroke rehabilitation, carpal tunnel syndrome, osteoarthritis, headache and asthma.

Although the panel lamented the paucity of well-designed clinical studies of acupuncture, it found that in many cases "the data supporting acupuncture are as strong as those for many accepted Western medical therapies."

Nonetheless, it said, larger, better and longer studies are needed to establish properly acupuncture's therapeutic benefits and limitations. A major barrier to mounting such studies is lack of financial support from commercial sources, which have no vested interest in a technique that cannot be patented.

Most presenters here focused only on the relatively few studies that met the "gold standard" for modern clinical research: those entailing random assignment of patients to treatment and control groups, and independent, well-documented assessments of the results. Even some of these studies were considered limited, a number of them because they involved too few or too infrequent acupuncture treatments, or even incorrect acupuncture points.

Further, a major problem in designing acupuncture studies is selection of a control treatment that does not prejudice the results. For example, most studies have used other, nearby points on the skin for comparison with the effects of manipulating real acupuncture points. But this "sham acupuncture" has some biological effects as well, and they make it harder to determine the true benefit of real acupuncture.

Jane E. Brody, November 1997

ACUPUNCTURE: WHAT'S IT GOOD FOR, MAYBE?

Misconceptions about acupuncture abound. While some believe that it is a highly effective pain reliever, others say it is nothing more than a glorified and expensive placebo lacking scientific proof for the many claims made in its behalf. The truth, according to nearly a score of reports made to a federally sponsored conference, lies somewhere in between.

Acupuncture researchers from this country and abroad were invited by the National Institutes of Health to summarize the best available evidence, pro and con, for the effectiveness of acupuncture in their fields. Their reports, which examined topics ranging from acupuncture's well-publicized ability to relieve pain to its potential effects on respiration, digestion, immunity and even fertility, more than anything begged for longer, larger and better-controlled studies to document carefully what acupuncture can and cannot do.

An independent panel of twelve experts who evaluated the reports concluded, however, that for certain common health problems, there was adequate evidence to warrant making acupuncture with manually or electrically manipulated needles a treatment option for Americans.

The panel was especially impressed with the safety of acupuncture when used by well-trained therapists following sterile techniques. Adverse side effects are far less common than those associated with most drug treatments and surgery.

The most convincing findings for the benefits of acupuncture presented to the panel involved the areas described below. But even for these areas, researchers emphasized that not everyone was helped by acupuncture, just as all patients do not benefit from drugs intended to treat their conditions. About 20 percent of people, including a few leading researchers as well as some experimental animals, are "nonresponders" who are not helped.

Further, they said, unless the correct acupuncture points are used and enough treatments are given, the technique is not likely to accomplish its goal. In general, they said, at least ten sites should be stimulated for at least ten treatments to determine whether acupuncture is beneficial.

For pain control, Dr. Ji-Sheng Han of Beijing Medical University in China reported that while "acupuncture by itself is not enough to produce complete anesthesia," half the amount of anesthetic drugs were needed when electroacupuncture was used during brain surgery, resulting in more stable blood pressure and respiration and faster recovery from surgery. The consensus panel found acupuncture to be definitely useful in treating postoperative dental pain and probably helpful in relieving pain after other forms of surgery.

But most patients who seek acupuncture suffer from chronic pain, like recurrent headaches, unremitting low back pain, osteoarthritis and fibromyalgia. Dr. Brian Berman of the University of Maryland School of Medicine in Baltimore concluded that ten well-designed studies of chronic pain showed that "acupuncture definitely performs better than an inert placebo," but a benefit was demonstrated in only half the studies comparing real acupuncture with sham acupuncture or with standard medical therapy.

Likewise, Dr. Daniel Cherkin of the Group Health Center for Health Studies in Seattle said a review of acupuncture studies for low back pain by the Dutch Health Insurance Board had uncovered only two well-designed studies showing acupuncture to be superior to sham treatments.

"Benefits of acupuncture may exist, but they are not yet proven," Dr. Cherkin concluded. "More scientifically rigorous studies are needed that compare acupuncture with existing treatments for low back pain and that evaluate both the short-term and long-term outcomes in terms of symptoms, functional ability and cost."

As for chronic pain in the head, neck and face, Dr. Steve Birch of the APT Foundation, a substance-abuse treatment center in New Haven, reported mixed findings. He cited several studies indicating that acupuncture, if used for at least ten treatments, could reduce the intensity and frequency of facial and neck pain and was better than a dummy medication and roughly equivalent to standard drug therapy for treating chronic headaches.

Like previous researchers, Dr. Gary Kaplan of the Medical Acupuncture Research Foundation in Arlington, Virginia, found most acupuncture studies of osteoarthritic and musculoskeletal pain to be seriously flawed. But a few good studies prompted him to conclude that "acupuncture is a viable treatment option that should be made available today to patients suffering from these painful problems." For example, in a study of patients with severe knee arthritis, 80 percent reported a lasting decrease in pain and disability and seven of twenty-nine patients canceled joint-replacement surgery.

For addiction, more than five hundred clinics in this country use acupuncture to help treat people dependent on drugs or alcohol. A leader in the field, Dr. Michael Smith at Lincoln Hospital in the Bronx, treats upwards of two hundred patients a day and has found, as have others, that acupuncture increases the likelihood that patients will become drug-free and stay in treatment.

Dr. Kim A. Jobst of the Gardiner Institute in Glasgow, Scotland, said eight well-designed studies of patients with asthma and other chronic respiratory disorders showed that "over all, there is a clear positive impact of acupuncture on acute and chronic symptoms of pulmonary disease." Benefits included less need for potent medications and "a significant improvement in subjective well-being." Fewer than 10 percent of acupuncture patients reported negative side effects, and many more reported positive ones like increased energy and strength and feeling warmer and more relaxed.

Immune responses can be impaired by trauma, including surgery, as well as the use of morphine to counter severe pain. Dr. Xiao-Din Cao of the Institute of Acupuncture Research in Shanghai described studies in laboratory animals and patients showing that electroacupuncture given for a few days could enhance the responsiveness of the immune system and "attenuate the immunosuppression induced by surgery and postoperative morphine."

Acupuncture was perhaps most effective in alleviating nausea, the consensus panel concluded. Dr. Andrew Parfitt of the National Institute of Child Health and Human Development described large studies showing that acupuncture could control the nausea of pregnancy and prevent nausea and vomiting following surgery and chemotherapy.

Dr. Janet Konefal of the University of Miami School of Medicine reported that acupuncture's ability to alleviate severe depression was comparable to the benefits of antidepressant drugs. Dr. Yu Jin of Shanghai University Medical Center described acupuncture's success in inducing ovulation in women who were infertile because of an inability to ovulate. Several became pregnant.

Dr. Margaret Naeser, a licensed acupuncturist at the Veterans Affairs Medical Center in Boston, described preliminary success in using the experimental technique of low-energy laser acupuncture for patients with neurological damage. In tests on a small number of patients, adults who had suffered a stroke and young children with cerebral palsy experienced decreased spasticity, and patients with carpal tunnel syndrome reported a significant decrease in pain and disability.

Jane E. Brody, November 1997

ACUPUNCTURE: MY JOB, DANCING
WITH DOUBTERS

I first came into contact with complementary medicine as a dancer. I saw therapies like pilates and yoga help dancers with their movement problems. When I got into physical medicine and rehabilitation training and found that these therapies were not widely used or known about, I found out as much as I could about how they could help people with medical problems. In addition, I've been interested in Chinese medicine since I was a little girl. I did my seventh-grade science fair project on acupuncture.

Now, as medical director of the Mind Body Center for Complementary Medicine at Morristown Memorial Hospital, I spend about half my time seeing patients. I also have to educate medical staff about complementary medicine. Doctors are a tough audience; they've seen fads come and go, so it's important to show there is evidence these are not quack therapies. In an acupuncture class, I make them practice the techniques on one another. Many come in skeptics and leave converts. I've heard many physicians say that learning acupuncture was the one course that changed their practice more than any other.

A fellow physician on staff with me at the hospital I used to work at had back pain that had not responded to physical therapy, oral medications or injections. After three treatments, his pain had subsided significantly. "I don't know if it was you or God," he said, "but I have to admit I'm a lot better." "Oh," I said. "I'm sure it was both. We try to work together whenever possible."

Treatment also makes believers out of patients. They are often nervous when they come in for acupuncture, so I give them a needle in one of a couple of spots, like the top of the head, and this usually calms them down right away. By the end of a session, because of the endorphin release prompted by the procedure, they can be pretty euphoric. We make sure they sit down a few minutes before leaving and that they have their coat and purse with them. I jokingly tell them not to sign any large checks or make any large purchases right after treatment.

One of my patients is a businessman with sarcoidosis, a connective tissue disease. He decided to get acupuncture, hoping it would relieve his symptoms of numbness and tingling in his feet. The day he came in, I had a resident following me around. She was a little nervous about watching all the needles go in. The patient was obviously nervous, too. I said, "I'm asking you all these questions, but what you really want to know is if this is going to hurt." Well, I stuck a needle in the top of his head. He immediately felt more relaxed. The med student was sitting there with big eyes. I thought, "Maybe I'll put a needle in her head, too." I did, she calmed down, and we all had a good laugh.

Ann Cotter with Michelle Cottle, December 1999

ACUPUNCTURE HELPS SOME QUELL COCAINE CRAVING

Acupuncture appears to help some cocaine addicts escape their dependence on the drug, according to a report by researchers at Yale University.

Experts on drug abuse say cocaine addiction is one of the most difficult forms of drug dependency to treat. And while many treatment centers have been using acupuncture for some time, usually in combination with other therapies, scientific studies of its effectiveness in treating cocaine addiction have been inconclusive.

In the Yale study, 53.8 percent of the subjects who had needles inserted in four acupuncture "zones" in the ear five times a week tested free of cocaine at the end of the eight-week study period. In comparison, 23.5 percent of control subjects given "sham" acupuncture treatments and 9.1 percent of subjects who watched relaxation videos tested free of the drug during the final week of the study. The report appears in the August 2000 issue of the journal *Archives of Internal Medicine*.

The study involved eighty-two men and women in the New Haven area who were addicted to both heroin and cocaine. They were receiving methadone treatment for the heroin addiction but were still using cocaine regularly. Thirty of the subjects, however, were dropped from the study after missing sessions.

The researchers called the findings promising but cautioned that the study was relatively small and that more research needed to be done to confirm the results. They also said that acupuncture was not a panacea and suggested that it should be used along with other therapies like counseling.

"These are a difficult group of people to deal with," said Dr. Herbert D. Kleber, the medical director of the National Center on Addiction and

Substance Abuse in New York and a professor of psychiatry at Columbia University, who is familiar with the study.

"We don't have medicine for treating cocaine addiction, and acupuncture appears to be a useful adjunct for decreasing dependence," Dr. Kleber said.

Dr. Arthur Margolin, a research scientist in the department of psychiatry at Yale's medical school and lead author of the report, said that among the benefits of acupuncture were its low cost and lack of side effects. And unlike pharmaceutical treatments, Dr. Margolin said, it can be offered to pregnant women. The study's findings are also encouraging, he added, because "they suggest that with the proper groundwork we can conduct rigorous trials of complementary or alternative therapies."

One obstacle that has confronted researchers trying to determine whether acupuncture works has been the difficulty of finding convincing "placebo" treatments to act as scientific controls. For the sham needle treatment, the Yale researchers inserted four needles along the rim of the ear, in spots that are not commonly used in acupuncture treatment and that had little effect when stimulated in preliminary tests. The relaxation tapes were used to control for the possibility that simply sitting quietly for forty-five minutes in a darkened room might itself produce an effect.

In the acupuncture treatment, the needles were inserted five times a week for about forty-five minutes per session, according to guidelines developed at Lincoln Hospital in the Bronx, and adopted by the National Acupuncture Detoxification Association. Urine samples were taken three times a week to test for cocaine use. All the subjects in the study, which was financed by the National Institute on Drug Abuse, also received psychotherapy as part of the treatment program.

Dr. Margolin said that scientists did not yet understand how acupuncture might work to curb addiction but that there were a variety of theories. For example, acupuncture has been linked to the release of opioids, the body's natural painkillers, which might help reduce the craving for cocaine. Or the procedure might stimulate the vagus nerve that runs through the center of the ear, producing a relaxing effect.

In Chinese medicine, Dr. Margolin added, the stimulation points used in the study are associated with a diagnosis called "empty fire." He said, "This is a pretty good either metaphorical or literal description of a cocaine-addicted individual."

Erica Goode, August 2000

MAGNETS EASE PAIN, SURPRISE SKEPTICS

No one was more skeptical about using magnets for pain relief than Dr. Carlos Vallbona, former chairman of the department of community medicine at Baylor College of Medicine in Houston. So Dr. Vallbona was amazed when a study he did found that small, low-intensity magnets worked, at least for patients experiencing symptoms that can develop years after polio.

Dr. Vallbona had long been fascinated by testimonials about magnets from his patients, and even from medical leaders. But his interest in magnet therapy became more serious in 1994 when he and a colleague, Carlton F. Hazelwood, tried them for their own knee pain. The pain was gone in minutes. "That was too good to be true," Dr. Vallbona said.

Dr. Vallbona knew that the power of suggestion can fool both patient and doctor. But he also wondered: could strapping small, low-intensity magnets to the most sensitive areas of the body for several minutes relieve chronic muscular and joint pains among patients in his postpolio clinic at Baylor's Institute for Rehabilitation Research? Valid studies could allow consumers to make informed choices. And if magnet therapy were found to be safe and effective, it could relieve pain with fewer drugs — and their unwanted side effects.

Endorsements from professional athletes are one reason Americans spend large sums on magnets to seek pain relief. But most doctors take a "buyer beware" attitude because many claims lack scientific proof or explanation of how they might work. The Food and Drug Administration has warned doctors and manufacturers about health claims for magnets.

Aware of the medical profession's skepticism about magnet therapy, Dr. Vallbona sought to conduct science's most rigorous type of study. Participants would agree to allow the investigators to randomly assign them to groups getting treatment with active magnets or sham devices. But neither the patients nor the doctors treating them would know what therapy was used on which patient.

First, Dr. Vallbona informally tested magnets on a few patients. One was a priest with postpolio syndrome who celebrated mass with difficulty due to marked back pain that prevented him from raising his left hand. After applying a magnet for a few minutes the pain was gone, Dr. Vallbona recalled, and "the priest said this was a miracle."

Then a human experimentation committee allowed Dr. Vallbona to test fifty volunteers with magnets that, at 300 to 500 gauss, were slightly stronger than refrigerator magnets. They were made in different sizes so they could fit over the anatomic area identified as setting off their pain.

It was difficult to design a system to prevent participants from learning whether they were being treated with a magnet or a sham. So Dr. Vallbona asked Magnaflex, Inc., a magnet distributor in Corpus Christi, Texas, to provide active magnets and inactive devices that could not be told apart. The devices were labeled in code.

As a further precaution, a staff member observed the patients throughout the forty-five-minute period of therapy to make sure they would not try to find out—by testing with a paper clip, say—what treatment they were receiving.

After the investigators identified the source of the pain and then pressed on it, the thirty-nine women and eleven men in the study graded the pain on a scale of 0 (none) to 10 (worst). Then after the experimental treatment, the participants rated their pain in a standard questionnaire. The volunteers were tested only one time.

The twenty-nine who received an active magnet reported a reduction in pain to 4.4 from 9.6, compared with a smaller decline to 8.4 from 9.5 among the twenty-one treated with a sham magnet.

The Baylor scientists emphasized that their study applied only to pain from the postpolio condition. Nevertheless, their report in the November 1997 issue of *Archives of Physical and Rehabilitation Medicine*, a leading specialty journal, shocked many doctors who had scoffed at claims for magnets' medical benefits.

In an article about magnet therapy for chronic pain published earlier in 1997, Dr. William Jarvis, a professor of public health and preventive medicine at Loma Linda University in California and president of the National Council Against Health Fraud, dismissed magnet therapy as "essentially quackery."

Now, Dr. Jarvis said in an interview, the Baylor study changed his mind. "But like any other pilot study, it needs to be replicated," he said.

Dr. Vallbona's findings have led him to try to carry out a larger study in several medical centers, and they are expected to lead other investigators to conduct their own studies.

Dr. Lauro S. Halstead of the National Rehabilitation Hospital in Washington, a pioneer in studying the postpolio syndrome, was among experts who said that further studies were needed to answer questions like: Will various strength magnets produce different degrees of benefit? How long does the pain relief last? Will the effect wear off after multiple applications? For what other conditions might magnets work?

At the University of Virginia, Ann Gill Taylor's team began recruiting 105 volunteers with fibromyalgia, a painful muscle condition of unknown cause, to test magnetic sleep pads.

Like the Baylor study, the volunteers and doctors were not told whether the subject would be sleeping on an active or sham magnet. Participants were told that if they tried to determine whether their treatment was with a real magnet or a sham one, it could ruin the findings of the study. But Dr. Taylor said there was no way to prevent cheating.

Dr. Taylor said she also planned to conduct studies of possible uses of magnets in relieving phantom limb and stump pain among amputees.

Dr. Vallbona said he did not know why magnets worked for many postpolio patients but not for all, or why some said they felt improvement in areas of the body far distant from where the magnet was applied.

Magnets' medical benefits have been proclaimed for centuries. So why has it taken so long to do studies to begin to answer the questions? The reasons involve economic, political, professional and human factors.

Many doctors criticize the lucrative magnet industry for not investing in studies the way drug companies often do. "They don't do simple research," Dr. Jarvis said, and "it is hard to imagine an easier study to conduct than a magnet one for pain."

Yet doctors share the responsibility to do such research, and only rarely have they reported undertaking the scientifically controlled studies needed to settle major disputes about reported therapies. In many such debates, doctors demand a biological explanation for a therapy's benefits. Without documentation that satisfies them, doctors may summarily reject the claims. Yet in their everyday practices, the same doctors may use other therapies that lack scientific proof for why they work.

Scientists working in nonprofit medical schools and university hospitals are strongly influenced by economics because they need government grants to pay for their overhead. Since scientific success is measured in part by the dollar amount of their grants, doctors tend not to pay for their studies, even if they are relatively inexpensive.

The Baylor study was exceptional. It was done without a grant. Had it been done with government aid, Dr. Vallbona said, it would have cost about $50,000. Magnaflex provided the active and inactive magnets free, the doctors donated their time and insurance companies were not charged for magnet therapy.

Until recently government agencies and the scientists who judge applications to them have tended not to support studies on magnets and other therapies on the fringe. The reluctance is well-founded. Over history, so many claims for popular remedies have failed to hold up that many doctors are reluctant to put aside a promising project of their own to study something that may well turn out to be a fad.

Scientists are heavily influenced by peer pressure. Senior scientists often discourage younger investigators from replicating another group's studies because doing so is less likely to advance their careers than making novel findings. But in an age of medical consumerism, patient demand is changing some research agendas. For instance, the National Institutes of Health has created an Office of Alternative Medicine, which is paying for the magnet studies at the University of Virginia.

In tackling fringe areas, scientists usually know that they are stepping in deep water, risking scorn from colleagues who believe that what they are studying is theoretically unsound at best and quackery at worst. Even so, many with the courage may not know how deep the waters are.

Lawrence K. Altman, M.D., December 1997

LEARNING PILATES, ONE STRETCH AT A TIME

It is called Pilates, and I had been hearing about it for some time but dismissed it as a faddish '90s workout. It fit the mold perfectly: it had the requisite exotic name (pronounced puh-LAH-tees), you had to go to a gym to do it and celebrities hailed it as a miracle workout that managed, with perfect '90s perversity, to give shapely women the bodies of twelve-year-old boys.

Pilates, I had heard, involved archaic equipment with names like "the reformer" and "the barrel," but that was about all I knew when I arrived at TriBeCa Bodyworks, a Pilates studio on Duane Street, determined to see if my bias was well-founded. A model-thin woman blew by me, a single line of sweat dripping down her radiant cheek. Great. I hated the place already.

Alycea Baylis-Ungaro, the owner of the studio, had instructed me to bring loose clothing and to wear socks. No sneakers were necessary. Showing me to the changing room, she whispered, "Even men do Pilates. We get a lot of them." It is true. During my workouts at least one-third were men. Besides, there is, as I soon learned, nothing feminine about Pilates.

The exercise method was invented by a man, Joseph Pilates, a boxer, acrobat and physical therapist from Germany. Obsessed with body conditioning, he developed the framework for Pilates while serving as a nurse during World War I. The goal of his program was to improve overall strength, flexibility and alignment by strengthening the abdominal and pelvic muscles.

So that patients could exercise in bed, he redesigned a hospital bed and developed simple exercises. Modern Pilates apparatus relies on the use of springs to provide resistance, much like weights, but easier on the body.

He opened the first Pilates studio in the United States in New York City in 1926, with his wife, Clara, and taught the method until his death in 1967. Coaching clients, he usually wore a bathing suit and often chomped a cigar and quaffed beer, while Mrs. Pilates dressed in a nurse's uniform.

A workout developed that long ago, when athletes smoked and tennis players wore long pants? Still, I signed up for three one-hour Pilates sessions. The first, Alycea said, would just be introductory. For $65, she would lead me through the fundamental exercises. Later sessions would get more intense, Alycea promised, at $55 a session. A bargain! I could not quite believe I was handing over this much money to exercise. I am a reasonable person. I live near a park. I own a pair of sneakers. Why not just put them on and run around the park?

The reason became clearer with each exercise. Alycea took me to the reformer, a long, low, bedlike apparatus with a flat, padded carriage that slid back and forth the length of the bed. It made a dentist's chair look friendly. Alycea had me lie faceup on the carriage, with my knees bent and my feet on a raised steel bar at the end of the apparatus. I was to straighten my legs as I pulled in my stomach.

The carriage, which is set on three long springs, was difficult to slide out, then snapped back against the end of the apparatus with a loud "Bang!" that echoed through the studio. Heads turned. Alycea did not look pleased. The next time, I was told, do it smoothly, no banging. And I was told to stop arching my back. Pilates exercises are designed to protect and strengthen the back.

"The more distance you put between your belly button and your spine, the more pressure you put on your back," Alycea said.

By changing the position of my feet on the steel bar and pushing, I worked different muscle groups in my legs while working my stomach muscles.

"It's a real New York workout because it's really efficient," Alycea said. "You have to use all your muscles at once." And you get it all in a neat and snappy sixty minutes.

We moved on to more complex movements, my least favorite being the "hundreds." Lying faceup on the reformer, I had to raise my feet six inches, suck in my stomach, squeeze my buttocks together and, holding a stirrup set on springs in each hand, keep my arms at my sides and bounce them up and down, one hundred times. With so many details to focus on, you hardly feel the pain.

I was beginning to understand why Mr. Pilates called his workout contrology. For every exercise that focuses on strengthening muscle, another stretches the body and encourages balance. And each movement—whether a derivative of the sit-up with legs jutting in the air, or lying flat and pulling on leather harnesses attached to springs—involves stabilizing the core of the body, the torso and buttocks, while moving the arms or legs. (This is the part that appeals to women: the movements are small and repetitions are short, so you tone muscle without bulking up.)

After about a half hour on the reformer, Alycea introduced me to "the Cadillac," which looked a lot like a gurney with harnesses and pulleys. After more stomach exercises, including sit-ups and leg lifts, Alycea had me lie on my back and put my feet into the harnesses. With my feet above my head and my back raised off of the mat, I was hung like a side of beef. Then, using my stomach muscles, I had to pull my body down to the mat against the resistance of the springs, curling my spine, vertebra by vertebra. It felt as if I was stretching every bone in my back. But there was no pain. Instead, I felt stress ebbing until it was gone. I could have done it all day.

But that was not the best part. Alycea had me sit up and stretch to touch my toes while she pushed and rubbed my back. I was forgetting about the $65. I left my first session with my stomach muscles dazed and confused, but I was still troubled that I had not broken a sweat. But when I arrived for my second session, Alycea reminded me that the reformer workout did not get longer, it got faster.

"And that's where the aerobics come in," she said.

And did they ever. I was more relaxed with the machines and my movements became smoother and faster. But when I slowed down, I heard about it.

At most Pilates gyms, you do individual sessions with a personal trainer to learn the movements—there are more than five hundred—until you get up to pace. After about thirty sessions, you can advance to what is called a duet—two people with a trainer—then to groups of three and four.

I had never employed a personal trainer, but I found that having one by my side was surprisingly comforting. I liked having someone there to coddle me while I suffered through the workout. Besides, it is far too easy and tempting to cheat with Pilates.

What is extraordinary about Pilates is its broad appeal. Some professional dancers do it to maintain flexibility and stay fit without adding excess stress to their bodies. And unlike running or aerobics, Pilates is good for the elderly, people with injuries, and even pregnant women.

"They do it right up to delivery," Alycea said.

As for me, Pilates was a revelation. I had not realized how tight my muscles had become working in an office, slouching over a computer keyboard. By the third session, I was a convert. I was getting the aerobic workout I wanted while regaining some of the flexibility I had lost.

But if I start to get that twelve-year-old-boy look, I just may have to ease off. For a while, anyway.

Amanda Hesser, November 1998

T'AI CHI: EXERCISING BODY AND MIND

Kenneth Powell of Brooklyn is a compleat athlete. He plays tennis, works out in a gym, skis and surfs. But in addition to these vigorous activities, two or three times a day this thirty-seven-year-old father of two preschoolers does t'ai chi, a Chinese exercise that is at once calming and strengthening.

You may have seen the people of China doing t'ai chi on television during President Richard M. Nixon's visit in 1972, but by now you have no doubt come across people in your neighborhood going through the slow, graceful, tranquil, dancelike motions of t'ai chi, a five-thousand-year-old form of mental and physical exercise. Though long touted for the emotional well-being it bestows, recent studies indicate that t'ai chi can also improve physical health. It helps tone muscles, combat fatigue and improve circulation. And because it is a gentle form of exercise, it is particularly helpful for people who are unable to perform more vigorous activities because of age, illness or physical disabilities. There are different styles of t'ai chi (some include martial arts), but their effects on health are quite similar.

Robert Parry, in a well-illustrated book, *Tai Chi Made Easy* (People's Medical Society, $16.95), said: "Tai chi is about generating and feeling energy through movement. It is not just about fitness." He added that it was "a special way of looking at life—a path of inspiration and a guide toward relaxation and health." Regular practitioners say it helps them deal with stress, unleashes their creative energy, counters depression and fosters self-confidence and optimism.

T'ai chi is, in one sense, a form of meditation. Unlike transcendental meditation, a focused inner peace is achieved through movement; unlike yoga, the movement is continuous and puts little stress on joints and muscles. Recent studies have established some expected health benefits and revealed some surprising ones. Researchers have shown t'ai chi to be especially helpful to the elderly, improving their sense of balance and reducing their risk of falls. But as Mr. Powell and millions of others have discovered, t'ai chi can be good for people of all ages and at all levels of physical prowess.

"T'ai chi has given me a knowledge of balance and centeredness that I can apply to every sport I do, even walking," Mr. Powell said. "I know how to breathe properly, how to lower my center of gravity, how to use my body efficiently, how to relax, all of which I can apply to my regular life." T'ai chi professionals report that daily practice of t'ai chi also reduces the chances of injury during other activities because it strengthens leg muscles and promotes coordination, proper posture and a natural flow to one's movements.

One of the best books on the subject, *Tai Chi for Health*, by Edward Maisel (Holt, Rinehart & Winston), was originally published in 1963 and was republished in an updated version in 1972. It is practical throughout and stripped of mysticism. Describing t'ai chi's advantages, Mr. Maisel wrote that it could be done anywhere, at any time, by anyone who could stand and move. It requires no special equipment or clothing, just something loose and comfortable, flat shoes or bare feet and a 4-by-4-foot space. Mr. Maisel wrote that people who became anxious or distracted could "simply move to a small spot, wherever they may find themselves, and perform their tai chi for its calming effect."

In a fifteen-week study sponsored by the National Institute on Aging and published in the *Journal of the American Geriatrics Society* in May 1996, Dr. Steven L. Wolf, a rehabilitation medicine specialist at Emory University School of Medicine in Atlanta, randomly assigned 215 people seventy and older to three groups. One took weekly t'ai chi lessons and practiced on their own twice daily. Another met to discuss issues important to the elderly and were told to continue their usual exercise. The third got balance training.

Among those doing t'ai chi, blood pressure fell and grip strength increased, and the participants' sense of control over their lives improved. But most important, when followed for up to seventeen months after the training period ended, the members of the t'ai chi group had reduced their risk of falls by nearly half. In another study, by researchers at the University of Connecticut, leg strength increased in people older than seventy-five who were trained in t'ai chi. One note of caution: some t'ai chi moves involve deep knee bends or squats, which are best avoided by people with arthritic knees or hips.

Though t'ai chi may look simple, as if moves were invented de novo by the practitioner, it is actually a highly programmed series of gentle movements, one flowing into another. It must be learned and practiced regularly (most experts say daily) to be beneficial. It usually takes six months to a year to learn all the moves, though you can learn as few or as many as you choose and do only one or a few moves in a single session.

There are now t'ai chi teachers all around the country. If attending a class is impractical, books like Mr. Parry's can help you learn the movements. He presents them with step-by-step descriptions and photos and diagrams, including some basic dos and don'ts: keep your spine upright and your breathing slow and rhythmic, move from the center of your body, maintain a low center of gravity, never lock elbows or knees, drop your shoulders, maintain space between your arms and your body, maintain a wide stance, keep moving at all times, step forward heel first, keep the forward knee over the toes and imagine your bodily tensions dissolving as you work.

Do your legs get tired standing in a museum or in a long line? That is because most of the time you are standing still on two planted feet, which impedes circulation and holds muscles in a state of tension. As one foot lands in t'ai chi, the other lifts. Muscles are continuously tensed and relaxed, and fatigue is not likely to limit your endurance. In fact, Mr. Powell says, just the opposite is true. T'ai chi, which he sometimes does for two hours at a time, is energizing.

T'ai chi can be done alone, in silence or (as some prefer) to soothing music, or it can be done with a partner, as depicted in Mr. Parry's book. Though t'ai chi can be practiced anywhere, most people prefer the outdoors, weather permitting, which is the true Chinese way. To find a t'ai chi instructor, check your Yellow Pages or inquire at local health clubs, Ys or hospital-based rehabilitation centers. Or if you see someone practicing t'ai chi in your neighborhood, wait until the workout is finished (no one doing t'ai chi wants to be interrupted) and ask where that person trained.

Jane E. Brody, July 1997

FALUNG GONG: A MYSTICAL EXERCISE REGIMEN DRAWS IMMIGRANTS AND THE DEEPLY CURIOUS

About ten to twelve people stand in a circle near a well-traveled path in Riverside Park at 6 A.M. every day and together they move their hands in smooth and deliberate strokes—up and down, in an arc and around again.

The joggers and dog walkers who pass barely give them a second glance. They, in turn, are oblivious to the city that is awakening around them. Their eyes are shut, their faces expressionless as they listen to the gentle strains of traditional Chinese music and the voice of their master, Li Hongzhi, a man the Chinese government has declared a criminal. Mr. Li's voice guides them through the exercises at the heart of Falun Gong, the spiritual movement banned in China in the summer of 1999. Officials arrested thousands of Falun Gong followers across China and announced that they planned to prosecute the movement's top leaders for subversion. In October 1999, thousands of Falun Gong members converged on Beijing to pressure the government to reverse its ban.

But even as the Chinese government continues its campaign to eradicate Falun Gong from Chinese society because of fears that it has gained cult status, the movement's popularity in the New York area has continued to grow among immigrants and Westerners alike. There are about two dozen loosely organized practice groups in the city of anywhere between five and sixty people each. And nearly six hundred followers showed up at an "experience sharing" conference in upper Manhattan earlier this month.

In many ways, the movement is benefiting from a wave of interest in qigong (pronounced chee-goong), a form of Chinese healing and physical strengthening that has thousands of years of history and thousands of different styles of exercise and meditation. Since the early 1990s, a growing number of qigong classes and centers have emerged across the region as an alternative to yoga or t'ai chi, or as a means for recent Chinese immigrants to socialize with one another.

Yet practitioners of the two spiritual imports find themselves in an awkward relationship. Followers of Falun Gong describe their practice as a more enlightened version of qigong. Practitioners of qigong, on the other hand, cannot seem to distance themselves from Falun Gong fast enough for fear of being labeled a cult. Still, the tension seems more rooted in nervousness over what is happening back in China—where members say they are being persecuted for their beliefs—than what is evolving here.

Local Falun Gong adherents like Hong Wei Wu, a computer programmer on Wall Street and an immigrant from Shanghai, are outraged by the actions of the Chinese government. "You know the Chinese government always wants to control everything," she said. "But they don't know we only want to become a better person and to improve our health with Falun Gong."

New Yorkers who practice Falun Gong, which combines elements of Buddhism, Taoism and qigong, are an eclectic bunch. About half the followers are Chinese, who learned about Falun Gong from friends and relatives in China, and the rest are a mix of white, black and Hispanic residents, who learned about the practices at health expositions or from friends. The movement's growing popularity has been aided by its easy accessibility. Groups often practice in public parks, and there are a number of Web sites where the curious can learn about it. (In fact, the founder, Mr. Li, lives in Queens, but he makes very few public appearances.)

Like qigong, Falun Gong teaches that exercise and meditation can harness the body's energy, an intangible force known in Chinese as qi, to improve one's health. Exercises often mimic the movements of animals, a tiger, a monkey or a crane, and are designed to help direct the qi in one's body to help clear "blockages." But Falun Gong also espouses a philosophy of life that includes a Falun, or "law wheel," that spins in the abdomen, drawing in good forces and expelling bad ones. It also suggests that advanced students can gain supernatural powers like X-ray vision and unusually long lives.

They describe their practices as an elevated, more enlightened version of qigong. "It's way, way above qigong," said Gail Rachlin, a media relations consultant who has tried other forms of qigong but now practices Falun Gong regularly in Riverside Park. "Qigong can help you physically but it doesn't stay with you and Falun Gong goes beyond the physical by helping you upgrade your thinking and mentality."

But many practitioners of traditional qigong are extremely wary of being confused with Falun Gong. They say Falun Gong's emphasis on morality and the cult of personality surrounding its founder separates it from traditional qigong, where the emphasis is on self-help and independence.

Dr. Effie Poy Yew Chow, president of the American Qigong Association and a consultant on alternative medicine for the National Institutes of Health, said that while Falun Gong followers are urged to stop taking medicine to cultivate themselves, "true qigong is about setting people free to make choices and not dropping everything just to do one thing."

Local followers of Yan Xin qigong, another enormously popular style of qigong in China and here, were so paranoid about being linked to Falun Gong and subsequently being targeted by the Chinese government that they refused to discuss their practices for publication. Nancy Chen, a medical anthropologist at the University of California at Santa Cruz who has closely studied qigong, said that some followers are probably fearful because the Chinese government's campaign to purge Falun Gong is neither its first nor likely its last effort at eradicating a specific brand of qigong.

The Chinese government created a commission in the early 1990s to try to regulate and contain the thousands of styles of qigong that had proliferated in the 1970s and 1980s. In the process, the government branded a handful of qigong masters as charlatans, just as it has Li Hongzhi. Many qigong masters, who develop their own style, have sponsored studies to try to show a scientific basis to their abilities. Some purport to use their qi to perform superhuman feats like letting trucks roll over their bodies without being injured or setting things on fire with a mere touch. Some claim they can shrink cancerous tumors and cure AIDS by projecting their qi into patients.

Lei Zhong, a doctoral candidate in immunology at a New York university who has been practicing qigong for five years, said he was drawn by scientific curiosity. "Traditional qigong is based on science that we don't fully understand," he said. "I think of it as a scientific challenge. How does it work and how can human energy be so powerful?"

Yi Wu and his wife, Rong-Er Shen, run classes and see dozens of patients each week at their qigong center in midtown Manhattan. At a recent healing session, Mr. Wu gathered his qi by going through the deliberate movements of his own style of qigong. Then, from across the room, he projected his qi out of his forehead toward his patient, Carl Peterson, a retired physicist who suffers from abdominal cancer. Mr. Wu never laid hands on Mr. Peterson, but he said his qi had created "a very strong energy field that allowed the patient to feel restful so that his body could then slowly repair itself." When Mr. Wu was done, Mr. Peterson said he felt as though the tension had been drained out of him and been replaced by "a sense of well-being." He added that he didn't go to Mr. Wu "looking for a cure for cancer. I came to build up my energy, and the energy is definitely coming back."

While millions in China seem to have turned to qigong starting in the late 1970s as they searched for new meaning and direction in post-Mao China, followers in the United States seem drawn to qigong mainly for what they see as its health benefits. And their ailments can range from insomnia and achy joints to cancer and other life-threatening diseases. Many experts say that qigong started to take off here shortly after Bill Moyers's 1993 public television series *Healing and the Mind*, which generated a best-selling book and which introduced Chinese healing methods to a wider audience.

"Before that people didn't know what qigong was, but the series explained that qigong is what makes acupuncture work," said Dr. Richard M. Chin, an acupuncturist and qigong master who has offices in Westport, Connecticut, and Manhattan. While acupuncturists use needles to manipulate and direct qi, he explained, "with qigong you can learn the breathing yourself and learn to relax so that you can heal yourself."

The American Qigong Association hopes eventually to create training standards and certification requirements for qigong, much like those now imposed on acupuncture. Those standards would be a move toward legitimizing qigong in the United States, which, in an odd way, would parallel the Chinese government's recent attempts to regulate the myriad of styles in practice there.

But, Dr. Chin stressed, "we're not talking persecution like what China is doing with Falun Gong. You can do any style you want; we just want to evaluate it."

Qigong's elusive qualities will make it difficult to create standards. "Qigong is a pure art, and you can't evaluate the part of it that is mystical," Dr. Chin said. "But you can make sure that the foundation is there and that there is an understanding of channels and how to do a diagnosis. We may not be able to produce masters, but we can at least produce good practitioners."

Vivian S. Toy, October 1999

JUST THE RIGHT SPOT: SPEEDY
SIDEWALK MASSEURS

Regina Bradford had seen them a thousand—who knew, maybe a million—times, but she had always been something of a skeptic. "Massage?" she would think when she passed them in SoHo or Central Park. "These guys? Whatever."

Then there was Wednesday, November 10—a bad day, an apocalyptic day. Her four-year relationship was on the rocks. Her beloved terrier, Samson, had just gone to the vet with mysterious retching. Ms. Bradford, a thirty-one-year-old jazz singer, was turned down for a lucrative gig. And to cap it off, she had developed a nasty little crick in her neck.

So when she came across the five Chinese massage guys clustered near Bethesda Fountain in Central Park, she tossed doubt to the wind and plopped down on one of their ergonomic chairs. Ten minutes and $10 later, she rose with a smile and—lo and behold—her aches and pains were mostly gone.

"You know, I feel pretty good," she said, giving her shoulders a gentle test roll. "It wasn't a miracle, but it was better than I thought."

Depending on whom you ask, the Chinese chair masseurs are either charlatans or chiropractic wonders. But they have undisputably moved beyond a minor sideshow role at festivals and street fairs, popping up in the city's parks and squares and on sidewalks wide enough to accommodate their padded chairs. There is no way to tell precisely how many of them are at work on the streets on a given day. They usually practice without city permits and, though they are required to file for state massage licenses, many do not, officials say, opening them up to criticism among professionals.

But in a metropolis where being stressed out might as well be an Olympic event, the mobile massage squads offer a possible dose of bliss to curious passersby or even longtime Swedish and shiatsu fans looking for a quick, convenient fix. The vast majority practice a brand of Chinese massage called Tui Na (pronounced twee-nah), a subset of the larger art of physical healing known as qigong (pronounced chee-goong), which attempts to harness the body's energy, an intangible force called qi in Chinese.

"They spend ten minutes, give you a little qi, and you feel better," said Michael Winn, president of the National Qigong Association, whose group has grown to four hundred members from one hundred members just two years ago. "They're actually meeting a need caused by a fast-paced life of tension and fatigue."

Take Li Xing, for example, a lanky man with veiny hands, who set up his chair in Central Park the other day. Though Mr. Li, who is thirty-nine, arrived in New York from China only last year, he already considers himself an important part of Manhattan's stress-reduction team.

"Everybody needs a massage—especially in New York," said Mr. Li, digging his elbow in a client's scapula. "People here work too long. Run around too hard, too much. Truthfully, they need to relax."

Somehow, though, outdoor Tui Na seems anything but relaxing. There is no padded table, no wafting scent of incense, no oceanic sound track or panpipe music drifting through the room. Instead, clients hunker down on duct-taped chairs, their foreheads pressed against circles of cracking foam. Police sirens often skirl in the background. Frankfurter smells float by. Sometimes, people stop to watch.

Nonetheless, under the fingers of masseurs like Mr. Li, tension slides from achy muscles, the back loosens up, the shoulders drop. Techniques vary: some practitioners knead the flesh, others slap or karate-chop. The focus tends to be the spine. But arms are shaken and necks are rubbed.

"My fingers are like acupunture needles," Mr. Li explains.

Typically, the masseurs will spend the morning and afternoon in one of the city's parks, then move on to evening spots like Prince Street or the northern fringes of Times Square. In spring and summer, they say, they often work on ten to twenty customers a day at the rate of a dollar a minute. Come winter, many abandon their chairs for jobs in Chinese restaurants or takeout stands. Though there are hundreds of qigong schools across the country, most of the street masseurs said they learned their craft from relatives in China or through informal lessons from friends in New York.

Before leaving the city of Shenyang five years ago, Jack Feng learned Tui Na from a pal in the military and eventually, he said, worked as the official masseur for the Chinese air force volleyball team. Now, he spends his weekdays serving clients in the park and his weekends charging up to $70 an hour to visit private customers at home.

"I have a dance teacher, a waiter and many, many businessmen," Mr. Feng, thirty-seven, said proudly as Mr. Li acted as his translator. "Some customers come here to Central Park and like me. Then, they give me their card."

A private practice is a cherished thing among the masseurs because, as they said, the police sometimes run them out of parks or plazas, issuing tickets and sometimes confiscating their chairs. "Two times this has happened to me," said Mr. Li. "Two times I have bought a new chair."

The masseurs also walk a fine line with state regulators, who require that they be licensed, said Dr. Kathleen Doyle, executive secretary of the State Board for Massage Therapy. "If they're actually doing what's considered within the scope of massage, they need a license," she said.

Lucy Liben, dean of the massage therapy program at the Swedish Institute, said Tui Na is a well-respected form of massage and is taught at her own school, but added that nearly all the street masseurs were unlicensed and could present a danger to the public.

"This creates a lot of frustration among our graduates who made a tremendous investment in their training," she said. "They often see customers being solicited on the streets by people with no guarantee that they have training in safety, hygiene or any of the other standards we hold ourselves to."

But a lack of official training on the part of the Chinese masseurs does not seem to keep people away from their chairs. Cheap, convenient and fast—the words were used again and again to describe why customers stopped for a massage.

"I used to get regular massages, but then my massage therapist moved to another club," said Madelyn Miller, an artist from the Upper East Side, after she rose from Wang Bing's chair. "It's basically chop-chop technique, but it definitely does the trick."

Leslie Walker, thirty-six, of the Upper West Side, was strolling through Central Park with her two-year-old daughter, Charlie, and stopped for a massage on a whim—no appointment needed.

"You're more relaxed on a table," Ms. Walker conceded, "but if I had to wait for that I wouldn't have had a massage just now."

Of course, the masseurs know that their livelihoods depend on caprice. But some, like Mr. Feng or Mr. Wang (who is forty-seven and learned Tui Na from his older brother in China twenty-five years ago), try drawing customers by offering thirty-second samples and by greeting everyone who crosses their path with a chipper, "Hello. Massage?"

Others, like Mr. Li, have trained themselves to spot potential customers from afar and so sit back, lying in wait. "I can see the customer, see his face," said Mr. Li. "And then I know it. I know he wants massage."

Alan Feuer, November 1999

RUBDOWNS ARE FINE. THEN AGAIN, THEY CAN GET A LITTLE TOO TOUCHY

Massage—it's a '90s kind of boom business. Be they aging, active, aching, stressed-out or simply indulgent, more and more Americans are thinking they could sure use a nice rubdown right—no, a little to the left, higher—Stop! There! *Oooohhhhhh! Aaaahhhhhh!*

Americans spend an estimated $2 billion to $4 billion annually on massages—in resort spas, storefront back-rub outlets, workplaces, therapists' offices and at home. With even some health insurance plans now covering massage, the industry is responding to rising demand. Since 1991, according to Martin Ashley, a massage expert, membership in the two largest professional associations for massage therapists in the United States has more than doubled (to 39,000) as has the number of massage-training schools (to more than four hundred).

You want variety? The scores of exotic-sounding types of massage available—from Aston-Patterning to Zero-Balancing—indicate that we're no longer talking karate chops by a guy named Sven anymore.

But one thing has been slow to change in massage, and that is its association with sex. Both massage and sex involve intimate touching. The former is often a prelude to the latter in romance—a path encouraged lately by a bumper crop of how-to-sex manuals and videos now on the market. And of course, massage parlors that front for prostitution continue to operate as massage goes mainstream.

Upshot: a lot of confusion. Professional associations that set standards for the industry say sex is never appropriate in massage—it's illegal—but people in the business acknowledge the blurry line between the two, and discuss it all the time. Here are excerpts.

In the guidebook *Massage: A Career at Your Fingertips* (Enterprise

Publishing, 1995), Martin Ashley, a lawyer and massage therapist, says requests for sex during massage most often come from men being massaged by women (roughly 75 percent of massage therapists are female). He provides this context for those aspiring to the business:

In many parts of the United States, a sexual massage is more common and easier to find than a legitimate massage. In some areas . . . the sexual massage ads in the Yellow Pages completely overwhelm the few listings for massage therapists. . . . Millions of men have had sexual massage experiences, and continue to have them today. As such, it is understandable that they would have some confusion about what it is you do. That is why you should be 1) nonjudgmental and 2) completely clear in your communications before beginning a massage.

If a client persists in seeking sex, Mr. Ashley advises, "terminate the massage immediately."

But not all massage practitioners say no, according to David Palmer, a former massage school director who made these observations in *The Bodywork Entrepreneur*, a 1990 collection of articles from his journal of the same name:

1. Sexual massage for pay is illegal and I know of no state where this is not true. While some of us may not like that fact, for the moment we do have to live with it. Therefore the only stance we can take as an emerging profession is that sexual massage is never appropriate and, consequently, is unethical.
2. Unethical is not the same thing as immoral. Whether you think that sexual massage for pay is immoral depends on your own personal value system.
3. Sexual massage pays very well. In fact, I have met people who have paid off their mortgages, put themselves or their children through college, and otherwise had normal suburban lifestyles while doing sexual massage professionally.

   Since clients often get the wrong idea, many legitimate practitioners prepare for the worst. Responding to a query sent via an Internet mailing list for massage therapists, some shared their tactics for heading off trouble:

- Best one I know of is to tilt the table and dump the offender.
- I have a fighting trophy from a contest that I casually show people who are trying to threaten me. The thing I don't tell them, though, is it was a third place out of three women.

In an interview in *The Bodywork Entrepreneur*, Daphne Chellos, an authority on sexual ethics in massage, was asked, "What is ethical? What if either the practitioner or the client has sexual feelings during a massage?" Her answer:

"It is okay to feel sexual during a massage. However, it is not okay to take that a step further and expect the client or practitioner to interact with those feelings. Sexual feelings can be channeled appropriately to enrich the massage experience. . . . Body work can fulfill a need for touch especially in people who are not currently in a relationship. As long as neither the client nor the practitioner feels adversely affected by these feelings, this is an appropriate benefit from massage therapy."

Tom Kuntz, March 1997

[7]

Prayer, Laughter, Meditation and the Power of Placebos

The Mind-Body Connection

Few people doubt that there is a connection between mind and body. How else to explain sexual arousal, or the pounding of the heart that begins the moment you realize your wallet is missing? Going beyond instantaneous reactions, it is widely believed (though not proved) that emotions, for better or worse, can have lasting effects on health. It is known that the power of suggestion, of having great faith in the doctor or the therapy being given—also known as the placebo effect—can sometimes play an important part in recovery from illness or injury.

The link between body and mind is not mystical. It has a physical basis: the nervous system influences the secretion of hormones by the endocrine system, and both of those systems also act on the immune system, which guards against infection and cancer. What is not clear is whether those transient effects can really have long-term consequences for health. Such questions have given rise to an entire field of study, known as psychoneuro-immunology.

Many people would like to think that the mind-body connection can be harnessed in the interests of health. More and more are turning to prayer, meditation and hypnosis to help them deal with pain and sickness, and the fear and frustration that ill health can bring. Often, doctors do not object, as long as those approaches are used along with conventional treatment and not in place of it. Indeed, many professionals welcome anything patients can do to find peace of mind, feel better and get through their illness and its treatment. And the medical establishment has begun to conduct rigorous studies of the placebo effect: many patients and some doctors feel that if a dummy pill or sham operation helps them feel better, with none of the risks or side effects of conventional therapy, and at a fraction of the cost, so what if it's a placebo?

But mind-body theorizing can have a dark side: it leads some people to blame themselves for their illnesses, and tempts some onlookers to accuse patients of making themselves sick and interfering with their own recovery by being angry, sad, scared or pessimistic, or lacking the will to fight their diseases. In a book published in September 2000, The Human Side of Cancer (HarperCollins), Dr. Jimmie Holland, who is chairman of the Department of Psychiatry and Behavioral Sciences at Memorial Sloan-Kettering Cancer Center in New York City, warns against the "tyranny of positive thinking" and the "myth of the cancer personality." It makes no sense to blame people for having cancer or to expect them to feel cheerful when they are ill, she says, citing numerous studies showing that stress, depression, grief and personality type do not bring on cancer or make it worse. "My view is that if a positive attitude comes naturally to you, fine," Dr. Holland says. But she says that many negative, pessimistic people also survive cancer, and adds, "I have seen patients who had no belief in the mind-body connection and who discounted the importance of their attitude completely, yet they survived."

SEEKING HELP FOR THE BODY IN THE
WELL-BEING OF THE SOUL

Early Sunday mornings in a chapel at Riverside Church in New York, a service begins with meditation enhanced by aromatherapy and music. The communion includes laying on of hands, an ancient rite for the sick.

Finally, congregants gather in the church's new Wellness Center, where they discuss topics like nutrition and cancer.

Most of the congregants are women. Whether for social or biological reasons or both, said the Rev. Diane Lacey Winley, the center's coordinator and a board member of New York City's Health and Hospitals Corporation, "women find it easier to use prayer and meditation to find energy, strength and healing."

But women aren't alone in exploring the connection between spirituality and health, nor are clergy members the only professionals who talk of healing and religion in one breath. Just as more and more churches and synagogues offer liturgies to promote well-being, some sixty American medical schools now offer courses on health, religion and "spirituality." Both the religious and medical establishments are aware of polls showing that most Americans think that faith and prayer benefit health and that doctors should discuss the connection.

This hybridization of science and spirituality combines two of the baby boomers' greatest enthusiasms. As their huge generation ages, their increasing health concerns, from menopause to breast cancer, seem almost as likely to elicit a spiritual quest as a search for the best specialist. There is no denying that religion can "heal," in that it can greatly comfort the sick. But despite the testimony provided by polls and best-selling books, tapes, courses and other healing industry products, spirituality's effect on health remains a more hotly debated issue in science than in the rest of society.

The simplest and best-documented evidence of religion's salubrious effects concerns longevity. California's Alameda County Study and the National Health Interview Survey, which was financed by the Centers for Disease Control and Prevention, have tracked the health of thousands of randomly selected people, the first for decades and the second for eight years. These well-respected studies show that, even when allowing for individual differences, like medical problems or smoking, subjects who attend services weekly—the most common gauge of religiousness—live longer than those who do not. In the national health survey, frequent "attenders" died, on average, at age eighty-three; those who never went to services died at age seventy-five. In the Alameda study, the relative risk of mortality for male attenders was 10 percent lower than for other men; for female attenders, however, the risk was 34 percent lower than for other women.

By many measures—frequency of prayer, attendance at services, value placed on spirituality—women are more religious than men. Whether their greater fervor confers extra health benefits remains in question. The National Health Interview Survey, for example, did not reveal a significant gender gap. But in the Alameda study, according to William Strawbridge, an epidemiologist and the Alameda project's director, religion was found to be nearly as good for women's health as not smoking.

That religious men and women tend to live longer does not require supernatural explanations. Not surprisingly, people who frequent churches and synagogues are likelier to avoid risky behavior like drug abuse and promiscuity. But, Dr. Strawbridge said, compared with people who do not go to services, even less straitlaced attenders are likelier to "clean up their acts" by quitting smoking, say, or by drinking less alcohol. Explaining the connection between longevity and religion, Dr. Strawbridge pointed to "the difference between hanging out with the church choir or the Grateful Dead."

Drawing a parallel to marriage's well-established contribution to well-being, Robert Hummer, a sociologist at the University of Texas at Austin, who has analyzed the National Health Interview Survey, said religious involvement could influence not only health habits but also relationships and the ability to cope with stress. "The general idea isn't that religion works instant cures or ensures that anyone who walks into a church will live to be eighty-five," he said, "but that it's linked with many factors that benefit health over a lifetime."

One Wednesday evening, about eighty people, some clearly frail, gathered for a healing service at Ansche Chesed, a synagogue on Manhattan's Upper West Side. Like the prayers and reflections, some simple songs gently acknowledged that, as Debbie Friedman, a composer and singer of Jewish spiritual music, said, "We all have to live with pain as well as joy." By the service's end, urban professionals had shed their reserve to sway together and sing.

Religion's potential health benefits are not limited to those who attend churches or synagogues. Herbert Benson, the director of the Mind-Body

Medical Institute at Beth Israel Deaconess Medical Center in Boston, which is affiliated with the Harvard Medical School, said spirituality promoted health in two straightforward ways. Research has shown that belief in the effectiveness of a placebo, or sugar pill, can relieve illness. Therefore, Dr. Benson reasons, "so can faith in the healing power of God—or nature, relationships or whatever resource the individual chooses."

And some spiritual practices, he said, have measurable metabolic effects. Whether produced by Zen breathing, Jewish davening (prayer) or reciting the Roman Catholic rosary, the quiet state that Dr. Benson calls the "relaxation response" can lower heart and respiration rates and slow brain waves. When performed daily, he said, this response acts as an antidote to the "fight or flight" response implicated in the stress-related ailments that motivate most visits to doctors and are resistant to drugs and surgery. The patient who combines standard medical treatment with this self-care, he said, "has all the bases covered."

Studies conducted by Duke University's Center for the Study of Religion, Spirituality and Health in Durham, North Carolina, indicate that deeply religious people are less likely to suffer from diastolic hypertension (high blood pressure when the heart muscle is relaxed) and depression, and tend to have lower levels of a protein called interleukin 6, which implies a strong immune system. "Religion offers powerful ways to cope with major life stresses, particularly health problems and experiences of loss," said Harold Koenig, a psychiatrist who is the center's director.

The idea that religion benefits health has its critics. Earlier this year, the prestigious British medical journal the *Lancet* published a report co-written by Richard Sloan, the director of the Behavioral Medicine Program at Columbia-Presbyterian Medical Center in New York. After reviewing hundreds of studies, he concluded, "There's no compelling evidence that religion affects physical health." It's not that religion could not do so, said Dr. Sloan, a psychologist. But with the exception of a few studies, like the Alameda survey, he said, "the vast majority" are flawed. Among his objections are poor matches between religious and control groups, as when nuns are compared with members of the general population.

Including spirituality in medical practice also raises ethical concerns.

First, Dr. Sloan said, there is the problem of "blaming the victim," or the patient who fares poorly. Then, too, "prescribing religion isn't the same as prescribing a low-fat diet," he said, adding: "There's lots of evidence that marriage is good for health, but doctors don't tell their single patients to wed. That area of life is too personal and private."

Even researchers who are convinced that religion promotes health often express reservations about studies that try to ascertain whether sick people who are unaware that others are praying for them do better than those who are not being prayed for at all. As a scientist, Dr. Koenig said, "I steer clear of that area." As a Christian, he finds the idea of a God who favors those who have others praying for them hard to reconcile with the image of a "Good Shepherd who will look for that one lost sheep."

Sometimes religion aggravates health problems. Alice Domar, a psychologist and the director of the Center for Women's Health at the Mind-Body Medical Institute in Boston, has found that very devout patients, particularly Catholics, Jews and women raised with a punitive image of God, find it harder to cope with infertility. "They're likelier to regard it as their own fault—even as punishment," she said.

In a process called "cognitive restructuring," staff members help patients substitute destructive thoughts about infertility with constructive attitudes. When a woman who had suffered recurrent miscarriages said God was punishing her, Dr. Domar replied, "So, God kills babies?" The shocked patient said, "Oh, no, God would never do that!" Only after logic replaced her fear could the woman see infertility as a physiological problem.

A few good surveys now indicate that religion fosters health. But as illustrated by the efforts to establish the effects of smoking or aspirin, Dr. Strawbridge said, "Numerous studies must replicate an effect before medicine regards it as proved." Meanwhile, many compassionate religious and medical professionals continue to draw from both spirituality and science in their efforts to heal.

The Rev. Barbara H. Nielsen, an Episcopalian minister and fellow at the Mind-Body Medical Institute, has found that some patients who believe their prayers go unanswered appreciate learning what she calls "a new way to pray": one asks for what one wants, accepts what will be and, finally, meditates. Then, Ms. Nielsen said, "one can listen for the real answer to prayers." She recalled how a Catholic infertility patient who used this method began to see that the identity of Mary wasn't limited to maternity, but, like her own, included work, marriage and good character. "This woman got the message that she's a fine person from Mary," Ms. Nielsen said, "once she listened."

Winifred Gallagher, June 1999

NO SWEET, NO SOUR, NO MEAT: IN DHARAMSALA, BREAST CANCER SURVIVORS SAMPLE TIBETAN MEDICINE

In fall 1998, when Dr. Yeshi Dhonden, formerly the personal physician to the Dalai Lama, came to New York, a friend called me. "He's specializing in breast cancer treatment," she said. "I think you should go see him." I was surprised. Not that the Tibetans were treating cancer, but that word of it hadn't got out on the cancer grapevine.

In eleven years as a breast cancer patient, I've watched as any hint, the slightest whisper, of a cure is instantly broadcast through the cancer community, thanks largely to the Internet. The online forums are giant bazaars that trade in information, some fantastically advanced, some fantastic. The headers on the bulletin boards could be an index to a book called *Every Oncological Proposition Ever Advanced: Bone Marrow Transplant, Shark Cartilage, Be Careful of Your Bras, Ladies*. But I hadn't seen one that said *Tibetan Medicine*.

Later, after traveling to the Tibetan Medical and Astrological Institute in Dharamsala, India, I would discover why. Wary of exploitation, the Tibetans are protective of their medical system, which is intricately linked to their culture. After centuries of fending off the Chinese, they are having no trouble dispatching the marauding vitamin companies that have come sniffing around, hoping to strike it rich with the next big alternative medicine trend.

There is another reason we're not seeing an abundance of cheesy advertisements for Tibetan medicine in the back of New Age magazines. It is gentle and slow-acting, entwined with Buddhist belief—the precise opposite of the quick, magic medical fix that Americans prize (and which I was half hoping for when I made an appointment with Dr. Dhonden last fall).

With his shaved head and maroon robes, Dr. Dhonden looked wonderfully out of context in the basement of a dingy Manhattan apartment. The examination was brief. He took my pulse, examined the vial of urine I'd been instructed to bring and, through an interpreter, asked about my medical history, including a few oddly pointed questions. Did I make frequent trips to the bathroom at night? Strangely, I had just seen a doctor for that complaint.

He then listed foods to avoid (barbecue, sugar, cantaloupe); provided me with four varieties of brown herbal pills (one of which had the distinct aroma of a barnyard); and, on my way out, barked one final observation in Tibetan. "Doctor says there's something wrong with your liver," the interpreter translated.

"The Tibetans always say it's the liver," my dinner companion at a party that night scoffed. After thinking it over, I joined her in smirking. At Memorial Sloan-Kettering Cancer Center in New York, where I was a patient, I was regularly scanned upside and down. If my liver was off, I would know.

But the next week, when a technician phoned with the results of my monthly blood work, he said: "Don't worry. Everything's fine. Well, except for one of your liver functions. It's a little high." I took the pills, and two months later, the test results were normal again.

When I was making plans to go to India with a friend, Connie Harris Nagle, I asked if she'd be interested in making the trek to the Tibetan Medical and Astrological Institute in Dharamsala, the former British hill station where the Tibetan government has established itself in exile. Ms. Nagle worked with Tibetan refugees for three years and is researching a book on Tibetan metaphor. She is also a breast cancer survivor. "Let's go," she said.

Before departing, I made inquiries about Tibetan medicine with several Western doctors, a few of whom were advocates. "It's one of the most profound medical healing systems on the planet, because its focus is so much on spiritual practice," said Woodson C. Merrell, a doctor who helped organize last year's First International Congress on Tibetan Medicine, in Washington, which drew specialists from about twenty countries to discuss aspects of the practice: herbology, meditation, moxibustion (the burning of herbs into acupressure points in the skin), spiritual right action (spiritually desirable behavior, according to Buddhist precept), subtle body channels that cannot be detected by modern science and incantations to the blue (the color of healing) Medicine Buddha, the particularly Tibetan incarnation of the deity.

"In the West, we have organ-based disease categories," said Dr. Mehmet Oz, a cofounder of Complementary Care Services at New York Presbyterian Hospital. "Their treatment is systemic. They don't just give everyone with diabetes the same herbs. Treatment is very different, depending on a person's 'humor,' on whether they have an imbalance of what they designate wind, bile or phlegm.'"

I also met a doctor who was not a wholesale proponent of Tibetan medicine. "People romanticize natural remedies," said Dr. Richard A. Friedman, the director of psychopharmacology at the New York Weill Cornell Center of New York Presbyterian Hospital. "They think that if it goes under the rubric of 'natural,' it must be good. But nature also brings tornadoes," Dr. Friedman said, adding that "with untested, natural treatments, there can be a big problem with drug interactions."

I also visited the one Tibetan doctor in New York, Choeying Phuntsok, a consultant at the Meridian Medical Center on East Thirtieth Street in Manhattan. "All disease is caused by ignorance," he said, when the conversation took a philosophical turn. "As long as you haven't achieved enlightenment, you're going to be driven by anger, ignorance and desire. Those three act on phlegm, bile and wind to produce illness."

And I phoned two educated observers. "Once all the legalities are sorted out, Tibetan medicine could be a very interesting boom," said Robert Thurman, the professor of Indo-Tibetan studies at Columbia University. Eliot Tokar, a lecturer on Tibetan medicine, said woefully: "It's the last great product line. The Gold Rush is starting. And as with any gold rush, it's bound to leave a few holes in the ground."

Any prospectors will have to contend with the trip to Dharamsala, which is winding, long and wearying. There are no flights in, no airport. After landing in Delhi at 10 P.M., we scrambled to board a bus leaving at 1 A.M., then sat bolt upright through the night as our driver, a washcloth draped over his head, sang loud Hindu chants and kept time with the horn. Through my window, smeared with the coconut hair oil of previous passengers, I could make out many holes in the ground, although they seemed like the product of disrepair, rather than any stampede. A few cradled nesting sacred cows. Eight hours later, after crossing the Punjab, we reached our terminus, Jalandhar. It was another three hours before we arrived at the foothills of the Himalayas, and Dharamsala.

Tibet was known as the "country of medicine," Terry Clifford notes in her book *Tibetan Buddhist Medicine and Psychiatry* (Weiser), and it doesn't take long in Dharamsala to realize that the exiles have reconstructed as much of the old country as possible. Once your eyes have adjusted to the astonishing color and sights—monkeys perched on low-slung roofs, maroon-and-orange-robed monks dodging rickshaws—you notice the signs everywhere for medical practices: Delek Western-style hospital, Dr. Sant Marwah Clinic. They're scattered up and down the hilly roads that lead to Men-Tsee-Khan, the sprawling white Tibetan Medical and Astrological complex that was founded in 1961 by the Dalai Lama. From our lodgings at the placid Kashmir Cottage, run by the Dalai Lama's younger brother, we could see the white prayer flags that fluttered from the roof.

The pungent smell of herbs drying, combined with the altitude, made me light-headed on our first morning's tour, through the room where our astrologers filled orders for star charts, through the clinic where nuns and students lined up beside a condom dispenser for free consultations, in the plain, sea green ward where six men lay on cots.

One's eyes were yellow with hepatitis. Another, a boy who had recently escaped from Tibet, was shaking with abdominal pain. "Doctor's planning to keep him for nine days," our guide, Tseten Dorjee, the assistant to the clinic's director, said. "If he doesn't get better, we'll move him across the street to Delek hospital."

"But what if it's appendicitis?" my friend whispered, and lagging behind, we considered the advantages of Western medicine.

The tour ended in Mr. Dorjee's office. On the computer behind him, three ovals with the Dalai Lama's face swirled on the screen saver. We talked about how knockoff artists were peddling bootleg "precious pills," the highly valued Tibetan mixtures of as many as 153 herbs and minerals, including gold. To try to thwart them, Men-Tsee Khan had begun stamping all containers with holograms of the myroban plant, Mr. Dorjee said. He pulled out a notebook fat with requests from drug and vitamin companies. So far, one pharmaceutical firm, Padma A.G., a Swiss concern, was making headway. Otherwise, "We say, 'Send us proposal,'" he said. "We say, 'We have to look into the legalities.'"

"There are not enough herbs for ourselves," he continued. "How can we collaborate with them?"

On the way out, we met with Tenzin Choedrak, the Dalai Lama's current personal physician. Dr. Choedrak, seventy-three, was stooped and looked frail. He had a cauliflower nose, bunched and flat. For twenty-two years, he had been imprisoned and tortured by the Chinese. After he escaped, he lectured about how he had survived psychologically. We spoke briefly, then made plans to meet the next morning for a medical consultation.

We arrived at nine. Outside, children shrieked in the courtyard. Inside, the air smelled like cloves. From his daybed, Dr. Choedrak motioned me to sit, clasped my wrist. "How long you stay?" he asked through the interpreter, and for a moment, I was worried that he was considering sending me to the ward. His voice was shaky, but the pressure of his fingers on my wrist was surprisingly firm.

No sweet, no sour, no meat, the interpreter informed me, before handing over packets of herbs, including one that contained six silk-wrapped precious pills. "To prevent chemicals and for sleep and for blood purification," she explained. "And to improve energy. Your hemoglobin is low." I raised one eyebrow. At Sloan-Kettering, they'd just recently detected mild anemia.

In context, the experience was impressive. But later I found myself reflecting on whether Tibetan medicine could be transported out of context, to the United States. One night we had dinner with Jempa Kalsan, the center's senior astrologer. "I forecast best time for treatment, when the best time to pick herbs is," he said, and I tried to imagine what the Food and Drug Administration's position on medical astrology would be.

But the differences between East and West became most apparent to me one afternoon during a conversation with Nawang Dorjee, a Fulbright scholar, director of education at the Tibetan Children's Village in Dharamsala, and an old friend of my travel mate's from her Tibetan Refugee Project days.

"When I was diagnosed with breast cancer six years ago," Connie said, catching Mr. Dorjee up on her life, "I went to a Tibetan doctor. 'Prepare for your death,' he told me. 'Prepare for your death!' But I've been fine."

"Oh, that's so Tibetan," Mr. Dorjee, who is not related to Tseten Dorjee, said, smiling. "What he meant was, stop collecting bad deeds. Start praying. Be at peace—because we believe in reincarnation. Become ready for your next life."

Not bad advice, we agreed.

"But can you imagine a doctor at Sloan-Kettering telling a patient that: 'Prepare for your death'?" I said, and the image made us laugh so hard we doubled over.

"Prepare for your death" became a running punch line for the rest of the trip. "Prepare for your death!" one of us would say, and the other would collapse in laughter. And maybe it was the pills, or maybe the magnificent rise of the Himalayas above us, but funny thing was, we both agreed, we'd never felt more alive.

Katherine Russell Rich, June 1999

LAUGHTER: WHY IT'S GOOD FOR YOU

Laugh, and the world laughs with you—whatever the country, whatever the tribe. Anthropologists have never encountered a culture where people do not laugh to express merriment and sociability; even deaf people sometimes laugh out loud. Babies begin laughing at the age of two or three months, said Dr. William F. Fry of the Stanford University School of Medicine, just when the parents are getting fed up with all the fussing. The rate of laughter picks up steadily for the next several years, until around the age of six or so, when the average child laughs three hundred times a day.

After that, social training and the desire to blend in with one's peers conspire to damp liberal laughter. Estimates of how much adults laugh vary widely, from a high of one hundred chuckles daily to a dour low of fifteen, but clearly adults lose their laughter edge along with the talent for finger painting. Some laughter authorities view that decline as a blow to the health of body and spirit. When you laugh robustly, you increase blood circulation, work your abdominal muscles, raise your heart rate and get the stale air out of your lungs; after a bout of laughter, your blood pressure drops to a lower, healthier level than before the buoyancy began.

Beyond such overt benefits, Dr. Lee S. Berk of the Loma Linda School of Public Health in California has also discovered subtler effects of laughter on the immune and neuroendocrine systems. He and his colleagues have learned that an hour spent laughing lowers levels of stress hormones like cortisol and epinephrine. At the same time, the immune system appears to grow stronger, the body's T cells, natural killer cells and antibodies all showing signs of heightened activity.

"It's no longer mystical," he said. "We've always heard that laughter is good for you, and now we're gathering the hard, serious stuff to show why this is so."

What remains to be demonstrated, though, is that any of these immune changes actually help fight or prevent disease.

Dr. John Morreall, a philosopher and laugh consultant who runs a firm called Humorworks out of Temple Terrace, Florida, tries to persuade businesses like Kodak and Xerox and, yes, also the Internal Revenue Service, of the financial value of laughter on the job. "It gets the creative juices flowing, it helps in problem solving, and it smooths the way during difficult times like annual evaluations or when giving criticism," he said. "The ability to think in funny ways and original ways can overlap." Punch lines and bottom lines likewise overlap: if you cannot afford to give your employees raises or job security, you can always give them the freedom to laugh.

Natalie Angier, February 1996

MEDITATION GAINS GROUND EVEN IN HOSPITALS

As her meditation session drew to a close, Mary Bryant found it difficult to get up from her chair. Not only was it hard to break the calming spell cast by her instructor, but Ms. Bryant was still stiff from running the New York City Marathon and pushing, for the whole twenty-six miles, a flower-strewn wheelchair dedicated to a late friend and fellow breast cancer patient.

Finally, the tall, slender Ms. Bryant summoned her resolve and managed to stand while repeating her teacher's suggested thought, "I am here now." She added her own twist, "I am here now, and I am cancer-free."

It seemed a fitting mantra for the inaugural meditation class at Memorial Sloan-Kettering Cancer Center's Integrative Medicine Service in Manhattan, where patients can also get massages, acupuncture, nutritional advice and a crack at playing Tibetan bowls. With its muted earth tones, river rock fountain and artfully lighted shelves of crystals, the center at 303 East Sixty-fifth Street, which opened on November 1, 1999, more closely resembles a spa in Big Sur than part of a huge hospital. Yet it is the latest example of a national trend in which conventional medical institutions are embracing healing methods once dismissed as alternative medicine and combining them with standard treatment.

Meditation, the discipline of directed attention that began in India about 2,500 years ago, is among the most popular techniques now going mainstream.

"It's not invasive, it has no side effects, it has tremendous benefits that are very well documented and it's something patients can do on their own so it doesn't cost anything," said Dr. Barrie R. Casselith, chief of the new program, who holds a doctorate in medical sociology.

"It's not a cancer treatment," Dr. Casselith quickly added. "It deals with quality of life and helps with symptoms. It can relieve pain, lower blood pressure and heart rate. It can make people feel calmer, it enhances mood. It does lots of good things."

Her counterpart at Beth Israel Medical Center, Dr. Woodson Merrell, called meditation "perhaps the most powerful tool for health."

In 1998, Congress gave the National Institutes of Health $10 million a year for five years to expand a network of mind-body research centers and provide training for health workers in a variety of meditative approaches. One of the most popular techniques used, though there are scores of styles, is a form called mindfulness meditation, in which the patient learns to be aware of sensations and thoughts and temporarily tune out everyday life.

"We cannot keep up with the demand of health professionals to learn this," said Dr. Herbert Benson, the cardiologist who coined the term "relaxation response" and founded the Mind/Body Medical Institute at the Beth Israel Deaconess Medical Center in Boston.

Dr. Benson, who helped popularize meditative techniques, whether they consist of prayer, exercise or more traditional Eastern meditation skills, first documented the physiological benefits of the techniques and their effect on stress nearly thirty years ago. Since then, he said, his findings have been repeatedly affirmed.

During a study presented by Harvard researchers in October 1999 at the annual meeting of the Society for Neuroscience, five people who had been meditating daily for at least five years were placed inside a magnetic resonance imaging scanner, or MRI. During a forty-two-minute period they were asked to stare at a dot on a screen, randomly to generate a mental list of animals and to meditate. The resulting pictures of their brains showed that the regions that process emotion and influence cardiorespiratory function were most active during meditation.

In other words, said Dr. Sara Lazar, an author of the study, they verify "what meditators have been saying all along: that they feel calmer and that meditating brings about specific, quantifiable changes in the body."

Still, skeptics view the current romance with meditation as inspired by money as much as by open-mindedness. "It's good marketing," said Dr. Richard Sloan, a psychologist and director of behavioral medicine at Columbia-Presbyterian Medical Center. "There's no doubt the relaxation response has an impact on the autonomic nervous system, but there's a question whether that translates into a health benefit or whether it's just ephemeral."

The Rev. Larry VandeCreek, director of pastoral research for the HealthCare Chaplaincy, cited a 1993 study published in the *New England Journal of Medicine* that found the general public was spending huge amounts of money on alternative medicine. "There's certainly some cynicism here, trying to capture or recapture a piece of the market," Mr. VandeCreek said. "But I think there may also be some sincere attempt to do what's best for the patient, and if some of these interventions are helpful, then they ought to be used."

Whether meditation is offered as a purely secular relaxation technique or a more spiritual exercise also remains a sensitive subject. At Columbia-Presbyterian's Center for Meditation and Healing, at 16 East Sixtieth Street, Dr. Joseph J. Loizzo, a psychiatrist, begins classes with the ritual ringing of silver Tibetan bells and recently led one pair of advanced students in a discussion of Tara, the Buddhist goddess of compassion. Tuition for an eight-week course is $950.

A practicing Buddhist and firm believer in the power of meditation to overcome depression and mood disorders, Dr. Loizzo nonetheless prescribes antidepressants when needed.

"He asked me the first time I met him, 'Are you spiritual?'" said a former patient who now studies with Dr. Loizzo once a week and meditates twice a day. The forty-one-year-old schoolteacher, who asked not to be named, had been hospitalized for depression and began meditating to wean herself from the drug Effexor. "I used to feel that depression was always out there and that I was one of the people it could get," the woman said. "Now I understand you can heal from within, that we have a lot of resources we can use."

At Sloan-Kettering, where administrators carefully discuss meditation in strictly nonreligious terms, Barbara Parisi, a patient, began meditating to stave off anxiety but said her daily practice had since gained a spiritual side. Ms. Parisi, fifty, who has lung cancer and meditates during her weekly chemotherapy sessions, likes to picture herself in her garden or floating among stars and clouds.

"To me, it's godlike, it's love, it's connection to other human beings and life," she said. "You feel so vibrant and so full and so good. It makes me feel that even if I don't win this battle, it will be all right because there's a sense of peace."

Ms. Bryant, a fashion model in her thirties who had a mastectomy and chemotherapy in the last year and is going through follow-up tests, talks about meditation in more practical terms. "The uncertainty is terrifying," she said. "We have the strength inside to handle it, but you have to clear your head to find the strength."

Sloan-Kettering spent $500,000 to renovate what had been a prostate cancer clinic, adding a small studio for meditating, yoga and exercise. Patients pay $80 for each hour they spend there. Insurance coverage varies greatly; some companies pay for some services, but Medicare does not. "It's evolving, and some insurance companies are more accepting of it than others," said Simone Zappa, the program director of the Integrative Medicine Service.

During its first meditation class, Dr. David Payne, a psychologist, led Ms. Bryant and two other women in an hourlong mental body scan in which they focused on their sensations from head to toe and were urged to "bring a sense of honor and respect" to their bodies. All three women were smiling broadly and sitting as still as statues by the end of the class.

"I do believe I'm cancer-free," Ms. Bryant said. "But I feel it's important to stay strong to keep my immune system strong to help fight the disease."

Leslie Berger, November 1999

HOW DO YOU STOP AGONIZING PAIN IN AN ARM THAT NO LONGER EXISTS? A SCIENTIST DOES IT WITH MIRRORS

The third time he lost his left arm, Derek Steen yelped with joy. He could not believe his good fortune.

The problem began ten years ago when Mr. Steen crashed his motorcycle, tearing all the nerves that attached his arm to his spine. The limb was hopelessly paralyzed, bound in a sling. He lost his arm a second time, so to speak, one year later when, deemed useless and getting in the way, it was amputated.

But Mr. Steen, a twenty-eight-year-old part-time worker in San Diego, continued to suffer. His phantom arm felt paralyzed, pressed against his body, and it ached horribly for ten years. Then, late last year he was cured. After a simple, three-week treatment involving mirrors, his paralyzed phantom arm suddenly vanished, as did the gnawing pain in his phantom elbow. In its place, Mr. Steen says, he has a much reduced phantom limb composed of his lower left palm and all five fingers, which he can now "wiggle" freely from the stump below his shoulder.

Dr. Vilayanus S. Ramachandran, a professor of neuroscience at the University of California at San Diego, who devised the treatment, said Mr. Steen's "body image" had been profoundly altered, much for the better.

Dr. Ramachandran described the finding—a rare example of successful treatment for phantom limb pain—at the second annual meeting of the Cognitive Neuroscience Society being held in San Francisco in March 1995.

Phantom limbs occur when the brain modifies its sensory maps after an amputation, he said. The brain region mapping an arm no longer gets input from the arm but it continues to be constantly stimulated by inputs from adjacent body parts. These stimuli fool the brain into thinking the arm itself is still there.

But sometimes, as in Mr. Steen's case, a phantom limb can be paralyzed. "The arm is in a fixed position, as if frozen in cement," Dr. Ramachandran said. "The patient can't generate the slightest flicker of movement, even though he can feel all the parts. I started thinking why."

The answer lies in the feedback loops in the brain that integrate vision, senses, body movements, body image and motor commands, Dr. Ramachandran said. In the first few weeks after the accident, Mr. Steen would try to move his injured arm, to no avail. His brain sent signals to his arm, commanding motion, but though his eyes confirmed the arm was there, it did not move.

In time, Dr. Ramachandran said, Mr. Steen developed "learned paralysis."

"His brain constantly got information that his arm was not moving," even though it was still there, Dr. Ramachandran said. After the amputation, he still felt it was there.

"Now if it's true paralysis can be learned, can you unlearn it?" Dr. Ramachandran said. "And how do you do that if you don't really have an arm?"

Simple. With mirrors. Dr. Ramachandran constructed a simple box without a lid and front and placed a vertical mirror in the middle. By placing his right arm into the box, Mr. Steen could see a mirror image of his missing left arm.

"I asked him to make symmetric movements with both hands, as if he were conducting an orchestra," Dr. Ramachandran said. "He started jumping up and down and said, 'Oh, my God, my wrist is moving, my elbow is moving!' I asked him to close his eyes. He groaned, 'Oh no, it's frozen again,'" the scientist said. "The box cost only five dollars, so I told him to take it home and play around with it."

Three weeks later, Dr. Ramachandran said, "he phones me, sounding agitated and excited." The conversation went like this:

"Doctor, it's gone!"

"What's gone?"

"My phantom arm is gone."

"What?"

"All I have is fingers and a lower palm dangling from my shoulder."

"Does this bother you?"

"No," Mr. Steen replied. "The pain in my elbow is gone. I can move my fingers. But your box doesn't work anymore."

The telescoping of fingers is common in phantom limbs, Dr. Ramachandran said. "But nevertheless I couldn't help think that I had permanently altered someone's body image."

The reason the arm disappeared and the body image changed probably has to do with tremendous sensory conflict, Dr. Ramachandran said. "His vision was telling him that his arm had come back and was obeying his commands. But he was not getting feedback from the muscles in his arm. Faced with this type of conflict over a protracted period, the brain may simply gate the signals. It says: 'This doesn't make sense. I won't have anything to do with it.'

"In the process, the arm disappears and the elbow pain goes away," he said. "The reason the fingers survive and dangle from the shoulder is that they are overrepresented in the cortex, much more so than the rest of the arm. So there may be a kind of tip-of-the-iceberg phenomenon going on here."

Dr. Ramachandran is now treating other kinds of phantom limb pain, including a clenching spasm of phantom hands. "People feel as if their fingernails are digging into their hands and say it is excruciatingly painful," he said. The mirror box has helped one such patient.

The new finding may also have relevance to stroke rehabilitation, Dr. Ramachandran said. In the early stages, some paralysis is due to swelling in the brain and learned paralysis could result. While destroyed tissue could not be revived, he said, other circuits might be reestablished with the use of the mirrors.

These ideas remain highly speculative, Dr. Ramachandran said. Moreover, pain is notoriously susceptible to placebo effects, so it may be difficult to prove that these brain-based therapies are effective.

Nevertheless, striking results are being seen with some stroke patients who lose the ability to talk. At the University of Iowa, Dr. Antonio Damasio and his colleagues are teaching American Sign Language to patients whose primary language areas have been partly damaged but not destroyed. By learning a sign for a concept, he said, they are often able to reconnect with the word for that concept—and in this way can learn how to speak once again.

Such plasticity or adaptability in the adult brain may be more common than most people realize, said Dr. Michael Gazzaniga, a neuroscientist who is an expert on split-brain patients at the University of California at Davis.

An effective treatment for severe epilepsy is to cut the bundle of fibers that connect the left- and right-brain hemispheres. Each half brain is conscious but does not know what the other half sees or does.

In such patients, the left brain "wakes up and starts talking," Dr. Gazzaniga said. The right brain usually shows no sign of language comprehension, and it certainly had no ability to talk—until a patient named Joe stunned researchers by learning how to talk with his right brain. Joe was like other split-brain patients for thirteen years, Dr. Gazzaniga said. Then his right brain started recognizing and saying words independently of the left brain. Now, fifteen years after surgery, Joe can name 60 percent of the stimuli presented to his right brain, Dr. Gazzaniga said.

"It could be that new connections have been made, or that others have been unrepressed," Dr. Gazzaniga said. "At this point we have no idea how or why it happens." But answers, should they be found, might be used for helping people overcome all sorts of brain injuries and neurodegenerative diseases.

Sandra Blakeslee, March 1995

YOUR CANCER ISN'T YOUR FAULT

Several years ago, I cared for a middle-aged doctor with colon cancer. The cancer was found in a routine physical examination. During an exploratory operation, the surgeons discovered that the cancer had spread to his liver. Like many cancer patients with no family history of the disease, the doctor experienced shock and disbelief. These emotions then gave way to a profound sense of guilt.

"I didn't take care of myself," he said. "Instead of salami and eggs, I should have been eating whole grains for breakfast."

Cancer patients often blame themselves for their illness. The idea that such an aggressive and life-threatening disease arises randomly runs contrary to our firm belief in cause and effect. When no other reason, like genetic predisposition, can be summoned, the mind weaves the most tenuous strands of information into an imagined cause.

I tried to shift my patient's focus from blaming himself to something more productive: pursuing treatment while preserving his quality of life. But the patient kept focusing on what he should have done. He, like all doctors, had been taught that high-fiber diets helped prevent colon cancer. This was based on observational studies in Africa, which noted that people there had diets high in fiber and correspondingly low rates of colon cancer.

I thought of this patient, and the tendency for many cancer patients to blame themselves for their disease, when I read the research results published this week in the *New England Journal of Medicine*. Two large studies found that dietary fiber is not a major factor in the development of colon polyps, the precursors of cancer. These studies, based on careful statistical analysis, stand in stark contrast to the observational reports that have been the prevailing wisdom of medical teaching for three decades. While diet may be important in colon cancer, it is not clear what aspect—a specific vitamin, chemical or cooking method—might explain the differences in risk across the globe.

We humans seem particularly prone to blaming ourselves for our illnesses. In some religions, disease is seen as a divine punishment for sin. And religious people often rationalize the seeming injustice of their malady by interpreting it as an appropriate form of retribution. Among some practitioners of alternative medicine, it has become popular to assert that there is a "cancer personality"—that people are more likely to develop cancer if they have low self-esteem, are frequently depressed or have unresolved anger. This theory, while conveniently explaining why ineffective alternative treatments, like laetrile and coffee enemas, fail, also allows a debilitating guilt to pervade the remaining days of a patient's life.

Even in the mainstream medical community, behavior is often used as a rationale for why cancer does or does not develop. For instance, until studies debunked the theories last year, it was widely believed that high-fat diets promoted breast cancer and that foods rich in retinoids, derivatives of vitamin A, helped prevent recurrent head and neck cancers.

Of course, diet and behavior are not irrelevant. Smoking has been directly linked to lung cancer, and a low-fat, low-cholesterol diet helps prevent cardiovascular disease. Yet given our self-destructive tendency to pin blame on our own behaviors, it is critical to marshal sound data rather than rely on unproven impressions.

Cancer is a complex disease, arising from the interaction of our genes with numerous factors in the environment. No single influence can completely explain its genesis. We must minimize our risk for cancer, but not blame ourselves if we develop it.

My patient with colon cancer died two years ago, before this new information on diet and colon cancer was available. The tragedy seems more profound: knowing that he didn't cause his cancer would have alleviated some of the anguish that he experienced.

Jerome Groopman, April 2000

PLACEBOS: THE BRAIN'S TRIUMPH OVER REALITY

Many doctors know the story of "Mr. Wright," who was found to have cancer and in 1957 was given only days to live. Hospitalized in Long Beach, California, with tumors the size of oranges, he heard that scientists had discovered a horse serum, Krebiozen, that appeared to be effective against cancer. He begged to receive it. His physician, Dr. Philip West, finally agreed and gave Mr. Wright an injection on a Friday afternoon. The following Monday, the astonished doctor found his patient out of his "deathbed," joking with the nurses. The tumors, the doctor wrote later, "had melted like snowballs on a hot stove."

Two months later, Mr. Wright read medical reports that the horse serum was a quack remedy. He suffered an immediate relapse. "Don't believe what you read in the papers," the doctor told Mr. Wright. Then he injected him with what he said was "a new superrefined, double-strength" version of the drug. Actually, it was water, but again, the tumor masses melted.

Mr. Wright was "the picture of health" for another two months—until he read a definitive report stating that Krebiozen was worthless. He died two days later. Doctors who know this story dismiss it as one of those strange tales that medicine cannot explain. The idea that a patient's beliefs can make a fatal disease go away is too bizarre.

But now scientists, as they learn that the placebo effect is even more powerful than anyone had been able to demonstrate, are also beginning to discover the biological mechanisms that cause it to achieve results that border on the miraculous. Using new techniques of brain imagery, they are uncovering a host of biological mechanisms that can turn a thought, belief or desire into an agent of change in cells, tissues and organs. They are learning that much of human perception is based not on information flowing into the brain from the outside world but what the brain, based on previous experience, expects to happen next.

Placebos are "lies that heal," said Dr. Anne Harrington, a historian of science at Harvard University. A placebo, Latin for "I shall please," is typically a sham treatment that a doctor doles out merely to please or placate anxious or persistent patients, she said. It looks like an active drug but has no pharmacological properties of its own.

Until fairly recently, nearly all of medicine was based on placebo effects, because doctors had little effective medicine to offer. Through the 1940s, American doctors handed out sugar pills in various shapes and colors in a deliberate attempt to induce placebo responses.

Nowadays, doctors have real medicines to fight disease. But these treatments have not diminished the power of the placebo.

Doctors in Texas are conducting a study of arthroscopic knee surgery that uses general anesthesia in which patients with sore, worn knees are assigned to one of three operations—scraping out the knee joint, washing out the joint or doing nothing. In the "nothing" operation, doctors anesthetize the patient, make three little cuts in the knee as if to insert the usual instruments and then pretend to operate. In a pilot study of ten patients, two years after surgery, those who underwent the sham surgery reported the same amount of relief from pain and swelling as those who had had the real operations. A larger study is under way.

A review of placebo-controlled studies of modern antidepressant drugs found that placebos worked about as well as genuine drugs. "If you expect to get better, you will," said Dr. Irving Kirsch, a psychiatrist at the University of Connecticut who carried out the review. His findings were met with a great deal of skepticism.

But there are many similar examples. A study of a baldness remedy found that 86 percent of men taking it either maintained or showed an increase in the amount of hair on their heads. But so did 42 percent of the men taking a placebo. Some studies are specifically designed to explore the power of placebos rather than drugs. On Coche Island in Venezuela, asthmatic children were given a sniff of vanilla along with a squirt of medicine from a bronchodilator twice a day. Later, the vanilla odor alone increased their lung function, 33 percent as much as did the bronchodilator alone.

And at Tulane University, Dr. Eileen Palace is using a placebo to restore sexual arousal in women who say they are nonorgasmic. The women are hooked up to a biofeedback machine that they are told measures their vaginal blood flow, an index of arousal. Then they are shown sexual stimuli that would arouse most women. But the experimenter plays a trick on the women by sending, within thirty seconds, a false feedback signal that their vaginal blood flow has increased. Almost immediately they then become genuinely aroused.

Placebos are about 55 percent to 60 percent as effective as most active medications like aspirin and codeine for controlling pain, Dr. Kirsch said. Moreover, placebos that relieve pain can be blocked with a drug, naloxone, that also blocks morphine. For a while, many scientists thought that placebos might work by releasing the body's natural morphinelike substances, called endorphins. But that is not the only explanation, he said. While placebos can act globally on the body, they can also have extremely specific effects. For example, a study was carried out in Japan on thirteen people who were extremely allergic to poison ivy. Each was rubbed on one arm with a harmless leaf but was told it was poison ivy and touched on the other arm with poison ivy and told it was harmless. All thirteen broke out in rashes where the harmless leaf contacted their skin. Only two reacted to the poison leaves.

Studies have shown, time and again, that placebos can work wonders. Like "real drugs," they can cause side effects like itching, diarrhea and nausea. They can lead to changes in pulse rate, blood pressure, electrical skin resistance, gastric function, penis engorgement and skin conditions. The question is, why? Explanations of why placebos work can be found in a new field of cognitive neuropsychology called expectancy theory— what the brain believes about the immediate future.

Like classical conditioning theory (Pavlov's dogs salivate at the sound of a bell), expectancy involves associative learning. The medical treatments you get during your life are conditioning trials, Dr. Kirsch said. The doctor's white coat, nurse's voice, smell of disinfectant or needle prick have acquired meaning through previous learning, producing an expectation of relief from symptoms. Each pill, capsule or injection is paired with active ingredients, and later, if you get a pill without active ingredients, you can still get a therapeutic effect, he said.

Such conditioning shows how expectations are acquired, Dr. Kirsch said. But it does not explain the strength and persistence of placebo effects. These responses occur almost instantly, with no apparent conscious thought, and are therefore wired firmly into the brain, he said.

Response expectations are strong because the world is filled with ambiguity. A long, thin object seen in dim light could be a stick or a snake. But it may not be safe to take the time to find out. So people evolved a mechanism to anticipate what is going to occur. This expectation speeds the perceptual processing at the expense of accuracy. As in the outside world, people's internal states have inherent ambiguity. That is why, when people in an experiment were given a drug that produced a surge of adrenaline, they interpreted the feeling as anger, euphoria or nothing at all, depending on what they had been told to expect.

Critics of alternative medicine say its enduring appeal is explained by the placebo effect. When conventional therapies fail to help chronic or poorly understood conditions, the acupuncturist, homeopathist or chiropractor steps into the breach with a potent belief system ready-made to help the suffering patient. "If a guy in a white coat or a guy dressed in feathers can induce a patient's immune system to fight back, who is to say which is better?" said Dr. Dan Molerman, a medical anthropologist at the University of Michigan at Dearborn.

Support for the expectancy theory emerged about ten years ago, when many scientists realized how closely the brain, the immune system and the hormone production of the endocrine system are linked. Chronic stress sets into motion a cascade of biological events involving scores of chemicals in the body—serotonin, cortisol, cytokines, interleukins, tumor necrosis factor and so on. Such stress lowers resistance to disease and alters gene expression. When people are under stress, wounds tend to heal more slowly, latent viruses like herpes erupt and brain cells involved in memory formation die off. The precise molecular steps underlying all these changes have been mapped out.

But what about the opposite? Can a thought or belief produce a chemical cascade that leads to healing and wellness? Researchers studying placebos think the answer is yes, and they offer several ways it might work:

- A placebo might reduce stress, allowing the body to regain some natural, optimum level called health.
- Special molecules may exist that help carry out placebo responses. For example, a study found that

stressed animals can produce a valiumlike substance
in their brains, but only if they have some control over
the source of the stress. People almost certainly have
similar brain chemistry.

- Placebos may draw their power from the way the brain
  is organized to act on what experience predicts will
  happen next.

Dr. Marcel Kinsbourne, a neuroscientist at the New School for Social
Research in New York, explains it this way: The brain generates two kinds
of activation patterns, which arise from networks of neurons firing
together. One type is set in motion by information flowing into the brain
from the outside world—smells, tastes, visual images, sounds. At the same
time, the cortex draws on memories and feelings to generate patterns of
brain activity related to what is expected to happen.

The top-down patterns generated by the cortex intersect smoothly
with the bottom-up patterns to inform us about what is happening, Dr.
Kinsbourne said. If there is a mismatch, the brain tries to sort it out, without necessarily designating one set of patterns as more authoritative than
another. The expectations that result are internally generated brain states
that can be as real as anything resulting purely from the outside world.
For example, recent experiments with monkeys show that if they expect a
reward like a sip of apple juice, cells in their brains fire twenty to thirty
seconds before they actually receive it. In other words, expectancies are
embedded in the brain's neurochemistry.

"We are misled by dualism or the idea that mind and body are separate," said Dr. Howard Fields, a neuroscientist at the University of California at San Francisco who studies placebo effects. A thought is a set of
neurons firing which, through complex brain wiring, can activate emotional centers, pain pathways, memories, the autonomic nervous system
and other parts of the nervous system involved in producing physical sensations, he said.

Morphine will alter brain patterns to reduce pain. So will a placebo.
Obviously, placebos have limits. Mr. Wright's miraculous remission aside,
most people cannot think, hope or believe their way out of cancer or AIDS.

As Dr. Howard Spiro, a gastroenterologist at Yale University, put it: Some diseases are unleashed with the power of a fire hose. Others unfold at a trickle, and perhaps those are the ones amenable to placebo effects.

Sandra Blakeslee, October 1998

PLACEBOS: THE DOCTOR'S ENTHUSIASM CAN GIVE PILLS AN EXTRA KICK

Though some people respond more strongly to placebos than others do, it seems that everyone responds at some time or other. And doctors seem to play a large role in the degree of that response.

"The thing that trumps everything is the enthusiastic physician," said Dr. Dan Molerman of the University of Michigan. For example, one study offered the same drug to patients with identical symptoms, with one difference. Some were told by their physicians, "This drug has been shown to work," while others were told, "I am not sure if this treatment will work—let's just try it." The first group of patients did much better, Dr. Molerman said. "The physician is an agent for optimism and hope and a great inducer of beliefs."

Physicians can even fool themselves. Years ago, researchers carried out controlled studies of a drug for angina, or heart pain, and found it was no better than a placebo, Dr. Molerman said. Once doctors knew that, its effectiveness fell. While doctors and patients affect one another's expectations, both are swept up into a wider context of culture and biology, said Dr. David Morris, an adjunct professor of medicine at the University of New Mexico in Albuquerque. The brain circuits through which placebos act, he said, are activated through the experience of living in a particular culture.

To explore the importance of cultural context, Dr. Molerman compared 122 double-blind placebo-controlled ulcer studies from all over the world. Doctors used the same techniques, the same drugs and the same placebo pills, and studied an image of the stomach lining before and after treatment to see what worked. The drugs worked 75 to 80 percent of the time, Dr. Molerman said, whereas the placebos worked from zero to 100 percent of the time, depending on the country. The placebo healing rate for ulcers in Germany was 60 percent, almost double the world average of 36 percent, which is about where the United States fell. But in Brazil, the mean placebo healing rate was a startling 6 percent.

"I don't have a hint of what is going on here," Dr. Molerman said. "I can only say that cultural differences affect ulcer treatments, even though ulcers are the same the world over."

Sandra Blakeslee, October 1998

HYPNOSIS FOR PAIN, FEAR AND BAD HABITS

When Michael Tracy learned at the age of fifteen that he had a form of cancer known as lymphoma, his world seemed to cave in. His father had just died of brain cancer, so as he dealt with the grief and fear, he faced a series of dreaded spinal taps, bone-marrow aspirations and chemotherapy treatments that would fill his weeks for the next two years.

"I'd be so nervous that I would walk into the hospital and just throw up before anything even happened," he recalled from his home in the Park Slope section of Brooklyn.

But Mount Sinai Medical Center, where he was treated, had recently added something else to its disease-fighting arsenal: hypnosis. Elsa Pelier, an art therapist and child-life specialist, used techniques of suggestion to help Michael relax. She then asked him to envision a "pain switch" during an injection. "I visualized a light dimmer that I turned down to make the pain less," said Michael, who is now seventeen and whose cancer is in remission. "I felt my whole body calm down. It made a huge difference."

Hypnosis, that mysterious but highly touted technique of tapping the unconscious to accomplish all sorts of things, is quietly enjoying a period of prolific use. Though practiced for two hundred years and officially recognized by the medical establishment in this country years ago, hypnosis has only recently been buoyed by the growing acceptance—

among doctors and patients alike—of the relationship between mind and body. Psychotherapists use it to try to snuff out phobias and addictions, while dentists employ it to tame the terror of drilling and filling. Hospitals from Mount Sinai to Memorial Sloan-Kettering Cancer Center find hypnosis valuable for beating pain, and even paramedics, like those in North Tarrytown, New York, are using hypnosis techniques to calm trauma victims.

"In the last ten years there has been a noticeable increase in the use of hypnosis for pain control and habit control," said Dr. Herbert Spiegel, a retired clinical professor of psychiatry at Columbia University who taught hypnosis there for twenty-two years. "There's more sensitivity to the fact that the mind has great therapeutic powers."

The Office of Alternative Medicine, a federal agency created in 1992 by the National Institutes of Health, is financing three studies on hypnosis. Bill Moyers's public television series *Healing and the Mind*, which generated a best-selling book in 1993, introduced a wide audience to such alternative approaches as hypnosis. And the enormous popularity of such spas as Canyon Ranch, which offers hypnotherapy at its resorts in Arizona and Connecticut, has exposed still others to the treatment.

Mary Mitchell, a thirty-two-year-old publishing executive who lives on the Upper East Side, first tried hypnosis while vacationing at Canyon Ranch. Having struggled with her weight most of her life, she hoped that hypnosis could help her eat more slowly and stop using food as a substitute for relaxation. The results were mixed. "I definitely noticed a difference in the beginning," she said. "There is some little alarm that goes off inside so that even if I don't stop eating, I stop and think about stopping. But it wasn't the magic bullet. Frankly, I was hoping it was."

That is exactly what most hypnotists, many of whom prefer the term hypnotherapist, want to get across: that what they do is not magic, that everyone has experienced a so-called hypnotic state before, for instance when lost in thought on an open highway, unable to recall what has just passed by. In fact, many people who have undergone hypnosis express near-disappointment at not feeling transformed or out of control, as they had expected. What they do experience, they say, is a state of profound physical relaxation, and a heightened mental awareness that makes it easy to focus on the suggestions of the therapist. While not everyone responds, some people report dramatic changes.

"The only thing you are making use of is a semidissociative state, which is a very creative one," said Dr. Marianne S. Andersen, a psychologist and clinical instructor at Mount Sinai and a fellow of the Society for Clinical and Experimental Hypnosis, a nonprofit organization in Indianapolis founded in 1949. "The magic lies within you, not in the therapist. You are not under anyone's control. All hypnosis is essentially self-hypnosis."

Another sign of its growing popularity is the number of medical professionals who are being trained in hypnosis. In 1990, when Dr. Andersen began conducting workshops at Mount Sinai for physicians, clinical social workers and psychologists, there were fifteen students; a more recent class had sixty. The New York Milton H. Erickson Society for Psychotherapy and Hypnosis in Manhattan, which offers a one-year program chartered by the New York State Board of Regents, has also had greatly increased enrollment.

But despite the great interest and the many studies conducted over the years, no one seems to know exactly how or why hypnosis works. "In terms of a real clear definition of hypnosis, we don't have it," said Dorothy Larkin, a registered nurse in Westchester County and president of the Erickson society. "It's a subjective experience. It's not really measurable."

Roughly 20 percent of the population are believed to be unhypnotizable, while another 20 percent fall readily into a hypnotic trance, although practitioners are not sure why some are more susceptible than others. Children nine to thirteen are considered the best subjects. "Children are of the world of pretend," Ms. Pelier said, "so you just join them in that world."

For Dr. Jeffrey M. Lipton, Mount Sinai's chief of pediatric hematology and oncology, hypnotic techniques are above all a way to make patients feel less helpless. "I don't think this is a substitute for analgesia and the new generation of antinausea and antivomiting medications," he said. "But it certainly allows us to rely less on those and to give children some control over what is going on."

Because of relaxation therapy and "hypno-analgesic" techniques like the pain switch, doctors can cut back on the amount of pain medication they require, whether general anesthesia or sedation, both of which pose a risk. "A spinal tap takes only five minutes," Dr. Lipton said, but he added that because of the pain medication, "the kid would spend the rest of the day—hours—asleep or not feeling quite right."

Harris A. Barer, a Manhattan lawyer, says he has long been a believer in the power of hypnosis. Twenty-five years ago, as he awaited surgery for a benign brain tumor, he was in so much pain that he fainted one night at the opera. Because the painkillers weren't working, Mr. Barer decided to try hypnosis. He saw Dr. Robert M. Naiman, a psychiatrist who champions the techniques. "I had two sessions with him and then I would go on the subway in the morning and reinforce it through self-hypnosis," he said. "In a period of three or four days, I was totally pain-free."

Dentists who use hypnosis by itself or in combination with anesthetics say it can calm even the most skittish patients. "It's really very gratifying to have a patient sit down in a chair and say, 'This is the only place in the world where I can relax,'" said Dr. Selig Finkelstein, a dentist in Pleasantville, New York, who has trained fifty other dentists in hypnosis.

In North Tarrytown, New York, several members of the Volunteer Fire Department Ambulance Corps studied hypnosis techniques during a workshop to improve their communication skills with accident victims. Michael Anzovino, the captain, used the techniques during two asthma-attack calls. In one case, involving a seventeen-year-old woman, he sped up his breathing to match hers and then slowly brought his breathing rate back down to normal, all the while asking the woman to follow along.

"I was skeptical at first," Mr. Anzovino said, "but it worked. The woman's breathing returned to normal before we reached the hospital."

Despite the growing use of hypnosis as a palliative, most people think of it as a last-ditch treatment for addictions, compulsions and phobias, from cigarette smoking to fear of flying. Rewiring the mind sounds appealing, but in reality hypnosis doesn't work that easily. People who respond the best, experts say, are those highly motivated to break their addictions and willing to practice self-hypnosis at home.

After receiving hypnosis for fear of flying, Virginia Pier, a forty-one-year-old fitness trainer, found that flights were less scary, but still unpleasant. "I noticed a big difference the first time I flew after trying hypnosis," she said. "I had a knot in my stomach, but it wasn't to the point where I felt I was going to die right then. Before, I would be clutching the seat the entire flight and turning colors and sweating."

It also meant continued effort. During a flight, she takes a deep breath and counts backward from ten, remembering images that relax her under hypnosis. "If I get sloppy and don't practice," she said, "I go right back into panic mode."

Hypnosis is not a regulated or licensed practice in New York State, and some therapists worry that its popularity has drawn charlatans into the field. But a professional in one of the disciplines the state does license, such as psychiatry or clinical social work, would still be subject to state scrutiny if a patient who had undergone hypnosis filed a complaint of negligence or fraud. Generally, patients should be wary of people billing themselves first and foremost as hypnotists, experts say.

"They should be trained as physicians, dentists or psychologists," said Dr. Spiegel, the Columbia professor, "and hypnosis should always be secondary to that. Anybody can call themselves a hypnotist. I know an electrician who took a weekend course in hypnosis and charges a lot to see patients. Any idiot can be taught how to induce a trance state, but what you then do to solve a patient's problems requires psychotherapeutic training."

Lisa W. Foderaro, February 1996

HYPNOSIS: CLOSE EYES. RELAX. TEN, NINE . . .

Before you can be hypnotized, you must first see whether you are hypnotizable. I was hopeful.

The hypnotherapist I chose, Dr. Marianne S. Andersen, is a psychologist and a leading figure in the field of hypnosis who practices out of a home office on West Fifty-seventh Street. I told her I wanted to focus on my eating habits. I described a roller-coaster history of weight control, a habit of eating about a third more than I should.

To test my ability to be hypnotized, I was asked to raise my eyes to the ceiling and close my eyelids. Dr. Andersen first counted down from ten, saying I would be going deeper and deeper into a state of relaxation. She then asked me to focus on the index finger of my left hand. I would feel a sensation on the fingertip, she said, and she asked me to nod when it appeared. I did feel a tingling, but wondered whether it was just my imagination. Then she counted to five and said I would be completely awake and alert. My ability to be hypnotized was above average, she said, a three on a scale of zero to four.

Okay. We were ready to begin. Again, roll the eyes toward the ceiling, close the lids. Relax. Ten, nine, eight . . . two, one, zero. Let yourself get more and more relaxed, she said. My body started to melt into the couch. I had never felt this relaxed. My mind was completely alert, though.

She had me envision a twelve-inch plate brimming with food and an eight-inch plate, also brimming. As I went deeper and deeper, I was to bring the image of the eight-inch plate with me, along with the words: one-third less. She said that in the coming week, I would leave behind about a third of the food on my plate. She said I would not feel deprived, but that it eventually might become an effort as the posthypnotic suggestion wore off.

I was ready to come out, she said. And on the count of five, I reluctantly opened my eyes.

Was that it? I hadn't entered the Twilight Zone. I remembered everything she'd said. "Trance" almost seemed a misnomer for what I had just experienced. Many people, it turned out, have the same reaction.

As for the results, I was able to leave food on my plate for a few days without a struggle. I admit that sometimes it was more like one-eighth than one-third. But three weeks later I must confess that I have no desire to leave something behind on my plate.

Lisa W. Foderaro, February 1996

EAST MEETS WEST: THE EXPERIMENTS OF DR. OZ

Joyce Donadio had arrived at the confluence of paradigms. She was a forty-nine-year-old, diabetic computer operator from Nutley, New Jersey, with a lifelong smoking habit and a blood-starved left ventricle. The extremity of her condition had been driven home a week earlier by a crashing heart attack. She was wheeled into Operating Room 21 at Columbia-Presbyterian Medical Center at 7:30 A.M. For the next eight hours her life was in the hands of blue-and-green-gowned nurses, physician-assistants, anesthesiologists and surgeons of various rank and experience who cut veins out of her legs, sawed her sternum in half, spread her ribs and then made way for Dr. Mehmet Oz, perhaps the most accomplished thirty-five-year-old cardiothoracic surgeon in the country. He strode into the arena in his rubber clogs, hands upraised, ready for a sterile towel, latex gloves and the delicate work of securing a future for Donadio's faltering heart.

At the invitation of Oz and his patient, there were two other people on hand in surgical gowns and masks: a second-year medical student named Sally Smith, stationed at Donadio's feet, and a fifty-two-year-old healer named Julie Motz, who was standing at Donadio's head. As volunteers in Oz's Cardiac Complementary Care Center, they worked for free through the operation, seldom moving except to reposition their hands. As Oz requested sutures and clamps and units of lidocaine, Motz called softly to Smith to move her hands from the small toe of Donadio's right foot to a point on the sole known as "the bubbling spring."

What they were doing no one else in the operating room knew how to do, or had ever seen done during a coronary bypass, or had ever thought worth doing, even as an experiment. In this ultimate theater of scientific medicine, the women were using their hands as kings once did to treat subjects with scrofula and as Jesus is said to have done and as shamans and mothers and Chinese qigong practitioners still do. They were using their hands to run a kind of energy, which science cannot prove exists, into Donadio's "kidney meridian," which also may or may not exist.

East does not easily meet West, especially when East is an unproven form of vitalist healing called energy medicine and West is a high-tech medical center where science is the one true God. Columbia-Presbyterian jealously guards its reputation as one of the top teaching and medical-research facilities in the country. Its doctors may not know exactly why or how an intervention works—the general principles of anesthesia, for example, remain shrouded in the mystery of consciousness itself—but most of the drugs and procedures employed have at least some footing in science, and have been proved safe and effective by quantifiable standards.

That's the kind of test most therapies in the realm of alternative medicine can't pass. While many therapies seem harmless enough, they are often premised on metaphysical philosophies beyond the scope of science, and their claims of efficacy are supported by testimonials, not controlled studies. All the same, Americans spend an estimated $13.7 billion annually on "unconventional" therapies, from hands-on healing to homeopathy, aromatherapy and biofeedback. This enormous interest seems to be based on the perception that mainstream medicine has become more enamored of fancy machines than of the art of healing and on the inability of scientific medicine to cope with the scourges of the times: heart disease, cancer, AIDS.

Popular fascination has finally begun to spur interest among practitioners of allopathic medicine; therapies long ignored in this country, or dismissed without investigation, are receiving new attention. The Office of Alternative Medicine at the National Institutes of Health is sponsoring research in many areas, and courses in alternative medicine are springing up in top-tier medical schools.

At Columbia-Presbyterian the presence of hands-on healers in an operating room is only the most dramatic example of a new willingness to venture into the terra incognita of healing. In November 1993 the College of Physicians and Surgeons at Columbia University accepted a $750,000 private grant from Richard Rosenthal, a retired utility executive and philanthropist, who, moved by the plight of ailing friends for whom doctors said nothing further could be done, wanted to finance a center to study alternative medicine.

"I discussed it with some colleagues, and my feeling was you can't not pay attention to this area," said Dr. Herbert Pardes, the dean of the faculty of medicine at the College of Physicians and Surgeons. "A university teaching hospital is exactly the place you can look at things that may be offbeat. We should bring a rational approach to these therapies. The public will be served."

At the moment, with a staff of four and a bare-bones budget, the biggest thing about the new Richard and Hinda Rosenthal Center for Alternative/Complementary Medicine is its unwieldy name. But the director, Fredi Kronenberg, who has a doctorate in physiology, has recruited a distinguished scientific advisory board and involved the center in a number of studies, including the effects of t'ai chi on the autonomic physiology of chronic pain.

The center met with a barrage of flak when it co-sponsored a course in alternative medicine at the medical college last winter. Dr. Victor Herbert, a Columbia medical-school graduate, professor of medicine at Mount Sinai and a board member of the National Council Against Health Fraud, threatened to join in picketing the center if some of the lecturers he considered "con artists" and "sociopathic liars" were not removed from the program. "I am nasty," said Dr. Herbert. "I call practitioners of fraud practitioners of fraud. It's my feeling that the Rosenthal center has been promoting fraudulent alternatives as genuine."

Controversy or none, the Rosenthal center brought a lot of doctors with an interest in unorthodox therapies out of the closet, Mehmet Oz among them. In his training and skill Oz personified the prowess of Western medical science; in his experience he understood its limitations. He could sew bypass grafts and implant new hearts, but he was hard-pressed to change the habits that put his patients on the operating table or to grapple with the emotional and psychological factors that might hasten their healing. Depression, for instance, has emerged as one of the major risk factors in the recovery of heart patients after surgery.

Oz wasn't interested in leading a revolution. Many notable doctors from Bernie Siegel to Deepak Chopra had been advocating alternative therapies for years. Dean Ornish's pioneering program to reverse heart disease through exercise, a vegetarian diet and daily meditation is now so respectable that some insurance companies have embraced it as a viable alternative to bypass surgery. If there were new approaches that might improve the quality of life of cardiac patients, Oz was willing to raise some eyebrows to evaluate them and do what he could to nudge a major medical center in new directions. More than willing—he felt ethically obliged.

Mehmet Oz is one of those rare beings who seem incapable of sloth. "He's doing a heart transplant right now," his secretary says on the phone, "and he's got a double-lung transplant waiting, and those are in addition to his two regularly scheduled open hearts, and then at three he's supposed to fly to Boston to deliver a lecture." So exceptional is Oz's energy that some of his colleagues use him as a benchmark, correlating their own vitality as a fraction of a "full Mehmet unit."

"He runs down lobs," sighs his tennis partner, mentor and department chairman, Dr. Eric A. Rose, who at forty-four is one of the top heart-transplant surgeons in the world.

To see what can be done on a full Mehmet unit, I waited in Oz's heavily trafficked office for the printer to disgorge his curriculum vitae. It seemed to take the better part of the morning: Harvard graduate, magna cum laude; medical school at the University of Pennsylvania, where he was class chairman and school president and also managed to squeeze in an M.B.A. from Wharton. During his residency at Columbia-Presbyterian he won the prestigious Blakemore research award four times. He holds a patent for a solution that preserves transplant organs and has two more patents pending, including one for an aortic valve that can be implanted without open-heart surgery. He's contributed chapters to 8 books, written 56 abstracts and 135 papers and performs about 250 operations a year. He has three children and lives with his wife, Lisa Lemole, an actress, in New Jersey.

What a resume can't convey is his enthusiasm and—no other word seems so apt—his openheartedness. "I used to bicycle to work across the George Washington Bridge, but my wife told me it wasn't professional," he said one day in his office. He shrugged cheerfully and laughed and reached into a drawer for a bag of Turkish apricots and almonds sent by a grateful bypass patient. Streams of colleagues and students wandered in to discuss cases, cadge almonds and rib him about a recent appearance on the evening news in which his work with mechanical hearts was accompanied by footage of the Tin Man from *The Wizard of Oz.*

Culturally speaking, Oz is something of a confluence of paradigms himself. He was born in Cleveland of Turkish parents, the oldest of three children, and he grew up in Wilmington, Delaware, where his father still has a thoracic-surgery practice. Oz grew up speaking Turkish as well as English. To retain dual passports and rights to family assets in Turkey, he had to take time during medical school to serve in the Turkish army.

It was his wife's family who piqued his interest in alternative medicine. His father-in-law, Gerald Lemole, was a member of the first heart-transplant team in Texas, but he had also been dubbed "Rock Doc" by *Rolling Stone* magazine for playing music in the operating room to relax patients. Emily Jane Lemole developed a special low-fat diet for her husband's cardiac patients; at one point she refused surgery for an inflamed gallbladder, preferring to handle it by modifying her diet. Her kids received penicillin for strep throats, but their bellyaches she treated with herbal tea, their earaches with garlic and olive oil, and for sore muscles, she rubbed their skin with arnica gel, a remedy Oz has found relieves his soreness after marathons.

"Most allopathic doctors think practitioners of alternative medicine are all quacks," Oz says. "They're not. Often they're sharp people who think differently about disease." Some colleagues of his father-in-law said they weren't going to refer patients if Dr. Lemole was going to put them on low-fat diets. Now low-fat diets are gospel.

The viewpoint in the Lemole household also reinforced lessons Oz had learned in Turkey, where families play a much larger role in the recuperation of sick relatives. "Ten years ago in this country, if you wanted a family member to stay in the hospital with a patient there was no way," Oz says. "In Turkey, you're not allowed to be left alone in the hospital. The nurse teaches the family how to do things, and somebody is always there with the patient."

When it seemed that the Rosenthal center didn't have the financial or political resources to undertake clinical trials, Oz set up the Cardiac Complementary Care Center. He mailed letters to one hundred cardiologists, outlining a study of therapies in four areas: diet, meditation and hypnosis, manual therapies like massage and energy medicine of the sort practiced by hands-on healers.

"I didn't feel there was a huge downside," he recalled. "I felt secure with my colleagues. If I kept doing what I am paid to do, the most they could do is caution me in a brotherly way. I would say to them, 'I know you think this is a little crazy, but I feel we are neglecting our patients in a crucial way.'"

For the first study, Oz wanted a project that would be a solid bet. Julie Motz, who was studying for a master's degree in public health and had been volunteering at the Rosenthal center, suggested a list of possible experiments, from hypnosis to aromatherapy. Gerard C. Whitworth, one of the perfusionists who operates the machinery in the heart unit, was interested in hypnosis. (Whitworth wanted to explore new approaches to cardiac care in memory of his father, who had died of inoperable heart disease.) Most doctors were familiar with hypnosis from medical school; it didn't entail any science-straining leaps of faith. The review board approved the study, and Oz and company set to work.

They obtained the consent of twenty-two patients scheduled for surgery at the hospital. Nine were designated a control group; the remaining thirteen were taught self-hypnosis. The instructors focused on helping the patients to relax their jaw and throat muscles in hopes of lessening the stress of having a breathing tube inserted down the throat. They suggested that the patients try to extend their hypnotic state to the surgery itself, in essence to program themselves to minimize their bleeding, maintain normal blood pressure and, in some unknown, subliminal way, reduce their experience of pain and discomfort. After their operations, the patients were to concentrate on healing quickly. The goal was to see how hypnosis changed the patients' quality of life— an outcome Oz and his colleagues assessed by having patients check off their levels of stress and depression on a standard psychological-mood inventory.

The results suggest that patients who were taught self-hypnosis were significantly less tense after the operation than patients who didn't have the training. Their scores for depression and fatigue were also lower. As Oz and others point out, many benefits arise from being able to reduce pain without medication: patients are spared side effects like constipation and stomach bleeding; they feel empowered, having participated in their own recovery; they can leave the hospital sooner.

Encouraged by the modest success of the hypnosis experiment, Oz wants to pursue further studies. For example, could Q-10, a substance found in the energy-producing units of all cells, help the heart function more efficiently? Ideally he would like to poll patients as they enter the hospital: What are their feelings about alternative therapies? Would they be interested in participating in random studies?

Like all medical schools, Columbia's is grappling with the high cost of specialized medical treatment. In part, this means putting more emphasis on preventive and primary care medicine. The trick is how to explore the field without damaging the reputation of the institution; many marketers of alternative therapies are quick to seize on any imprimatur of legitimacy. Yet mainstream medicine can be criticized for overselling its own scientific legitimacy. "It's reasonable to say that much of existing medicine has not met the standards that alternative medicine is being asked to meet," says Clyde Behney, an assistant director of the Congressional Office of Technology Assessment. "But it still gets a lot more scrutiny. The data and record keeping are better, and the peer-review process is better."

Probably the most experimental work Oz and the cardiac-study group have done is in the field of energy medicine. Motz has assisted in a number of transplant cases. As popular as she is with patients and as careful as she is not to make any sweeping claims for her work (similar to the therapeutic touch practiced in many hospitals by about fifty thousand nurses), mainstream medicine remains leery of her beliefs. And she is still feeling her way into the institution, where anything from a floppy hat to a lack of deference can close people's minds.

She now has her surgical sea legs under her, but the first time Motz observed open-heart surgery, she had a shaky debut. She had been standing at the patient's head, outside the sterile field, periodically telling Oz what changes she was able to sense in the patient's energy. The patient was obviously not awake but probably had some awareness, most likely smell and perhaps hearing. (Open-heart patients are often fitted with headphones and provided with tapes to "listen" to, including, if they want, Oz's own specially recorded Sufi trance music.) For the bypass team, it was quite a novelty to hear Motz report that she was registering the patient's moods in her body—various states of fear, anger or satisfaction perceived as roughness in her chest or turbulence in her stomach. At one point, seeing that Motz was not looking so good herself, Oz asked a burly assistant to take her outside for some air. When the assistant returned he said: "I sense a change in my stomach. It's a tenseness. . . . No, it's a growling. No, wait a minute. . . . I'm just hungry."

Probably the most painful part of Joyce Donadio's heart surgery was at the beginning, when a catheter was being inserted into the jugular vein in her neck. "Now, Mrs. Donadio," said the anesthesiology resident in a saccharine voice. Donadio gripped Motz's hand and rolled away from the pain of the needle. Motz spoke soothingly to her. You did not have to know anything about energy medicine or subscribe to the belief that a field of unmeasurable energy flows in and about the body to see what it meant to one person to be able to hold the hand of another at T minus zero.

A week later, Donadio was sitting in her hospital room with her husband, Joe, a parking-enforcement officer. She'd climbed a set of stairs and washed her hair. Her appetite had returned. The zipper wounds on her chest and left leg were mending nicely. Oz and Motz and Smith stopped by to see her. Oz said she'd be going home soon. He lingered for a bit, then ducked out to check on other patients. "She's euphoric now," he said. "I want her to get greedy. Her purpose is not just to survive; it's to go out and do great things."

The two women stayed a while longer. Donadio said to Motz, "I was so afraid, and you made me feel relaxed. At last somebody wasn't telling me what was going to hurt but what was positive. I told my girlfriend about it on the phone, and she said, 'What is she?' And I said, 'I don't know.'"

Donadio looked at the two women and then at her husband. "If I have to go for an operation ever again, I'm calling them, I swear to God."

Chip Brown, July 1995

AYURVEDIC MEDICINE:
ANCIENT CURES FOR OPEN MINDS

One of the surest ways to bring a luncheon conversation to a halt at the National Institute of Mental Health in Bethesda, Maryland, is to suggest that phlegm, bile and wind are neurotransmitters. So why then did the institute send biomedical scientists to India in 1997 to confer with Ayurvedic physicians, who still believe that ill-sorted humors of the body cause unbalanced minds?

Despite some recent concerns over government funding of research on alternative therapies and scoffing by skeptics, an estimated one-third of Americans are using these treatments, despite their doctors' disapproval. Humoral medicine is a case in point. Although it was discredited in the seventeenth century in the West, it has made a comeback in spas, health food stores and healing centers across the country, in botanical extracts, aroma therapies, purges and holistic diets.

There is even a curiosity among some NIMH scientists, who are concerned about the high cost of drug development and who acknowledge the prevalence of psychosomatic illness. They are reevaluating alternative medicine as a body of knowledge rather than dismissing it as quackery.

Humoral medicine had a long run in the West, starting in ancient Greece. In 159 A.D. sick gladiators sought out Galen, who drew on medical theories from the time of Hippocrates. Here is a decoction of the doctrine: There are four basic humors of the body (phlegm, black bile, yellow bile, blood), four basic qualities of sensory experience (hot, cold, wet, dry) and four basic ingredients of things going in and out of the body (fire, air, water, earth). Health means harmony, and fine-tuning is possible. If the body is dry, make it wet. If it is hot, cool it off. You are what you eat, and also what you excrete.

The essence of humoral thinking, according to the historian R.M. Yost Jr., is the idea that the human body contains juices and fluids whose ratios regulate health. When there is an excess of some humoral sap, the body heats up, reduces substance, separates the boiled from the unboiled parts and evacuates the stewed remains. The aim of the humoral physician is to assist this natural culinary process with warmers and coolers and to facilitate the evacuation process with purges, emetics and bleedings.

Although Hippocrates is often described as the father of medicine, Agnivesa, Susruta and several other ancient South Asian physicians could easily win a paternity suit. Their brainchild, Ayurvedic medicine (the science of life), is an even older version of humoral thinking. The oldest surviving Ayurvedic text, the *Caraka-Samhita*, probably dates from the sixth or seventh century B.C. Buddha's doctor was an Ayurvedic physician. So was the doctor of Morarji Desai, the Indian prime minister in 1979.

Official support for humoral medicine in South Asia has waxed and waned over the centuries, just as it has in the West. News of its demise at the hands of English scientists spurred its regenesis in India. Indian nationalists in the early twentieth century proudly rejuvenated the science of life as proof of their intellectual automony. Since Indian independence in 1947, the medical wisdom of the ancients has been turned into a growth industry with government subsidies.

There are Ayurvedic medical schools, journals, pharmacies and drug companies. Lotions, potions, massages and purges are used by hundreds of millions of Hindus, for everything from wrinkles, backaches, asthma and hair loss to impotency, senility, diabetes and schizophrenia. The old remedies, preferably prescribed in Sanskrit, are thought to be closer to the truth, and are popular in contemporary Indian society, even among the Westernized elite.

In recent decades the elites in the West have been catching on, once again. One measure of this is a recent scientific mission organized by Dr. Stephen H. Koslow, director of neuroscience and behavioral science at the National Institute of Mental Health. Dr. Koslow led an expedition of Western psychiatrists and pharmacologists to India to examine Ayurvedic medicine as a potential source of knowledge.

The NIMH delegation took a trip to Kerala to visit the Arya Vaidya Sala (the Pure Ayurvedic Doctor's Clinic), which uses Ayurvedic methods. There, hysteria and chronic headaches are treated by streaming medicated milk onto the patient's forehead. Asthma, inflammations of the vertebrae and other afflictions associated with dryness, desiccation and an excess of wind are counteracted with a gentle wet massage.

In the gardens of the clinic the medicinal roots and shoots of the jungle are cultivated by a botanist, who expounds the doctrine of signatures, which he attributes to Galen. "God created plants," he says, "as a provision for the health of human beings, and left a sign on them—some feature of their shape, color, habitat or behavior—for human beings to decipher." He points to a plant shaped like an ear that is a cure for earaches.

In the factory of the Kerala clinic an Indian nuclear physicist oversees a major industrial apparatus where they distill, standardize and mass-produce 2,500-year-old legendary decoctions. An M.B.A. from the Wharton School of Business takes care of the accounts. As the West lies down with the East, there are not enough beds in the clinic's nursing home to accommodate the international demand for its medical regimes.

Why is it now that humoral medicine, with its antique remedies from out of our past, has returned in the United States? It is the bet of some neuropharmacologists at NIMH that Ayurvedic practitioners know something about barks, roots, leaves and other botanical provisions for human beings that they can no longer afford to overlook. It is also a response to recent research on the power of mind-body effects. It is the bet of some psychiatrists at the institute that Ayurvedic healers know a lot about the salubrious reality of placebo cures.

And what do they say in India when the institute comes knocking on their doors? They say it is good to experiment with things to touch, smell and eat that are tailored to your own personality, that are less biologically shocking and invasive than a wonder drug. Any medical tradition that is 2,500 years old, they say, and has half a billion enthusiastic clients must be doing something right.

Richard A. Shweder, October 1997

[8]

Menopause, Breast Cancer and Wrinkles: A Lucrative Market

Women and Alternative Medicine

If menopause did not exist, dietary supplement manufacturers might well have invented it. It is hard to imagine a better target for their products — a natural process, but one accompanied by hot flashes, bone loss, wrinkles and other signs of aging, as well as other changes that most women do not find pleasant, to say the least. Supplement makers have projected that by the end of the year 2000, 10.2 million American women will be in menopause, with about 8 million having symptoms.

Although estrogen replacement therapy can help to ease the transition, many women turn to supplements instead, because they fear the hormone, which has been linked to an increased risk of breast cancer in some women. And aside from the fear of breast cancer, many women dislike the idea of taking prescription drugs for what is, after all, a natural part of life. Somehow, the idea of "natural" products has more appeal. To some women, small doses of phytoestrogens — plant estrogens found in flaxseed, some herbs and soy products, and weaker than human estrogen — sound gentler and less risky than what the doctor prescribes. Manufacturers know it, and market every imaginable manner of product to menopausal and "perimenopausal" women, from pills and powders to teas and tonics and face creams.

But are the supplements safe? And do they work?

The products get mixed reviews. Wild yam products, touted as a source of the hormone progesterone, actually do not provide it in a form that the human body can use. Some scientists call the marketing of the products the *"yam scam."* Red clover, said to be a source of estrogens, has raised concerns among doctors, who say it has not been studied enough to know whether it is safe and effective. There is simply not enough evidence to justify giving up the known benefits of estrogen replacement therapy. Soy products, initially embraced as a cure-all, have triggered warnings, particularly with regard to supplements that contain high levels of soy isoflavones, a type of phytoestrogen. The concern is that some studies have suggested that the isoflavones may promote breast tumors. And so doctors offer the tried and true, though unexciting advice: moderation.

A study in 1999 gave troubling insights into the factors that lead some women with breast cancer to seek alternative therapy along with conventional treatment. The researchers found that the women using supplements tended to be unusually worried and depressed, and perhaps in need of counseling. The results came as a surprise, because a previous study had showed women using alternative therapy to be stronger and better adjusted than those who did not. Some doctors took the study as evidence that conventional medicine fails to address the emotional needs of women with breast cancer, who may then turn to the health food store to find relief for their fear, frustration and uncertainty about the future.

MENOPAUSE: THE WILD NEW FRONTIER FOR ALTERNATIVE ENTREPRENEURS

Every day Marcie Rothman, who is fifty-one, takes three Body Wise Female Advantage nutritional capsules—an arsenal of twenty-two ingredients marketed as the natural answer to menopause.

The capsules contain soy protein, thought to be a selective estrogen-response modifier able to help stabilize a woman's suddenly dwindling supply of estrogen; along with black cohosh root, it is now a popular way to fight hot flashes. Another ingredient, Mexican yam, is a trendy natural source of the hormone progesterone; and passionflower, valerian root and kava are supposed to ameliorate mood swings. Also among the ingredients are evening primrose oil and flaxseed for essential fatty acids, as well as gotu kola and alphaketoglutaric acid, both of which are supposed to keep the brain sharp. Add vitamin pills, a calcium supplement to fight osteoporosis, exercise, a no-smoking policy and a low-fat diet, and Ms. Rothman figures that she has done everything she needs to do.

In fact, Ms. Rothman is helping to support a $4 billion alternative-remedy industry by dosing herself with nontraditional treatments. Twenty years ago she would have been at the fringe of consumer society. Today, she is a foot soldier in a revolution that includes members of the medical establishment, like Dr. Susan M. Love, who co-wrote *Dr. Susan Love's Hormone Dilemma*, and Dr. David Heber, the director of the Center for Human Nutrition at the University of California, Los Angeles.

Women, who buy the majority of medicines and medicinal treatments, have a dizzying array of products at their disposal, from vitamin supplements like the Body Wise line, with its scientific-sounding claims, to pulverized Chinese herbs. What these products do not have yet is quantifiable proof of either quality or effectiveness. No regulatory agency enforces quality control of these supplements, and there are not nearly enough scientific data to confirm that their ingredients do what they profess.

"There is a resurgence of a romantic idea about nature," said Dr. Richard A. Friedman, the director of psychopharmacology at New York Hospital–Cornell Medical Center. "Like all ideology, it's dangerous. The bottom line should be, If it works and it's safe and effective, what does it matter where it came from? Molecules are molecules."

Before 1994, the government categorized dietary supplements as food additives. Companies had to prove their products' safety to the Food and Drug Administration, which could yank an item off the shelf. But the 1994 Dietary Supplement Health and Education Act put the burden of proof on the FDA, which lacks the resources to police a growing industry. Even proponents of these treatments worry that women will end up with poor-quality products.

"My practical advice for right now is, go with one of the big herbal companies," said Dr. Heber. "Big companies have big insurance liabilities."

Dr. Friedman added, "It's buyer beware. You might get a treatment, a potentially toxic substance or a placebo. It's Russian roulette."

Ms. Rothman, a former magazine researcher who now writes about food and nutrition, spent two years using her professional skills to select what she considered a high-quality line of supplements manufactured in a plant that adheres to FDA pharmaceutical standards.

Not every product is as reassuring. A walk down an aisle in a large Los Angeles natural-foods store is truly a magical mystery tour stocked with tall canisters of soy-protein powder from four competing manufacturers; a line of herbal solutions promising that the herbs are suspended in organic alcohol; and seven kinds of ginseng. The menopause preparations take up two shelves: supplements comprising different ingredients and several pots of wild-yam cream, none that list the amount of wild yam in the preparation. There are remedies in the food aisles, primarily tofu meals that include barbecue-flavored snacks. And at the checkout counter, sixty-pill packs of Remifemin offer "nutritional support for women experiencing menopause." These same women can then repair to a nearby coffee boutique for a soyccino.

The standard alternative approach to dealing with the long-term effects of menopause—bone weakness, cardiovascular problems and skin dryness—depends on natural sources of depleted hormones, along with specific remedies for short-term discomforts like hot flashes. It usually involves a progesterone cream, of which Progest is the oldest and most popular brand, and a phyto- or plant-derived estrogen. Soy-protein powder is the phyto-estrogen of the moment. Women usually mix it into fruit juice or milk twice a day, though many who take it look forward to the day when an equivalent batch of isoflavones is packed into a flavorless capsule.

Then there are mavericks like Dr. Uzzi Reiss, a Beverly Hills gynecologist and antiaging specialist who says he has a "booked practice, early morning to late at night" concocting custom hormone cocktails for his patients. If the herbalists and nutritionists believe that Premarin is unnecessary, Dr. Reiss and his colleagues believe it is outmoded.

Menopause is the wild frontier for alternative entrepreneurs, with 1.3 million women very likely to be entering menopause this year. But even established companies, like Transitions for Women, which sells Progest cream and is based in Oregon, depend more on patient testimonials than on research.

Ms. Rothman's personal proof of efficacy is straightforward: she began taking supplements five years ago, when her stress level spiraled because of her parents' illnesses and a fractured romance. "I haven't had as much as a sore throat since," she said. Nor any menopausal symptoms.

The medical community prefers a broader sampling and has finally acknowledged public interest by beginning to research popular products.

Dr. Love includes soy-rich foods and herbs in her daily regimen. While "we need more randomized, controlled double-blind studies," she said, referring to the "gold standard" in which half the subjects receive an alternate remedy and half a placebo, she points out that women are frequently prescribed drugs for which such studies were not conducted.

"The requirement for gold-standard studies has to be seen in perspective," she said. Meanwhile, she keeps an eye on the emerging data. She had been taking 25 grams of soy powder every day, for example, until a recent double-blind study suggested 40 grams was optimal. "I bumped it up to forty," she said, "and the hot flashes disappeared."

Dr. Heber mixes four scoops, about 30 grams, of soy protein in a drink twice a day because studies on animals suggest there is a cancer-fighting, or antioxidant, effect.

But there is much trial and error in dosage and effectiveness; for all the popularity of topical progesterone preparations, for example, the FDA has yet to limit the progesterone content. What works is often a matter of experimentation and individual perception.

Dr. Friedman said the most hopeful sign was that the National Institutes of Health has an Office of Alternative Medicine currently doing studies. He said, "You have to ask: If I'm going to put this in my body, is it safe? What does it mean if a lot of menopausal women say they're feeling better on something? Did it work, or did they feel better because of the placebo effect?"

Women are generally disinclined to wait for official answers and prefer to apply their networking skills in an informal menopause information exchange. There are several reasons. This generation's distrust of authority has been heightened by managed care—having promised everything, medicine has delivered far less. "Skepticism is the inheritance doctors have gotten over the last century," Dr. Friedman said. "The more sophisticated medicine has become, the more the American public expects. That intersects with managed care, which has been a disaster in terms of the public trust." Expectations were very high, Dr. Friedman added, "but the results were less than people hoped for," so they have become "disillusioned with medicine."

This generation also has a global perspective. Thanks to an enhanced ability to travel abroad or search the Internet, women can learn about other cultures and treatments. "Baby boomers are a major revolution, seventy-seven million of us thinking we can change the world and live to one hundred and twenty," Dr. Heber said. "An internationalization of economies means we're getting an influx of information from cultures that like natural remedies. In China, they don't take Premarin."

The irony is that the baby boomers' curiosity, combined with their mistrust of the pharmaceutical-medical establishment and the torrent of data, has made the current menopause generation more responsive to promotions for products that are, for the most part, untested and unregulated.

That is not to say pharmaceutical companies ignore profit projections. But drugs, unlike "cosmeceuticals," undergo rigorous clinical trials to win FDA approval.

The danger is that women are doing their own informal clinical trials, and that most doctors cannot keep up with them. "We were all taught in medical school twenty-five years ago that drugs were good, vitamins were bad and supplements were dangerous," Dr. Heber said. "It's the younger doctors who are usually open to this and will do the research on their own."

Most doctors receive information about new treatments from drug-company representatives toting brochures and samples. These companies are not interested in alternative remedies so far. Since natural remedies cannot be patented, a successful product only guarantees increased competition.

Sharon MacFarland's father, Bruce, began selling Progest cream twenty years ago. Eight years later, Ms. MacFarland began the company's new division, called Transitions for Women. Today, she said, the company sells about a million tubes of Progest annually at $30 each through its catalogue and health food stores. That means more than 83,000 customers are using about a tube a month, enough to attract other companies with competing preparations.

Practitioners who recommend alternative remedies therefore urge women to find what Dr. Love calls a "guide" who knows which companies make the best products and how they are supposed to work. "You can't just take two of these and three of those," Dr. Love said. "You have to go to a herbalist, a naturopath, a traditional Chinese doctor and have them match the herbs to your needs. You hear what a friend takes, and you try that? Not a good idea. So go to someone who knows what they're doing. That's your only safeguard."

Karen Stabiner, June 1998

WORDS OF CAUTION ABOUT A HOT POTATO

At health food stores, tiny tubs of wild yam cream sell well, despite their price ($20 or more). The lure is wild yam's reputation as a source of natural progesterone, a hormone that proponents of alternative medicine consider a palliative for menopausal discomforts. Natural progesterone creams have also become a hot commodity. In recent years, sales of wild yam salves, pure progesterone creams and hybrids containing both have accounted for a large chunk of the mushrooming $600 million market in natural remedies for menopause.

Many women believe these products replenish their dwindling progesterone. Satisfied users say they have fewer hot flashes and more supple skin, and think they are also protecting themselves from osteoporosis and uterine cancer. Natural progesterone is widely perceived as safer than progestin, its synthetic cousin and a common ingredient in hormone replacement therapy. This conviction was bolstered by the debut in

December 1998 of the first prescription natural progesterone for menopausal women.

But do these products live up to the glowing testimony? And is the new oral prescription drug superior? Yam balms cannot supply the body with natural progesterone, said Gail Mahady, an authority on plant medicine at the University of Illinois in Chicago. "Only a pharmaceutical laboratory can convert the compounds in yams into progesterone," Professor Mahady explained.

Natural progesterone creams are not always what they seem to be, either. Aeron Life Cycles, a diagnostic testing company in San Leandro, California, screened twenty-seven products and found that fifteen of them contained no or little progesterone. The rest contained dosages that might be useful, but only if they were adequately absorbed—a big "if."

In fact, a report published in 1998 in the *Lancet*, the British medical journal, concluded that Progest, a relatively high-dose cream that is a top seller in the United States, does not raise blood progesterone levels sufficiently to protect the uterus from the cancer-inducing effects of taking estrogen alone; currently, that is the only use for which progesterone has been clinically approved. Many doctors find this result disturbing, because some women are substituting creams like Progest for the progestin normally prescribed in hormone replacement therapy. There is also little or no evidence to support the use of progesterone cream by itself to fortify bones or douse hot flashes, menopause experts said.

By contrast, the new prescription progesterone, a capsule sold under the brand name Prometrium, may offer genuine benefits to users of hormone replacement. While comparable to progestin in preventing estrogen's cancerous effects on the uterus, Prometrium is believed to offer better protection against heart disease. In clinical trials, it was better than progestin at preserving estrogen's positive effect on cholesterol levels.

Some women may also tolerate Prometrium better than Provera and other synthetic progesterones. But even though Prometrium is identical to the body's own hormone, it causes dizziness, headaches, sore breasts and other adverse reactions in 9 percent to 16 percent of women.

The drug is not cheap, either. A bottle of one hundred capsules (roughly a seven-week supply) sells for $54, though most insurers will cover some or all of the cost.

Kathleen McAuliffe, June 1999

HALTING HOT FLASHES, WITHOUT ESTROGEN

Hot flashes are a staple of menopause jokes, but there is nothing funny about them, and certainly nothing imaginary. They are experienced by at least 75 percent of American women at some point in menopause, including just before and just after. (They can also be brought on by the popular breast cancer drug tamoxifen and by the bone-building drug raloxifene.) They can vary from occasionally annoying to life disrupting, and they can last for as little as a few days or as long as ten years or more.

Hot flashes are especially disruptive for women awakened repeatedly with night sweats, leaving them unable to get restful sleep. A desire to suppress hot flashes is the main reason many women start hormone replacement therapy; estrogen in appropriate doses can eliminate them.

But there are millions of menopausal women who cannot or will not take estrogen. Many have had breast cancer or know they are at high risk for developing this disease, and because breast cancer cells can be stimulated by estrogen, these women and their doctors are reluctant to risk it. Other women experience unpleasant side effects from hormone replacement or are simply uncomfortable with the idea of dosing their bodies with hormones that nature has turned off. For such women, there are a number of simple, safe ways to reduce—and sometimes even eliminate—hot flashes without having to take hormones.

Hot flashes occur because the brain decides that the body is overheated. It sends out signals that dilate outer blood vessels and induce sweating, which results in heat loss. Skin temperature may rise as much as 8 degrees Fahrenheit. To a bed partner, a woman having a night sweat may feel like a radiator. Typically, a hot flash is felt most intensely in the upper body, especially in the face, neck and back. A woman may experience a feeling of intense heat for a minute or more or, in more severe cases, she may become very flushed and dripping wet. Her heart may beat faster, she may experience palpitations and, in rare cases, she may faint. Hot flashes may occur a few times a day or six or more times an hour.

Contrary to what some people think, susceptibility to hot flashes is unrelated to a woman's emotional, mental or physical well-being, although these factors may aggravate the problem. Nor are flashes the sole result of estrogen deficiency, since there are many women equally estrogen-deficient who get few or no hot flashes. Studies by Dr. Robert Freedman and colleagues at the Wayne State University School of Medicine in Detroit suggest that women with and without hot flashes are distinguished by differences in their body's thermostat, which is controlled by the central sympathetic nervous system in the brain.

In women with hot flashes, Dr. Freedman found, the central sympathetic nervous system is more active and, as a result, the brakes on the body's heat dissipation response fail to work properly. He noted that the drug clonidine, which suppresses central sympathetic nervous system activity, reduces hot flashes, whereas the herb yohimbine, which stimulates this system, provokes hot flashes.

Furthermore, Dr. Freedman's studies found that in menopausal women without hot flashes, as well as in younger women, there is a range of body temperatures—a neutral zone of about 0.4 degree Celsius, or 0.7 Fahrenheit—within which they neither sweat nor shiver. But in women with hot flashes, there is no such range. Thus, the slightest rise in body temperature—as little as 0.1 Celsius, which may occur, say, after drinking a hot cup of coffee or eating a big meal—can provoke a hot flash as the body tries to lower its internal temperature. And if the hot flash drops the body temperature too much, these women then shiver.

Women who suffer from hot flashes are advised to keep a diary for a few days, recording the time and circumstances surrounding each flash. Every woman is different, and what provokes a hot flash in one may not do so in another. Still, the following measures are effective in reducing the frequency and intensity of hot flashes in many women:

Diet

Limit or avoid caffeine (in coffee, tea, soft drinks and chocolate), alcohol, spicy foods, very sugary or salty foods, hot liquids and very large meals. Add soy-based foods to your diet; they contain weak plant estrogens, which may be helpful in reasonable amounts (one or two servings a day) and are not harmful to a woman who has had breast cancer. Ground flaxseed is also a good source of plant estrogens; it can be added to cereal, muffin mixes and bread dough.

Clothing

Avoid synthetic fabrics that do not breathe, like polyester and nylon, especially in blouses and dresses. Stick to natural fibers: cotton, rayon and silk. Make sure bedsheets are 100 percent cotton and blankets are a natural fabric as well. Avoid turtlenecks and long sleeves (except in an outer garment you can remove). Learn to dress in layers so you can easily take garments off and put them on again as your body temperature shifts.

Smoking

Don't. Nicotine constricts blood vessels, which can intensify and prolong a hot flash.

Exercise

Although intense exercise can cause a rise in body temperature that may provoke a hot flash, over all, women who are physically active tend to have fewer and less intense hot flashes, perhaps because their bodies become more tolerant of temperature extremes and more effective at cooling down.

Room Temperature

The warmer the room, the more hot flashes you are likely to have. Lower the thermostat at home to less than 70 degrees during the day and 65 degrees at night. Sleep with a window open even in winter, and in hot weather, use a fan or air conditioner.

Cooling Devices

Keep a thermos of ice-cold water nearby at all times, and take a cold drink as soon as you feel a flash coming on. Carry a battery-operated fan that will fit in your purse, or use a paper folding fan to cool yourself down.

Relax and Visualize

Stress is a common inducer of hot flashes. That's why women sometimes become drenched in sweat while making a business presentation or speech. Practice meditation techniques to calm yourself and keep you from overreacting to stressful situations. As you feel a hot flash coming on, imagine yourself in a cool or cold situation or picture the heat escaping through your hands and feet.

Slow, Deep Breathing

In studies supported by the National Institute on Aging, Dr. Freedman has shown that hot flashes can be cut in half by consciously reducing breaths to six or seven a minute, letting the abdomen rather than the chest expand with each inhalation. Practice the slow-breathing technique for fifteen to twenty minutes twice a day and use it when you feel a hot flash coming on.

Herbs and Vitamins

Anecdotal reports attest to the ability of vitamin E, at doses of about 800 international units a day, to reduce hot flashes. B vitamins and vitamin C may also be helpful. Claims about herbs are based mainly on small, poorly controlled studies and sometimes simply on folklore. One exception may be black cohosh, which German tests have found effective and which is now being tested in a well-designed study at New York Presbyterian Hospital. Although it has estrogenlike effects, it does not raise blood levels of estrogen, according to the lead researcher, Dr. Victor R. Grann, an oncologist.

Drugs

Two are effective: megestrol acetate (Megace) and clonidine (Catapres). Megace is a synthetic progesterone used to treat breast cancer;

possible side effects include weight gain and menstrual bleeding. Catapres, which lowers blood pressure, reduces the activity of the sympathetic nervous system and cuts hot flashes by about 50 percent. Possible side effects include drowsiness and dizziness if blood pressure falls too low. It is best taken orally at bedtime.

Jane E. Brody, November 1999

HORMONE REPLACEMENT THERAPY: WHY THEY DO IT, OR AVOID IT

For many menopausal women, the question of whether to take hormones is one of the most crucial health decisions of their middle years — and one of the most confusing.

Yes, the hormones relieve the hot flashes and the night sweats that plague many women during menopause, and they protect against brittle bones. But do they prevent heart disease as researchers have long believed, or do they make no difference to a woman's heart disease risk, as some studies now suggest? And what about breast cancer? With some studies indicating long-term use may slightly increase a woman's risk and others failing to find any increase, where does the truth lie, and how much should women worry? Then there are the questions of weight gain and mood swings. While many women believe that estrogen replacement makes them gain weight but soothes their moodiness, these effects are not found in scientific studies.

"You find yourself trying to decide which is the lesser of the evils," said Beryl DuMont, fifty-five, an office administrator from North Hanover, New Jersey, and one of a half dozen women who recently discussed their feelings about hormone replacement therapy.

"Do you take estrogen to prevent one problem and risk getting another one that you don't have and might otherwise never get?" Mrs. DuMont wondered. She stopped her first hormone treatment because of a bad reaction but is considering a second.

Estimates of the number of women who take or have taken hormones for the symptoms of menopause range from 10 percent to more than 40 percent, with factors as diverse as education and geography playing roles. One study published in 1999 in the *Annals of Internal Medicine* found that college-educated women and those living in the South and West were significantly more likely to use hormones than those living in the Northeast and Midwest. But according to the American College of Preventive Medicine, only about a third of women who use hormones take them as prescribed, something that may reflect women's fears about the side effects of such medication.

What is known is this: In the short term, hormone replacement therapy controls the hot flashes, night sweats and vaginal dryness experienced by many women during menopause. In the long term it also decreases a woman's risk of osteoporosis, the brittle-bone disease that can lead to life-threatening fractures. Estrogen also appears to increase a woman's level of good cholesterol and reduce the bad, but it promotes blood clotting, which can contribute to heart attacks.

Numerous studies have pointed to a link between a slightly higher risk of breast cancer and hormone use, and two reports published in 2000 suggest the risk is greatest in women taking both estrogen and progestin, as opposed to estrogen alone. That came as a surprise to many researchers who had believed estrogen was the primary culprit in the breast cancer–hormone link. It also was demoralizing because progestin is given in combination with estrogen specifically to lower the risk of endometrial cancer, a risk that increases more than tenfold when a woman takes estrogen alone.

Also in 2000, one of the most widely held assumptions about hormone replacement therapy—that it helps prevent cardiovascular disease—was called into question. Researchers reported that estrogen did nothing to slow the progression of heart disease in women whose arteries had already been partly blocked by it. Whether estrogen prevents heart disease remains unanswered.

More definitive results will come in 2005, when results from the first large-scale, long-term study of hormone use become available. But that comes as small comfort to women now trying to decide whether to take, or continue taking, hormones. Some try to circumvent the issue by experimenting with estrogens derived from plant sources, believing that these so-called natural estrogens are less likely to cause long-term side effects than synthetic estrogens. Yet there is little research to prove either effectiveness of the herbs or the lack of side effects, said Dr. Lila Nachtigall, a professor of obstetrics and gynecology at the New York University College of Medicine and one of the nation's leading experts on hormone replacement therapy.

"Women think that if it's over the counter or herbal or called a nutrient, that means it's safe," Dr. Nachtigall said. "They don't realize that it doesn't have FDA approval; they don't know that it can be sold without quality control, without science."

In the end, the decision a woman makes can involve any number of factors: her personal and family health history, her physical symptoms, her feelings about taking medication, her doctor's opinion and how much she trusts it, what friends have told her about their experiences during menopause.

What follows is what some women had to say.

Beryl DuMont, Fifty-five

North Hanover, New Jersey, Office Assistant, Scottish Widows Investment Management

I get migraines, which have always been linked to my period. It used to be three a year, but when I started menopause last year, I started getting them every week.

My gynecologist said estrogen might help and rattled off a whole ream of other benefits, too: it's supposed to help your bones, your general well-being.

I was concerned because seven years ago I had a breast lump removed; it was benign, but at that time, the surgeon said to me, "Under no circumstances go through any form of hormone replacement therapy."

When I asked my gynecologist about it, though, she said that just because I started taking hormones didn't mean I had to stay on them. That was a good point, and probably why I finally said, "Yes, I'll try it."

She prescribed the estrogen patch; I was supposed to use it for three or four weeks, then add progesterone. But when I read the brochure that came with the package, I got nervous. It talks about breast cancer and endometrial cancer, which scared me because I have endometriosis. But I thought, "My doctor knows my medical history, and she's still recommending that I try it, so I guess it must be okay."

The problem was, I didn't feel better while I was taking it. I was irritable, even more tired than I had been, and I kept waking up at night, although whether that was because of the estrogen itself or because I was afraid of it, I'm not sure.

Finally, after a month, I got a migraine that didn't go away for five days; my hands were also swollen and tingly. I called the doctor's office and they said I was having a reaction and that I should stop.

Now I'm in limbo. I just do not know what to think about this stuff. I'm supposed to go back to the doctor next month, and I haven't ruled out giving hormones another try.

But in the meantime, I'm going to talk to my pharmacist; he's big on alternative medicine, and I thought I would ask him for something herbal. I know it's unproven, but so many people are doing all right with it; maybe it will help me, too.

Diane Hill, Fifty-two
Monroe, Louisiana, Lawyer

I started taking hormones five years ago. My doctor was the one who brought it up. It was the first time I'd gone to her, and when she took my history, she asked me about symptoms of estrogen loss. At the time, I was having hot flashes; they weren't keeping me up at night, but I was waking up in a pool of water.

My doctor said she recommended hormone replacement therapy, and gave me some samples. After I tried them for a while, I went ahead and filled the prescription.

I do feel better physically, but the truth is, I'm concerned about taking this drug. I'm not a person who readily takes prescription medicine for anything, and when I first got the samples, I read all the package inserts and looked it up in medical journals, so I'm aware of some of the medical dangers of taking hormones. On the other hand, estrogen loss seems to be a precursor for osteoporosis and some of the other deficiency ailments of the aged, and therefore I think there are some benefits to having [supplemental] estrogen in my system.

Actually, I don't take it as prescribed. I take it three days a week, and on the other days, I'm using soy and herbs—black cohosh specifically—which I learned about in my reading. I feel better about herbal supplements, because they're natural, not synthetic. They do help, but not enough for me to completely cut out the hormones.

I've haven't told my doctor exactly what I'm doing; I don't think she'd approve. All I've said is that I'm not taking the hormones every day, but that I am taking them regularly. I think she suspects, but she doesn't ask questions.

I hope that I will be able to drop the usage to one to two days a week, but right now I'll stay on them. It's probably been a year since I've fiddled with it. I seem to have a good combination now, where I can take it three days a week and go about my business.

I'm still experimenting with my body to see what I need, and I'll probably continue the estrogen until I find some other way of accomplishing my goals—of feeling as healthy as I did twenty years ago.

Ann Landy, Fifty-eight
Oakton, Virginia, Senior Associate with Caliber Associates, a Behavioral Research Firm

In a lot of ways, the choices were easier a decade ago, when I started taking hormones. Back then, it wasn't "Should we or shouldn't we?"; it was, "Oh my God, there's something that can help!" The recommendation from my physician was "Take this." So I did.

Now, there's so much information out there that it's gotten very confusing. For instance, there's heart disease in my family, and for a long time I thought I was protecting myself against it by taking hormones. I've been very disappointed to read the latest studies that say that may not be the case—although I'm still not convinced we have the full picture. Earlier this year, I went off hormones for three months; I was concerned because my breasts were always swollen and tender, and I weighed twenty pounds more than I did when I started.

Almost immediately, the tenderness and swelling went away, and I dropped four pounds. But the night sweats and hot flashes—one of the reasons I started taking hormones in the first place—returned with a vengeance.

Not long after that, I had to take a business trip, and I was miserable. Every two hours, I had a hot flash. I perspired so much that my suit was soaked; I was so embarrassed. I thought, "Enough already!" and went back to the doctor.

He gave me a prescription for Prempro, and I started taking it again—but only every other day, which seems to control the hot flashes without causing other symptoms. That's something I decided to do on my own, though. The prescription is for every day, and I haven't been back to the doctor to say, "Is this okay?"

There are probably good reasons for me to be taking this. Around the time I started menopause, I had a bone density study that showed some loss. But I still worry. I recently had a Pap test that showed atypical cells. Even though a repeat didn't find any sign of a problem, I can't help being concerned. Is there a connection to the hormones? Should I get off this stuff?

I haven't made up my mind as to how long I'll stay on hormones. I'd like to try discontinuing them periodically to see what the impact is. In the meantime, I just hope I'm doing the right thing.

Valerina Quintana, Fifty-one
Tucson, Arizona, Director of the University of Arizona Career Development Center

I'm not a person who likes taking medication. I keep a small bottle of aspirin in my medicine chest, but it usually expires before I get through it. So when I started menopause two years ago, I thought, "Okay, this is a natural part of life. I can get through it naturally."

My problem was the mood swings. Outside, I was the picture of calmness and coolness, but inside, I was going crazy. I'd go to social functions and have to leave, because I felt weepy. Once, I was driving and I couldn't remember how to get where I was going. Another time, I forgot the name of a colleague I had worked with for eight years.

My primary care physician gave me a prescription, but I put off getting it filled because I didn't like the idea of taking synthetic hormones. Then I went to a lecture by a naturopath about natural hormone replacement therapy. I really liked what I heard. Afterward, she gave everyone a free thirty-minute consultation. She told me, "You look healthy; you should be able to go through this with herbs." She suggested chaste berry and dong quai, but when I tried them, I felt like I needed something more. So I went to a compounding pharmacy [a pharmacy that makes up its own drugs from approved ingredients]. The pharmacist asked about the frequency of my symptoms and came up with a prescription based on that; she called my doctor to get his okay.

Now I take a daily troche containing tri-estrogen with progesterone, but they're natural, plant-based phyto-estrogens, instead of being molecularly altered so they can be copyrighted. I also use a testosterone cream that I rub into my arms; it's also from natural sources, not artificial ones.

Within a month, the mood swings started evening out and the hot flashes went away, although I will admit that my memory hasn't improved as much as I'd hoped; I recently started taking ginkgo biloba to see if that would help. The best part is that I don't have any side effects. My friends who are taking synthetic hormones say their breasts swell, and they sometime have spotting, but I don't have any of that.

I feel really good about what I'm doing. I like the fact that my prescription is based on my symptoms, so it's uniquely my own; when you go to a doctor, they give you the same prescription as everyone else, and we're all different.

Cathy Goldman, Fifty-nine

Forest Hills, New York, Retired

There's one simple reason I'm not taking hormones: family history.

My brother died of prostate cancer, and my mother, who's eighty-nine, had breast cancer. I have her body: we're both short, broad-boned women. When I look at her I think, "What happened to her could happen to me." Plus, I'm at high risk because I got my period at a very early age and never had children. So why take more chances?

I've talked it over with my doctor, but she's never pushed me one way or the other. The last time I went in, I was having a lot of mood swings; I told her, "I can't stand this; maybe I should go on hormones." She said she had no objection to my trying it for six months as long as I had a mammogram before and after. She gave me the prescription, but I just didn't have the guts to fill it.

My sister-in-law was on hormone replacement therapy; she got breast cancer. My sister-in-law's sister was on hormone replacement therapy; she got breast cancer. I thought: "What do I need this for? It's not worth the risk."

One gynecologist—a friend, not the one that I go to—said that if I were at risk of osteoporosis, it would be a different story. But when I had a bone scan, probably about five years ago, my doctor laughed and said, "There are people who would kill for your bones," because they're so thick and heavy.

Heart disease is a very big issue for me because my father died of it, but I have been increasing my aerobic activity, going to the gym and doing things like that to counteract that risk.

I'm also lucky because hot flashes have never been as much of an issue for me as they are for some women. I hate them, but when one hits, splashing my face with ice water is usually enough to relieve it. I know one woman who had to take a change of clothes with her to restaurants, because she'd get drenched. My whole outlook on hormones might have been different if that had happened to me.

The other good thing is that I was retired by the time I started menopause, so I could tough it out in private. I sold advertising for one of the networks, and it would have been very difficult meeting with clients and dealing with hot flashes at the same time.

Debra Lang, Fifty-four

Huntington Woods, Michigan, Assistant Superintendent for Elementary Education, Bloomfield Hills School District

I've been on hormone replacement therapy for six or seven years. What drove me to it were the hot flashes. You're burning up from the inside out, turning beet red, and you get horrible sleep disturbances. I have a demanding job, and I can't perform in peak condition when I'm exhausted. Within a few weeks [of starting on hormones], the hot flashes stopped. But the real surprise was how much it improved the quality of my life in ways I hadn't expected.

I'd been having memory problems; I'd forget words or switch them around, which was debilitating, since I give a lot of speeches as part of my job. But I never associated the problem with menopause until I started taking estrogen and realized that I was no longer having trouble.

The other problem I hadn't attributed to menopause was depression. I chalked it up to my kids growing up and leaving home. But as soon as I started on hormones, that disappeared, too, and my energy returned. I did have problems with breakthrough bleeding, which isn't something you want to deal with after you haven't had your period for a while. They tried a D and C, then increased my progestin, but I gained a lot of weight. I seriously considered going off hormones because of that, but I kept coming back to how much better it made me feel. Now I'm taking a new drug, femhrt, which is a synthetic and has a smaller dose of progestin. I'm feeling much better.

But I will admit the breast cancer piece is worrisome. The only person in my family who had it was my maternal aunt, and I decided she was far enough removed in the family tree to not make that a major factor in my decision.

But my friends and I talk about the risk a lot. We can get really philosophical that more of us are going to die from heart disease, but the truth is, we still worry, and all of us are going to wonder if we made the right decision if we get breast cancer.

The way I've dealt with it is to step back and look at the whole picture. I've concluded that my quality of life is so good I'm not willing to give that up for what may be in the future. Instead, I try to get mammograms regularly, do monthly self-examination—and stay on top of the literature.

Laura Muha, September 2000

CAMPAIGNS FOR SUPPLEMENTS
FOR THAT MIDLIFE EVENT

An upstart Australian company hopes to capitalize on two trends—the aging of female baby boomers and the growing popularity of dietary supplements—to promote a new herbal treatment for the symptoms of menopause.

Novogen Ltd., a medical research company based in Sydney, introduced Promensil, a supplement for menopausal women made from red clover, in the United States in April. According to Novogen, the red clover from which Promensil is made is a source of four plant estrogens that can replace the ovarian estrogens, or hormones, that decline in menopausal women.

Warren Lancaster, vice president for North America at Novogen, said the number of women forty-five years and older in the United States who are on the verge of menopause was expected to grow from 9.1 million in 1996 to 10.2 million in 2000 and 13.5 million in 2010. Of the 10 million or so women in this country now undergoing midlife changes, he said 8 million had symptoms and 2 million of them were taking prescription drugs to manage the symptoms.

"We want to establish Promensil as the leading brand in the market, and we've got to get the message of the health benefits of plant estrogens out there," he said.

Novogen, which is 8.5 percent owned by Protein Technologies International, a subsidiary of DuPont, is not alone in its efforts. According to the Competitive Media Reporting unit of the Dutch publisher VNU N.V., Enzymatic Therapy, a privately held distributor of dietary supplements based in Green Bay, Wisconsin, spent more than $800,000 in the first quarter of 1998 to advertise Remifemin, a product made from the black cohosh plant, which Enzymatic Therapy says provides "nutritional support to women experiencing menopause."

Amerifit of Bloomfield, Connecticut, another privately held dietary supplement company, is also promoting a treatment for menopause, Estroven.

Mark Blumenthal, the executive director of the American Botanical Council, a nonprofit herbal research group in Austin, Texas, said the concept of using dietary supplements, rather than prescription drugs, to treat menopause "is getting to be a hot topic." Mr. Blumenthal called Novogen's $5 million budget a "big chunk of change," but said, "No one knows their product, and people don't know how compelling their research really is. Promensil's research is not as solid from a clinical point of view as Remifemin's," he continued.

Doctors specializing in menopause were even more critical of campaigns by Novogen and its competitors for their supplements. Complaints have increased since the Food and Drug Administration regulation of supplements advertising was eased in 1994 with the passage of the Dietary Supplement Health and Education Act.

Dr. Wulf H. Utian, the director of obstetrics and gynecology at University Hospital in Cleveland, said he was bothered by contentions made in the supplements' advertising for efficacy, "claims based on limited or nonexistent scientific scrutiny."

"I hope consumers will not discontinue an effective treatment for menopause and take something that has not yet been proven," which could put them at risk, he warned.

Dr. Sadja Greenwood, a primary care doctor in San Francisco and the author of *Menopause, Naturally*, said she was worried about potential side effects of taking Promensil. "Red clover is a foreign food for humans, and you have to be cautious about introducing it into the diet," she said.

Jane L. Levere, August 1998

"NATURAL" REMEDIES FOR MENOPAUSE: PROCEED WITH CAUTION

A growing number of postmenopausal women are trying to sidestep the decision about whether or not to take replacement estrogen by choosing another route. They have turned to "natural" alternatives to hormone replacement, including foods and herbal supplements containing plant estrogens, phyto-estrogens, which have estrogenlike effects when taken by humans. They are also using creams made with the hormone progesterone, and cocktails made up of vitamins, minerals and herbs.

At low doses, most experts say, most of these natural remedies are probably safe. But they worry that some women are being overzealous in their self-treatment and taking supplements in unsafe doses. The greatest concern is for women with estrogen-dependent breast cancer. They are advised not to take hormone replacement because the estrogen in it may feed breast cancers, but some are taking large doses of these phyto-estrogens that may be just as harmful.

"What worries me is how women are not willing to go on hormone replacement therapy, but willing to go on a supplemental medicine, without any information but hearsay that it's safe," said Dr. William Helferich, an associate professor of nutrition at the University of Illinois.

Indeed, sales of supplements for menopause have risen greatly in recent years. In 1999, sales of soy isoflavones, the phyto-estrogen in soy, rose to $21 million in supermarkets and drugstores, more than triple 1998 sales. Sales for all-in-one menopausal formulas were $36.20 million in 1999, an increase of 197 percent, according to Spins and ACNielsen, market research firms. Sales of other popular herbs used to treat symptoms of menopause, like black cohosh, flaxseed, red clover, dong quai and wild yam, are also on the rise.

Eating soy and isoflavones is the most popular natural way to increase estrogen. Soy has estrogenic properties, and like hormone replacement, appears to lower cholesterol and reduce bone loss in postmenopausal women, though studies have not shown that it reduces hot flashes. Some studies suggest that soy foods may prevent cancers. This research, largely based on population surveys, has found that women in Japan, who eat a lot of soy, also have a low incidence of breast cancer, although the relationship is far from proven.

Laboratory and animal studies have found conflicting results, with some studies finding that soy isoflavones act as anticancer agents and others finding that the isoflavones may promote some breast tumors. Or it could be that isoflavones do both. Some scientists theorize that when eaten early in life, as in Japan, foods with soy in them may help prevent cancer.

"The way it may be protective in young women is that the phyto-estrogens may hasten the maturation of breast cells, and once they're mature, they're less susceptible to the effects of carcinogens," said Dr. Margo Woods, associate professor of medicine at Tufts University School of Medicine, who specializes in diet, hormones and breast cancer.

Soy, when added to the estrogen that is normally present in young women, may make breast cells mature at a much faster rate and protect against cancer. However, researchers believe that girls who menstruate early, and also are exposed to added estrogen, are not similarly protected, because without soy, levels of estrogen are too low to help mature breast cells. But many American women are introducing soy into the diet late in life, or are bypassing the tofu and going directly to supplements that contain concentrated doses of soy protein or isoflavones. This high-level, late-in-life intake, these scientists say, may promote cancer.

"It's wise to use soy foods, like soy milk and tofu, in moderate amounts in your diet," said Dr. Sadja Greenwood, an assistant clinical professor of obstetrics and gynecology at the University of California at San Francisco. "But to use the isolated soy proteins or the isolated isoflavone pills is very unwise, as we don't know the effects of them."

Isoflavones are a hundred to a thousand times less potent than the estrogen used in hormone replacement, but one can easily consume hundreds of times more of them in the supplements on the market—far more than what Japanese women consume. Some capsules contain as much as 500 milligrams of isoflavones, while the average daily intake in Japan is 25 to 50 milligrams.

Proving most promising for relieving hot flashes is black cohosh, an herb long used in American Indian cultures and studied in Germany for more than fifty years. It is the most thoroughly studied herb for treating symptoms of menopause, and research has found it fairly effective against hot flashes, mood changes and vaginal dryness, said Dr. Varro E. Tyler, professor emeritus of pharmacognosy at Purdue University. It may be the safest too. No studies have found any known phyto-estrogens in the herb.

"We don't know how it works—it may have unknown phyto-estrogens or it may work in some other way to reduce hot flashes," said Dr. Fredi Kronenberg, director of the Richard and Hinda Rosenthal Center for Complementary and Alternative Medicine at Columbia University College of Physicians and Surgeons. "I think the jury is still out on whether this is okay for women with breast cancer or not."

Moreover, black cohosh, like other supplements, is being sold in higher and higher doses in the United States, encouraging women to consume more than what has been used in traditional cultures. Capsules today contain as much as 250 milligrams; in Germany, where herbal remedies are regulated, the recommended dose is 40. And in Germany, women are advised not to take it for more than six months, because there are no long-term studies.

Women are taking a number of other herbs that, unlike black cohosh, are known to contain phyto-estrogens, like dong quai, red clover and flaxseed, to relieve hot flashes, but there is little research on their effectiveness and safety. Dong quai has been used in combination with other herbs in traditional Chinese medicine to treat hot flashes, but many Americans are taking it alone, though one controlled study found it ineffective on its own. Red clover, a potent phyto-estrogen, has not been used to treat menopause symptoms in traditional cultures, so little is known about its safety and effectiveness. Flaxseeds are even less studied.

Those women hoping to lower their risk of heart disease by taking phyto-estrogens may want to reconsider the strategy. Two studies have challenged the long-held belief that taking estrogen protects against heart disease. One study found that undergoing hormone replacement therapy with estrogen and progestin (a form of the hormone progesterone) for four years failed to lower the risk of heart attacks in women who already had heart disease. A second study that measured the arteries of women with heart disease found that taking hormones did not slow the buildup of cholesterol in their arteries.

Women who are taking high doses of these phyto-estrogens also need to consider their risks for endometrial cancer, a cancer of the uterine lining. More than two decades ago, a form of progesterone was added to the estrogen in hormone replacement therapy, because taking estrogen alone was found to increase the risk of this cancer.

So should women taking phyto-estrogens also be taking progesterone? "We just don't know," said Dr. Kronenberg.

Some women use creams derived from plants like wild yams, which some have thought acted like progesterone, to try to counter the risk. But in fact, wild yams have been found to neither relieve symptoms of menopause nor prevent endometrial cancer.

"We call it the yam scam," said Dr. Tyler. Wild yams can be converted to progesterone in the laboratory, but not so in the body.

Taking vitamin E is another approach to alleviating hot flashes. Studies have found some minor benefits when women take high doses—about 800 international units, known as IUs. (A report in 2000 from the Institute of Medicine, part of the National Academy of Sciences, warned that higher does of vitamin E could be harmful.) And many women have turned to the all-in-one menopausal pills, which seem to contain low doses of every supplement and herb that have ever been used in the same sentence with the word *woman.*

"They're putting subtherapeutic doses of everything in these capsules, but we don't know if subtherapeutic A plus subtherapeutic B equals an effect, or if it's useless because it's not enough of anything," Dr. Kronenberg said.

Postmenopausal women who are worried about their risk of heart disease and osteoporosis can lower their risks through lifestyle and diet. To minimize bone loss, postmenopausal women are advised to do weight-bearing exercise and take calcium and vitamin D supplements. To lower risk of heart disease, women should exercise, not smoke, keep weight in the normal range and eat a healthy diet.

Laurie Tarkan, June 2000

IN BREAST CANCER, ALTERNATIVE THERAPY MAY BE A SIGN OF SADNESS

Women with breast cancer who seek alternative therapies like herbs or acupuncture in addition to standard treatment may be unusually worried and depressed and in need of extra help in coping with their fears about the disease, researchers say.

Doctors should ask patients whether they are using alternative treatments, and patients who say yes should also be questioned about anxiety and depression, said Dr. Jane C. Weeks and Dr. Harold J. Burstein, cancer specialists at the Dana-Farber Cancer Institute in Boston. They said that although some distress was only natural when a person was given a diagnosis of cancer, patients who seem exceptionally troubled should be offered psychological counseling.

Their study, published in June 1999 in the *New England Journal of Medicine,* included 480 women with early-stage breast cancer, 28 percent of whom began using alternative therapies for the first time after their cancer surgery. The researchers found that women who began the alternative treatments, compared with women who did not, reported a lower quality of life, more depression, more fear of recurrence of cancer and less sexual satisfaction. They may have turned to alternative therapy for help in coping with their stress, the researchers suggested.

"We hope it will spark a dialogue and spur doctors to identify patients who might be more vulnerable and benefit from earlier interventions," Dr. Burstein said in a telephone interview. "These are things patients and doctors have historically been somewhat reluctant to talk about."

The 480 women in the study were treated from 1993 to 1995 in Massachusetts hospitals. Three months and twelve months after surgery, they filled out surveys that included questions about their emotional states before and after cancer was diagnosed and their use of alternative therapies like herbs, megavitamins, massage, homeopathy, special diets, relaxation techniques, self-help groups, spiritual healing and hypnosis.

The women used those treatments in addition to standard therapy, and not as a substitute for it. But three months after surgery, those who had tried the alternative methods for the first time were more depressed and fearful than those who had not. A year after surgery, all felt better, but those who had used alternative therapy still reported less sexual satisfaction and more fear of recurrence.

The results came as a surprise, contradicting earlier perceptions of patients who use alternative therapy, said Dr. Jimmie Holland, chairwoman of the department of psychiatry and behavioral sciences at the Memorial-Sloan Kettering Cancer Center in New York. Dr. Holland wrote an editorial that accompanied the journal article.

"I was not expecting this," Dr. Holland said in a telephone interview, explaining that a previous study had found that patients who used alternative medicine were better adjusted than those who did not, sought more control and hoped to add to their treatment. "But in this group it looks like these were the more vulnerable women who were having more problems in coping."

In her editorial, Dr. Holland wrote that the women in the study "were not psychologically strong" and that they "turned to alternative medicine to alleviate their distress." Dr. Holland said cancer centers were not doing their job if patients felt they must "get their psyches treated in the alternative world."

"We should be treating the whole person," she said. "The problem in health care today is that visits are so short that patients often don't tell a doctor or nurse how distressed they are, and doctors have no time to ask." Ideally, Dr. Holland said, doctors should notice when patients feel exceptionally troubled about their condition, and refer them to a psychologist, social worker or chaplain. But patients rarely bring up the subject, because they fear it will be seen as a waste of time or will result in their being labeled neurotic or unstable. Doctors should bring it up and ask patients how they are faring emotionally, Dr. Holland said.

"Our busy oncology clinics should be able to ask, 'Are you distressed? How much, on a scale of one to ten?'" she said, asserting that this works very accurately with pain and that it should work with distress, too.

Dr. Burstein said he and Dr. Weeks hoped patients would not be offended by their conclusions, which he said applied to the women taken as a group but not necessarily to each individual patient. "We've been very concerned that some might feel this is pejorative or that we think it somehow dysfunctional," he said. "But it's not a diagnosis. It's an entree for doctors to start talking to patients."

Dr. Holland said: "I think some patients are going to be furious. They'll say, 'How could you say such a thing about me? I'm fine. I'm not distressed.' And that may be true. This is one study."

Fran Visco, president of the National Breast Cancer Coalition, a patients' group, called the researchers' conclusions "almost patronizing," and said they might backfire and lead women using alternative therapy to hide it, to avoid being viewed as depressed or anxious. "It's very disturbing to me that scientists would automatically assume based on this small study that they know how to intervene with these women," Ms. Visco said. "The only conclusion they should jump to is that the distress comes from the fact that we don't know how to cure breast cancer."

Denise Grady, June 1999

SLATHER YOUR FACE WITH MULBERRIES AND GREEN TEA, FOR JUST $50 AN OUNCE

Somewhere in the middle of the 1990s, taking care of ourselves became a virtue. This may be why a man I know who is promiscuous, a chain smoker and a junk-food addict, considers himself health-conscious because he religiously takes powdered shark-fin capsules.

None of us wants to confess to anyone, least of all ourselves, that we are not doing all we can to be hale and hearty. But we tend to choose the primrose path, and ignore the steep and thorny way. For women, especially, our ally in self-delusion is the beauty industry. Once principally concerned with giving us powders and paints to trick the eye, it now mimics the health industry by striving to make us feel well. But where medical science can be painfully slow, beauty "science" is fast.

If a study hints that a substance or practice may be good for us, beauty science creates a product with warp speed. Creams and lotions promise to nourish every inch of skin. Salons want to cut our hair, and heal us as well. Even scents tout therapeutic properties. And it's all so much fun!

At Sephora, the Home Depot of cosmetics, skin care is in the "well-being" area, a clinically white environment designed to comfort and soothe. One entire wall is devoted to "cosmeceuticals": products developed by and for dermatologists and normally available only through them. Merely walking through the department will make a person feel as righteous as if she's given up smoking for the day.

The new face cream labels not only list multivitamins in the ingredients, but also boast of grocery cartfuls of herbs, vegetables and fruits. I myself confess an addiction to Vitalmine from Christian Dior. It contains vitamin C, magnesium and some B vitamins as well as E, but what I love is its orange-smoothie color and citrus smell. At $45 an ounce, it's more expensive than orange juice, which I don't always have time for in the morning. (But I never miss my Vitalmine.) Caroline Geerlings, the senior vice president for marketing at Christian Dior, says the color, texture and scent were designed to foster well-being, and predicts that Vitalmine will spearhead a trend toward products that look, smell and feel as healthful as they purport to be.

In my gym locker there's a jar of Vibrant from Prescriptives. Promoted as a cocktail for stressed skin, it's face cream with microscopic light-reflecting particles to make the complexion glow. But that's only the beginning. Supposedly, unseen spheres deliver purified water to the skin for eight to twelve hours. The ingredients include vitamins C, E, B_5, B_{12} and pro-vitamin D_3, not to mention mulberry, grape, whey protein, green tea, orange and lavender. With all that going on my face, I often feel that it's okay to have a candy bar lunch.

For added nourishment I use makeup. Face paint used to be a way of hiding dark circles and blemishes, the fruits of decadence. Now it can be considered a treatment. At least two companies known for skin care have brought out makeup that promises therapeutic properties, thanks to the inclusion of vitamins and hip herbal remedies like ginkgo biloba and rosemary. Even mascara comes in multivitamin varieties that promise to protect, nourish and strengthen lashes. I've been known to skip the workout and just tone my eyelashes.

Mary Tannen, June 1999

[9]

Skeptics, Misadventurers
and Charlatans

Cautionary Tales

In March 1998, a twenty-two-year-old man collapsed while lifting weights at a gym. By the time paramedics arrived, he had stopped breathing and had suffered cardiac arrest: his heart was in ventricular fibrillation, an abnormal rhythm in which it quivered instead of beating, and could not pump blood effectively. Although he was resuscitated, he spent several weeks in a vegetative state and then needed a month and a half at a rehabilitation center, before finally being released with "substantial residual neurologic impairment"—brain damage.

What could have caused this catastrophe in such a young man? His doctors cast part of the blame on his habit of drinking three 18-ounce bottles a day of a supposed energy booster, Ripped Force, which contained caffeine and additional stimulants known as ephedrine alkaloids, extracted from the plant ephedra, which is also called ma huang. Ephedra is used in popular supplements that promise to help people lose weight and gain energy, and it is also added to over-the-counter cold, sinus and hayfever medicines. Teenagers have taken it hoping to get high, imagining that it's a kind of herbal "speed" or "ecstasy." But the alkaloids, which include the compounds ephedrine and pseudoephedrine, can cause marked increases in heart rate and blood pressure in some people, increasing the risk of heart attack and stroke. The cardiologist who treated the young man suspected that the ephedrine alkaloids in Ripped Force, combined with prescription medicines the man was taking for asthma, had caused the abnormal heart rhythm that led to cardiac arrest.

The young man's story was one of several alarming cases described in an article about ephedra posted in November 2000 on the Web site of the New England Journal of Medicine. The authors had reviewed 140 adverse events linked to ephedra, including ten deaths and thirteen cases of permanent disability, that were reported to the Food and Drug Administration from 1997 to 1999. Ephedra, the authors concluded, had "no demonstrated benefit" and could be dangerous to some people. Their article was released on the Internet more than a month ahead of its actual publication date because of its "potential public health implications," the journal said.

The FDA had been trying for several years to rein in ephedra; it had proposed warning labels, limits on the dosage in various products and a ban on combining ephedra with caffeine or other stimulants in any one product. But the regulatory efforts were thwarted, in part by the 1994 law that protects supplements, and in part by protests to Congress from the supplement industry. A spokeswoman for the FDA said that the agency was nonetheless continuing to try to create new rules for ephedra, perhaps by the end of 2000.

The history of ephedra highlights the dangers of herbs and other supplements that are poorly controlled and vaguely labeled despite their powerful effects on the body. Although some supplements may be potentially beneficial, inadequate research and weaknesses in regulation make it difficult or impossible for consumers to distinguish reliable products from those that are unsafe or useless. Pregnant women are advised not to consume large amounts of ginger, which contains compounds that, theoretically, could cause birth defects. Some Chinese herbal mixtures have been found to contain toxic metals like lead and arsenic or a toxic herb that has caused kidney failure and cancers of the urinary system. Other products, like fat-trapping pills, fat-dissolving soap and salt water marketed as a vitamin, are completely worthless, and constitute cynical attempts to separate gullible people from their money. The abuses have earned the supplement industry *a legion of strident critics who condemn virtually every form of alternative therapy.*

Recent studies have revealed that Saint-John's-wort can interfere with drugs used to treat HIV patients and transplant recipients, and that other supplements, taken before surgery, may interfere with anesthesia or cause bleeding problems. Ginkgo biloba can lead to hemorrhaging in people who are already taking blood-thinning drugs like coumadin or aspirin. In September 2000, the National Center for Complementary and Alternative Medicine at the National Institutes of Health announced that it would spend about $4 million in 2001 to investigate potentially adverse interactions between prescription or over-the-counter drugs and herbal products.

ON THE FRINGES OF HEALTH CARE, UNTESTED THERAPIES THRIVE

From green algae pills to coffee enemas, from acupuncture to aromatherapy, alternative medical treatments have grown into a big business and a powerful force in modern medicine, alarming many in the medical establishment and largely escaping scrutiny from regulators.

Although folk remedies have been around for centuries, often coexisting with the treatments offered by orthodox medicine, medical experts say that during the 1980s and 1990s more people turned to more kinds of alternative therapies than ever before. A national telephone survey, published in the *New England Journal of Medicine* in 1993, found that one of three Americans used unconventional therapies, which can range from taking vitamin C for a cold to going to Mexican clinics for outlawed cancer treatments. The survey also found that Americans spent $13.7 billion in 1991 on such treatments.

Another national survey, published in 1994, found that 60 percent of doctors had at some time referred patients to practitioners of alternative medicine. The highly prestigious Beth Israel Hospital in Boston, which is associated with Harvard Medical School, set up a center for alternative medicine, as did Columbia University. And in 1991, the federal Office of Alternative Medicine was established as part of the National Institutes of

Health to provide the public with information on alternative treatments and to find out what works.

A growing number of health insurance companies, which increasingly set the standards for care, now cover once obscure treatments like naturopathy. Practitioners of naturopathy say that disease arises from blockages in the flow of a life force through the body and that cures follow from treatments like acupuncture and homeopathy, treating patients with infinitesimal amounts of substances that in larger doses might produce symptoms of disease. Meanwhile, many makers of alternative remedies have been reporting record sales. This financial growth is a direct result, analysts say, of a 1994 federal law curbing the regulation of the industry by the Food and Drug Administration.

Many doctors, scientists and government officials sharply criticize the practice of alternative medicine, saying that at best it does no harm and at its worst can present real danger. While conventional medicine adopts procedures that are consistent with established scientific hypotheses, and drugs must be stringently tested and approved by the FDA, alternative medicine practitioners can use therapies based on whims or discredited science, and their methods have not undergone rigorous tests.

The critics of alternative medicine point to reports about the dangers posed by some alternative treatments. Herbal preparations like ma huang, used in dietary supplements and in widely available mood-altering products, have caused deaths, as have coffee enemas, said to treat cancer and other diseases by detoxifying the body. The National Heart, Lung and Blood Institute has documented cases of kidney failure and death in people who have had chelation therapy—the intravenous injection of the synthetic chelating agent EDTA—advertised as a treatment for heart disease and ailments like Parkinson's disease, Alzheimer's and sexual impotency.

The very name "alternative medicine" is Orwellian newspeak, implying that it is a viable option, said Dr. Marcia Angell, executive editor of the *New England Journal of Medicine*. "It's a new name for snake oil," she said. "There's medicine that works and medicine that doesn't work."

Dr. Arthur Caplan, director of the Center for Bioethics at the University of Pennsylvania, said, "Some say, 'Look, why not let desperately ill people do what they want? Why stand between them and the latest piece of shark cartilage?'"

But he disagrees. Dr. Caplan is gravely concerned, he said, that because of alternative medicine, some patients will reject reliable mainstream treatments. Practitioners of alternative medicine, he said, encourage patients to think that "somehow, just by being out of the mainstream, nothing is risky or really dangerous or has side effects." It is, he said, "ridiculous to say that chemotherapy can cause side effects but chelation therapy or coffee enemas, that's completely without risk."

Alternative medicine encompasses a range of treatments outside those commonly accepted by the medical establishment. Generally, such treatments have not passed clinical trials. Although many medicinal herbs have pharmacologically active components, the focus of alternative medicine is not to isolate and test those ingredients.

Alternative medicine includes therapies offered by chiropractors, acupuncturists and homeopaths. Also included may be treatments like aromatherapy, the use of aromatic oils for relaxation, which is also promoted as a cure for hundreds of diseases. Alternative medicines include herbs, taken for various ills; green algae pills, said to foster alertness; and shark cartilage, promoted as a natural cure for cancer.

The regulation of alternative practices varies. All states license chiropractors, but only some license acupuncturists, naturopaths, homeopaths and practitioners of Chinese medicine. Some practitioners are M.D.'s, or have D.O., doctor of osteopathy, degrees, but others come from a broad range of backgrounds, ranging from correspondence courses to academic programs in schools that specialize in the field.

Some supporters of alternative medicine say that it offers a much needed antidote to high-tech, impersonal, cost-driven health care, and that even if the treatments are not cures, they could have powerful placebo effects. They say it emphasizes a different view of health, one based on natural healing and nontoxic interventions. Dr. Andrew Weil, author of the best-selling book *Spontaneous Healing* (Knopf, 1995) and director of the program in integrative medicine at the University of Arizona College of Medicine, said that alternative medicine "resonates with the spirit of the times."

But the critics point to reports of people with serious illnesses who have failed to pursue standard treatments in favor of alternative therapies that have not worked.

Anita Gergasko, of Hazlet, New Jersey, was fifty-eight when she died in a hospice from metastatic breast cancer, which she had fought for seven years. She had a mastectomy, her husband, Gerald Gergasko, said, but refused her doctors' urging that she have chemotherapy, treating herself instead with massive doses of vitamin C and herbs. When the cancer later spread to her brain, she agreed to chemotherapy but also took megadoses of vitamin B_{12}, which can counteract the chemotherapy drug she was taking.

"On her deathbed, she made me promise that I would see to it that nobody else in her family and none of her friends would get involved with this stuff," Mr. Gergasko said.

The rise in alternative treatments can be explained in part by the limits of modern medicine. Even though conventional, science-based medicine has reached unsurpassed heights of technical sophistication, it is still far from perfect. For many ills, it has nothing very effective to offer; doctors can seem hurried and brusque, and conventional treatments can be costly or painful.

But alternative therapies, unlike conventional ones, have not passed rigorous scientific tests showing that they are safe and effective. Generally, the only assurance patients have that alternative treatments will work is anecdotal evidence from other patients and practitioners. That dismays leaders of conventional medicine, who say that such evidence is not reliable because patients and their practitioners fervently desire success and are inclined to judge a treatment as more promising than it is.

Dr. Weil, of the Arizona program, said he realized that alternative medicine treatments had not met scientific standards for efficacy and safety. But "a great many things in standard medicine are not proven either—we just do them," he said.

Doctors do sometimes find that conventional treatments are ill-advised. For example, doctors no longer advise stress reduction to treat ulcers. Even reducing the amount of salt in the diet is increasingly in question.

But Dr. Caplan said Dr. Weil's response blurred the distinction between conventional and alternative medicine. "Medicine at least has a tendency to be self-correcting and self-critical," he said. "In lots of areas of alternative medicine, I haven't seen anybody even admit to the possibility of error."

Dr. Weil said that as a practitioner, rather than a researcher, he was satisfied with "a different standard of proof," like reports of patients who say they were helped. For disorders with no known cure, Dr. Weil said, "If I am faced with an immediate need for a treatment that might alleviate suffering or possibly promote a cure, and if I can assure myself that a treatment is safe, it is reasonable to try it."

But Dr. Richard A. Friedman, director of psychopharmacology at New York Hospital–Cornell Medical Center, said, "Not only is it impossible for Dr. Weil to know if an untested treatment is safe; he also cannot know if it is dangerous." Untested treatments, Dr. Friedman said, "range from harmless placebos to deadly poisons, and the consumer has no way of knowing which is which."

Dr. Weil and others who support various forms of alternative medicine say it represents the rediscovery of a different way of thinking about health, one that forsakes rigid medical models and looks instead to natural ways of helping the body heal itself.

Dr. David Eisenberg, who directs the new alternative medicine center in Boston and who conducted the national telephone survey on alternative medicine, said in an interview that for many people, alternative medicine might be a way of taking charge of their health or finding a practitioner who will take the time to listen to them. For many, the only harm is to their pocketbooks.

But in a study published in 1991 in the *New England Journal of Medicine*, Dr. Barrie R. Cassileth, an adjunct social psychologist at the University of North Carolina who studies patients' experiences with alternative cancer therapies, found—to her surprise, she said—that terminal cancer patients treated with coffee enemas and other alternative treatments were more miserable than those treated with chemotherapy and radiation and that their survival time was the same.

Dr. Stephen Barrett, a retired psychiatrist and a board member of the National Council Against Health Fraud, sees another danger in the growth of alternative medicine, which he calls "quackery."

"Quackery isn't necessarily about selling products and services—it's about selling misbeliefs," Dr. Barrett said. "For a quack to thrive, he has to promote unwarranted distrust. If you can convince someone that the government is not going to give you accurate information on any health matter, that doctors and researchers cannot be trusted, then that person will be damaged. If you are not sick, these misbeliefs may not cause you serious harm. But if you are sick, they may kill you."

Still, several voices within orthodox medicine have softened their criticism of alternative practices, though often for reasons that do not include a belief in their efficacy. At the American Cancer Society, a spokeswoman, Susan Islam, said the term *unproven methods* had recently been replaced by *complementary and alternative methods* because of a concern with "political correctness." The term *unproven*, she said, "is not P.C."

In 1994, Congress passed the Dietary Supplement Health and Education Act, which essentially did away with regulations on alternative medicines that called themselves foods or dietary supplements. Virtually overnight, it revolutionized the industry.

Under the law, products like herbs, shark cartilage or vitamins can be sold and promoted to enhance health as long as product labels do not claim that the products can prevent or treat disease. Before, manufacturers could make no health claims that the FDA had not approved.

The leading supporter of the act was Senator Orrin G. Hatch, Republican of Utah, a state whose dietary supplement industry has sales of $1 billion a year. Dietary supplements include vitamins and formulas for gaining weight, as well as herbs, shark cartilage and melatonin.

Critics of the new law say it has exposed cancer patients to outrageous claims for useless treatments. Dr. Charles Myers, director of the cancer center at the University of Virginia, says the law has "opened Pandora's box."

But Mr. Hatch, who takes dietary supplements, is proud of his role in getting the law passed. "These products have worked for people and helped people," he said. "You show me a doctor who says they haven't helped, and if you do, I'll show you a prejudiced guy."

Some alternative treatments are not regulated because they existed long before there were any regulations. Homeopathic medicines, for example, have never been subjected to testing for effectiveness because they were around before the FDA had laws requiring that. They can stay on the market because the FDA considers them safe.

Other treatments are permitted because practitioners use a legal product; chelation therapy uses EDTA, which is approved for lead-poisoning therapy. Treatments like coffee enemas and juice diets for cancer are not regulated by the FDA because they do not involve drugs.

By all accounts, the alternative medicine business has grown explosively in recent years, following passage of the 1994 act. In 1995, the stock of publicly traded dietary-supplement companies increased in value by 80 percent, said Matthew Patsky, an analyst with the Boston firm Adams, Harkness & Hill and a specialist in the dietary-supplement business.

After the 1994 act became law, Mr. Patsky said, "there was a recognition that there was not much risk in selling dietary supplements." So investors became interested, and that "has created an opportunity for these companies to go ahead and raise money in the public markets," he added.

Gina Kolata, June 1996

THE DESPERATE SEEK HOPE IN A CANCER "CURE" MADE FROM URINE

Ryan Smith, a seventeen-year-old from Waycross, Georgia, has been told by his doctors that he is dying of a brain tumor. They say the standard treatments of surgery, chemotherapy and radiation cannot save him. And so he sits, slouched on a soft leather sofa here in Houston, in the waiting room of Dr. Stanislaw R. Burzynski, his mother at his side, hoping for a miracle.

That miracle, he and his mother believe, is a cure that Dr. Burzynski says he has discovered: chemicals that the doctor calls antineoplastons. Dr. Burzynski says these chemicals are found in blood and urine, and when taken intravenously, through a catheter in the chest, can cure cancer and many other illnesses.

But the Food and Drug Administration has never approved of Dr. Burzynski's remedy. Established authorities in science and medicine say there is no evidence that it works. And in November 1995 the doctor was charged in a seventy-five-count federal indictment with introducing an unapproved drug into interstate commerce and using the mails to mislead insurance companies to pay for the treatment.

Dr. Burzynski's career is a prism through which to examine one of the fastest-growing challenges to modern medicine: the rise of alternative therapies that have not been scientifically proved to work. The medical establishment is arrayed against Dr. Burzynski, and laws against the use of unapproved drugs would seem to be barriers to his practice. But for nearly two decades he has eluded prosecution by both state and federal authorities, because of the slowness of the legal system, his persistent and determined use of apparent loopholes in Texas law and the pressure exerted by his many supporters.

Dr. Burzynski has argued that his treatment is not alternative medicine at all. But it is considered so by mainstream groups, like the American Medical Association and the American Cancer Society, and he is included in leading guides to alternative medicine. He was also a featured speaker at the First International Congress on Alternative and Complementary Medicine in 1995 in Arlington, Virginia.

He is certainly successful financially. The indictment claims that the gross income of Dr. Burzynski and his institute from 1988 to 1994 was $40 million, and that he took home $1 million a year. His practice is solely devoted to antineoplastons, and his clinic is the only one offering the treatment in the United States. He has been the subject of features in newspapers and national magazines like *Good Housekeeping*, as well as on national television shows like *Sally Jesse Raphael*, *48 Hours*, *CBS This Morning* and *Nightline*. Throughout the country, towns hold fund-raising events to help send dying patients to him.

His case has been brought before Congress in hearings on accusations that the Food and Drug Administration has abused its powers. And his case has been cited by Representative Peter A. DeFazio, Democrat of Oregon, to support a law that would allow doctors to treat patients with unapproved drugs. Hearings on a similar Senate bill were planned but then postponed indefinitely.

To many of his desperately ill cancer patients who have not found help through conventional treatment, Dr. Burzynski remains a hero despite his legal troubles. On a recent visit he presided over his clinic and showed no trace of modesty. Short, stocky and frenetic with crinkly blue eyes and a mustache, he compared himself to Einstein and Pasteur. "I am doing this," he said, "because I am trying to help humanity."

And patients, like Ryan Smith, keep coming. Ryan's mother, Marlene, said his troubles began last year when he inexplicably could not lift his right hand from a slice of pizza on his dinner plate. It turned out to be the first sign of an astrocytoma, she said, a malignant brain tumor.

The boy's treatments with surgery, chemotherapy and radiation were terrible, Mrs. Smith said, and Ryan suffered enormously. In January his neurosurgeon "looked at Ryan point blank and said, 'I have not cured anyone of this,'" Mrs. Smith said, adding: "He told the boy: 'It will grow back. You have three or four years to enjoy life.'"

She took refuge in prayer. Five weeks later, three people she knew gave her articles about Dr. Burzynski. She hesitated. She and her husband, a director of nurses at a nursing home, had already spent all their savings on Ryan and she had quit her administrative job to take care of him. How could she afford to pay for Dr. Burzynski? But friends and acquaintances began raising money. In March, Mrs. Smith told Ryan's neurosurgeon that she was taking her son to see Dr. Burzynski.

"He tried to talk me out of coming," Mrs. Smith said. "He implied I was wasting Ryan's good time by trying to find a cure that wasn't there. But I told him that I believed that this was something ordered by God and I was afraid not to come. And I also told him that Ryan was just seventeen years old and he wanted to fight. How can you live waiting to die?"

Dr. Burzynski, fifty-three, received his medical degree from the Medical Academy of Lublin, Poland, in 1968 and came to the United States in 1970 as a research assistant at the Baylor College of Medicine in Houston. In 1977 he opened the Burzynski Research Institute and began treating patients with the chemicals he calls antineoplastons.

In an interview Dr. Burzynski seldom mentioned his patients but bragged about his discovery of antineoplastons, which he claims are a natural and nontoxic substance that constitute the body's own defense system against cancer and other diseases. To obtain antineoplastons for treatment in Houston, he said, he originally isolated them from urine—his own, his wife's and even urine from public urinals. He said he now synthesizes them chemically.

These drugs, Dr. Burzynski asserts, can cure a variety of diseases, including cancer, arthritis, multiple sclerosis and lupus. He has even suggested that they might cure some types of baldness. He also claims that some people who were infected with the AIDS virus have taken the drug and then tested negative for the virus. He said that one cure could work for all these diseases because they all involve "disorders of information processing inside the cell."

His theories pose basic scientific puzzles. Dr. Saul Green, a retired cancer researcher for Memorial Sloan-Kettering Cancer Center in New York, said it was unlikely that there was one underlying cause and one cure for all these unrelated diseases. "That's like saying every mammal that's alive on earth breathes oxygen and therefore every mammal on earth is the same," Dr. Green said.

Dr. Green reviewed Dr. Burzynski's claims under a grant from the National Cancer Institute and later consulted for a law firm representing Aetna Insurance Company in a continuing suit against Dr. Burzynski. He said in an interview that the theory and chemistry behind antineoplastons are "gobbledygook." First, he said "there is no evidence that the body has a natural biochemical surveillance system against cancer, AIDS, and other diseases." Beyond that, he added, Dr. Burzynski's chemistry "makes no sense" and antineoplastons are not even peptides, as Dr. Burzynski claims.

Asked about these charges Dr. Burzynski defended his theory and said he now knew that antineoplastons "are amino acid derivatives and other compounds."

The FDA has not approved antineoplastons because Dr. Burzynski has never completed clinical trials, controlled tests involving patients taking a new drug intended to prove whether a drug works and is safe.

The indictment of Dr. Burzynski states that "between 1983 and March 24, 1995, Dr. Burzynski had enrolled and treated only two patients under FDA-authorized clinical trials."

Dean Mouscher, who is directing the clinical trials for Dr. Burzynski, said Dr. Burzynski was too busy treating patients, running an antineo-plastons manufacturing plant, and conducting his own research to enroll patients in clinical trials to satisfy the FDA. Mr. Mouscher said he himself had a bachelor's degree in French and "no medical background."

Pressed by the courts, Dr. Burzynski has put about four hundred patients in clinical trials approved by the agency, Mr. Mouscher said.

"We saw the handwriting on the wall and started putting everyone in clinical trials," Mr. Mouscher said. The details of clinical trials of new drugs are considered proprietary, the FDA said, but Mr. Mouscher said the agency was allowing Dr. Burzynski to give his drug only to patients for whom all other therapies had failed.

Dr. Burzynski said he already had evidence from his patients' experience. Some see their tumors shrink and others are cured, he said. And, he said, he can provide doctors who will back him up.

One doctor he suggested, Dr. Bruce Cohen, a neurooncologist at the Cleveland Clinic, said that at the request of an insurance company he had a single session with a boy who had gone to Dr. Burzynski in lieu of receiving chemotherapy for a brain tumor. "His tumor did shrink on the therapy he received from Dr. Burzynski," he said. That was four years ago, Dr. Cohen said. And, he added, "that was the first and last time I saw that child."

Mr. Mouscher also suggested Dr. W. Byron Smith, an oncologist in Walnut Creek, California. But Dr. Smith said, "I'm a doubter about this drug, and I'm not convinced it works."

Dr. Burzynski says his patients prove that antineoplastons work. Asked for the best example of a patient who was cured with antineoplastons, Mr. Mouscher said it was Pamela Winningham, who is forty-four and lives in Skillman, New Jersey.

In an interview, Mrs. Winningham said she was told that she had an astrocytoma, a malignant brain tumor, in 1987, when she was thirty-five, and that after surgery and radiation therapy, her doctor told her she had six weeks to six months to live.

She went to Dr. Burzynski and within two months, she said, "the tumor had stopped growing," and six months later, "there was no tumor, only scar tissue." Although, she said, her doctor "did not really believe that the medicine was doing it," she is absolutely convinced that it cured her.

Mrs. Winningham's doctor declined to be interviewed or identified, saying he has been under such an unrelenting attack by Dr. Burzynski's supporters that he fears further publicity.

Most researchers who find a promising treatment publish their results in a prestigious medical journal. Dr. Burzynski said he had submitted a paper to the *New England Journal of Medicine*, but that it had been rejected. "So to hell with them," he said.

Dr. Burzynski said that as with Einstein and Pasteur, history will prove him right. Cures like this, he said, "have never happened before in medical history, so if the *New England Journal of Medicine* refuses to publish my paper, why should I waste my time with these fools?"

Dr. Burzynski's treatment has been questioned by the National Cancer Institute, the American Cancer Society, the Canadian government, the Texas Board of Medical Examiners and individual researchers who investigated his claims.

Dr. Patrick Kelly, the chief of neurosurgery at New York University Medical Center, said that he had reviewed some of Dr. Burzynski's cases, at the request of a supporter of the doctor, and that he had seen nothing that would indicate efficacy.

And yet, he has seen patient after patient with brain tumors go for the treatments, "throwing money down a rat hole," Dr. Kelly said, adding, "This might be money they saved up for a working lifetime."

Dr. Burzynski said the National Cancer Institute agreed that his treatment worked. "They found that tumors decrease and disappear as a result of antineoplastons," he said.

Dr. David Parkinson, the acting associate director of the cancer therapy evaluation program at the cancer institute, said that in 1991, the institute, under congressional pressure to look into alternative medicine, sent a team of doctors to Houston. The doctors said in a report that they had reviewed scans showing tumor size from 7 patients selected by Dr. Burzynski as his best cases out of the more than 2,500 patients, or less than 0.3 percent of the number he had treated. The group wrote that "antitumor activity was documented in this best-case series."

But, Dr. Parkinson said, "No one from the NCI ever has or ever would from that criteria claim that the treatment is active." Ordinarily, he said, the cancer institute does not deem a new treatment promising and warranting further clinical study unless tumors significantly shrink in more than 10 percent of a group of patients with the same ailment. And that itself is only the first hint of effectiveness, with further study required. The reason for this caution, Dr. Parkinson said, is that measurement errors and inaccuracies in measurement can erroneously show tumor shrinkage in 10 percent of patients whose tumors did not shrink.

In 1988, two oncologists working for the Texas Board of Medical Examiners, Dr. Phillip Periman of Amarillo and Dr. Fred N. Ekery of El Paso, reported on their review of records of twenty-six patients that Dr. Burzynski selected. Dr. Periman concluded, "In the eleven patient records I reviewed, no patient had a beneficial therapeutic response that could be ascribed to any of the antineoplaston treatments." Dr. Ekery reported on his review of sixteen patient records, "There was, in my opinion, little evidence of objective responses to the use of antineoplastons in the charts that I reviewed."

In November 1982, under pressure from patients who wanted the Canadian national health service to pay for antineoplastons, the Ministry of Health of Ontario sent two cancer specialists to Houston.

They submitted a report in early 1983, concluding that there was no evidence that Dr. Burzynski's treatment had helped even a single patient and that "the only patients who are still alive either had slowly growing tumors or had received effective treatment before being referred to Houston."

They wrote: "We were left with the impression that either he knows very little about cancer and the responses of different cancers to chemotherapy or else he thinks that we are very stupid and he has tried to hoodwink us."

Dr. Burzynski dismissed their report, saying the Canadians were "hired guns," sent by their government to find an excuse not to pay for his treatment. "If you'd like to find somebody who will lie, who will cheat for money, it's these guys," he said. For nearly two decades, first the Justice

Department, and then Texas, have been waging a campaign to stop Dr. Burzynski from treating patients with antineoplastons.

He has also battled insurance companies, which usually do not pay for experimental drug treatments, and at least two have filed fraud suits against him.

Dr. Burzynski has benefited in his legal battles from the inevitable slowness of legal proceedings and from having supporters in Congress, like Representative Joe L. Barton, Republican of Texas. Mr. Barton held three hearings in 1995 and 1996 on whether the FDA had abused its power, where Dr. Burzynski's patients provided a poignant note by testifying that the agency wanted to deprive them of a lifesaving drug.

John Robertson, a law professor at the University of Texas in Austin, said such powerful support has to influence state judges, who are elected. Another factor, he said, is that state laws can make it "exceedingly difficult for a state to limit a doctor's practice or discipline them if they want to fight."

Federal law, which covers drugs in interstate commerce, is clear enough. Doctors can only prescribe drugs approved by the FDA, although with its approval they can give patients experimental drugs as part of clinical trials to test safety and efficacy.

The agency began its warnings to Dr. Burzynski in 1978, informing him that he was violating federal law by providing antineoplastons to patients outside of clinical trials. In 1984, the Justice Department obtained a permanent injunction to prevent him from shipping antineoplastons across state lines. But it was not until 1995 that the Justice Department finally brought Dr. Burzynski before a grand jury, requesting, and receiving, a seventy-five-count indictment for mail fraud with intent to commit insurance fraud, shipping an unapproved drug across state lines and violation of FDA regulations.

The Texas Board of Medical Examiners has also been fighting the doctor in the courts, but that case is more complicated. It has bounced from court to court since 1986, and after Dr. Burzynski lost a round he asked the Texas Supreme Court to hear his case. He is arguing, among other points, that patients have a right to the treatment of their choice.

Patients waiting in Dr. Burzynski's office say that they know he is controversial but that they do not care. They have banded together to raise money for his legal defense, packed courtrooms in federal and state proceedings and given tearful testimony before Congress that if they cannot have antineoplastons they will die. They have written to President Clinton, their congressmen, their senators and the head of the FDA, seeking a reprieve for Dr. Burzynski, whom they see as their only hope.

Children, bald from previous chemotherapy, pushed in wheelchairs by grieving parents, chanted, "FDA, go away, let us live another day," in a protest in front of a federal courthouse in Houston. In interviews, they angrily proclaim that the FDA has mounted a vendetta against their doctor.

But not everyone remains a believer. Lydia Borek of Avalon, New Jersey, took her seventeen-year-old son to see Dr. Burzynski in 1991, after his doctors had told her that there was nothing more they could offer for his bone cancer beyond pain relief. She signed a contract with Dr. Burzynski, agreeing to pay $5,000 up front, and was charged more than $16,000 in three weeks according to copies of bills she provided. She says she paid more than $10,000 in all.

"I would have gone out and stood naked in traffic," Mrs. Borek said. "I would have died in his place if that were possible. I would have done anything to make this child live." Dr. Burzynski, she said, "offered us a thread to cling to."

When she and her son Brendan were in Dr. Burzynski's office, she said, "a very interesting thing happened." She explained: "I got caught up in this whole thing with all these sick people, people coming and saying they were cured. I feel so stupid even talking about it because I am intelligent and educated and so is my husband."

She believed in Dr. Burzynski, in spite of herself, she said, because "this beautiful child is dying and here's this person who may possibly have something."

Mrs. Borek said that Brendan was the first to have doubts, then she and her husband became disillusioned, deciding that there was no evidence that the treatment worked and that they had wasted three weeks of Brendan's precious time chasing an illusion. She took Brendan back to New Jersey, where he died six months later.

"It's fine to say Dr. Burzynski offers hope," Mrs. Borek said, "but you have to have hope in something that's not ephemeral."

Gina Kolata, July 1996

In March 1997, proceedings in the seventy-five counts against Dr. Burzynski and his institute in Federal District Court in Houston ended in a mistrial. The judge issued a directed verdict of acquittal on the thirty-four mail fraud counts, leaving one count of contempt and forty counts of introducing an unapproved drug in interstate commerce. When a new trial began in May 1997, all counts were dropped, except for the contempt charge. And on May 27, 1997, a federal jury acquitted Dr. Burzynski of that one last charge.

"Antineoplastons" never were approved by the FDA, but Dr. Burzynski continues to treat cancer patients.

THE UNWHOLESOME TALE OF THE HERB MARKET

Some people assume that what is natural is good for you, or at least harmless. That assumption, as it turns out, is a great marketing ploy but a dangerous motto for living.

So far, at least fifteen people have died in the United States after taking herbal products containing ephedrine, also known as ephedra or ma huang. And yet, this herbal drug is still on the market along with other untested herbs and so-called food supplements, including vitamins, amino acids, melatonin and "natural" birth control pills from yams.

Dr. Richard A. Friedman, a psychiatrist who directs the Psychopharmacology Clinic at New York Hospital–Cornell Medical Center, wanted to test the limits on what kinds of herbs could be sold without approval from the Food and Drug Administration. So he called the FDA. Suppose, he asked, he wanted to sell hemlock tea, the deadly poison that Socrates drank. Would there be any way for the FDA to stop him before his tea was on the shelves in health food stores and groceries across the nation? The answer was no. The FDA, he learned, "couldn't stop me from selling hemlock tea until the bodies piled up."

Why? There is a law that prevents the FDA from regulating herbs and other food supplements. In 1994, tens of thousands of Americans, responding to an intense lobbying campaign by the food supplement industry, wrote, faxed and telephoned members of Congress, urging them to deregulate the industry.

Mitchell Zeller, the deputy associate commissioner for policy at the FDA, who was, at the time, a congressional staffer, said that Congress received more mail in 1993 urging it to deregulate supplements than it received on any other issue that year, including health care reform or NAFTA.

And Congress responded. In 1994, it passed the Dietary Supplement Health and Education Act. As a consequence, makers of supplements no longer have to demonstrate that their products are safe before marketing them. The burden is on the FDA to show they are unsafe—after they have been marketed. The law also enables the companies to make unrestrained and unjustified health claims.

While Nassau County, New York, said last week it would ban the sale of stimulant herbs containing ephedrine, an amphetamine-like stimulant, other cities across the nation are still selling these herbs, with names like Cloud 9 (not to be confused with the health food candy bar of the same name), Ultimate Xphoria and Herbal Ecstasy. Stores are marketing the herb as a "natural" substance to promote euphoria or increase energy. Under other names, the herb is sold to promote weight loss or as an aid for bodybuilders.

One product marketed to bodybuilders combined ephedrine with kola nut, Mr. Zeller said. "It was a combination of nature's version of speed and nature's version of caffeine," he said. And some people who took it had strokes, heart attacks and psychotic episodes. Some even died.

One of the recent ephedrine deaths was that of a twenty-year-old Long Island man, Peter Schlendorf, who died shortly after taking eight Ultimate Xphoria pills while he was on spring break in Florida last month.

When the ephedrine casualty reports surfaced this month, the FDA decided to set up a toll-free telephone number to solicit adverse reactions to the herbs. The first day, the agency received 1,200 calls. Although some of the callers simply wanted more information about the herbs, many were alarmed by what had happened to them or to their friends.

The widespread shock about these deaths reflects two popular misconceptions of herbal products, experts said. First, said Dr. Friedman, there is the conviction that anything that is "natural" is also safe.

"There is a suspension of any critical disbelief," he said. By contrast, he added, many people view the pharmaceutical industry with great suspicion and search out supplements to replace prescription drugs. At the same time, many Americans are unaware that the FDA has no power to regulate food supplements. "Everyone alive today has come to expect that the products they buy are at least safe," said Dr. William Jarvis, director of the National Council Against Health Fraud. "They believe there is this powerful regulation going on. People are always talking about how the FDA is such a hard-nosed Gestapo organization. They feel we're overprotected." But, he added, "of course, that's not true when it comes to health care products."

Not all dietary supplements are dangerous, of course. In many cases, the worst that happens is that people waste their money. Dr. David Eisenberg, director of the Center for Alternative Medicine Research at Beth Israel Hospital in Boston, said, "I think that by and large the evidence is that many herbal products are safe.

"All have the potential to be dangerous," he said, but added that "the same is true for conventional medicines and drugs."

The difference is that the risks of conventional drugs must be established before they are marketed. And their benefits must be shown to exceed their risks.

In the case of herbs and other food supplements, Dr. Jarvis said, even doctors may have trouble deciding whether a person's symptoms have anything to do with a supplement. "Information on some herbal drugs or on their interactions with prescription drugs may be obscure or unavailable," he said.

Dr. Friedman tells a story about the dangers of herbs and the public's ignorance of them. One of his patients, an elderly woman, was taking drugs for manic depression. She went to a "natural" doctor, who gave her a drug to soothe her moods.

Dr. Friedman was concerned and called the other doctor, asking what he had given her. It was an herb from Romania. Dr. Friedman said that when he looked it up, "I almost died." In combination with the Prozac that his patient was taking, the herb could have killed her.

Dr. Friedman called the natural doctor and insisted he telephone the woman and urge her to stop the herb immediately.

The doctor who prescribed the herb wasn't incensed by the psychiatrist's intrusion. "He thanked me," Dr. Friedman said.

Gina Kolata, April 1996

"NATURAL, DRUG-FREE" HERB MAY BE ANYTHING BUT

Whatever it is you may seek—a memory boost, weight loss, stress relief, immune enhancement, mood elevation, sexual stimulation or therapy for your ailing heart, there is an herb being sold as the "natural, drug-free" answer to your prayers. But experts warn that an ill-informed foray into the ever-expanding world of botanical medicines can end up causing more problems than it solves.

Herbal products—which are sold as dietary supplements, not drugs— are virtually unregulated, leaving the fox (in this case, the manufacturer) to guard the henhouse. While many companies are conscientious about providing high-quality products free of dangerous contaminants and containing what the label lists—no more, no less—others market cheaply made products that contain little or none of the stated ingredient or, worse, too much. One study of sixty-four "pure" ginseng products found that 60 percent of them were so watered down with cheaper herbs as to be worthless.

Other products on the market are known health hazards. For example, sassafras, still widely available in health food stores, contains a carcinogen, safrole, that was banned decades ago by the Food and Drug Administration from use in foods.

Furthermore, hundreds of botanical products now sold in the United States have been tested and found wanting or have never been adequately tested to determine their effectiveness or safety, especially if used for more than a few weeks. Although health claims cannot legally be made on product labels or in advertisements, hundreds of articles, books, pamphlets and newsletters attribute all kinds of poorly documented medical benefits to herbal products. Even without the prospect of insurance reimbursement, herbs sell widely to gullible consumers desperate for a simple solution to their complex health problems and concerns.

Finally, different parts of a plant or different methods of preparation can yield different effects. As *Consumer Reports on Health* has pointed out, dandelion root acts as a laxative while its leaves contain a diuretic. An herb prepared as a tea may contain none of the active ingredients if those ingredients do not dissolve in water.

Therefore, anyone who is considering joining the seventy million Americans now using herbal products had best learn as much as possible about the herb's effects, side effects, drug interactions and conditions in which its use is inadvisable—as well as check on the producer's reputation.

Choosing a good product may be the greatest challenge faced by a potential consumer of medicinal herbs. First, how can you tell what a product may do for you? By law, labels can state only how an herb may affect bodily structure or function. They cannot claim any direct medical or health benefit. Does the statement "promotes prostate well-being" mean that the product is useful for men with symptoms of an enlarged prostate, i.e., the need to urinate frequently and urgently? Or does it imply that the product may help to prevent prostate cancer?

Also, because no specific health claims are made, labels are not required to carry health warnings. Without some independent research, you may be unable to tell whether it is safe to use a particular herb if, say, you have heart disease or diabetes.

Because the label is of little help, turn to reliable sources of information about herbs. I recommend two books by a university-based pharmacognosist with no financial ties to the herb industry: *Tyler's Herbs of Choice*, by Dr. Varro E. Tyler and James E. Robbers, and *Tyler's Honest Herbal*, by Dr. Tyler and Steven Foster, both published by Haworth Press in Binghamton, New York. (Although Dr. Tyler does not have equity interests in makers of herbal products, he has been paid by a number of herbal companies as a consultant and lecturer.)

Next, find a reliable manufacturer. Although there are no guarantees, you are likely to get the best products from large companies that have been in business for many years. Ask the proprietor of your pharmacy or health food store for recommendations. Don't shop for bargains, especially for costly herbs like ginseng. You're likely to pay good money for a bad product.

Although again it is not a guarantee of quality, look for standardized products that state the amount of active ingredient in each dose. Avoid dried herbs, as in teas, bulk herbs or powdered herbs in capsules. They deteriorate rapidly and are likely to be inactive. The most potent products are made from fresh herbs: liquid and solid extracts, tinctures and freeze-dried herbs in capsules. Before you buy any herbal product, check the expiration date.

If you are thinking of trying an herbal remedy for a known or suspected health problem, start by obtaining a diagnosis from a qualified doctor. Do not rely on an herbologist, naturopath, chiropractor, pharmacist or proprietor of a health food store to diagnose the problem. Many of the anecdotal reports of effective use of herbal products come from people who did not have a health problem in the first place. In other cases, people have unwittingly self-treated serious diseases with useless herbal products and thus delayed a correct diagnosis and effective medical care.

Always consult your doctor before you start to use an herbal product. It may have adverse effects on an underlying health problem or interact badly with other medication you take. Also, if a problem develops while you are using an herbal product, stop taking it right away and see your doctor.

Herbs contain drugs that can cause side effects, allergic reactions and hazardous drug interactions. For example, garlic, which acts as an anticoagulant in foods or botanicals, can add to the activity of a blood-thinning drug and cause excessive bleeding. Or someone taking medication to control diabetes could experience a dangerous reduction in blood sugar if ginseng was used.

All suspected adverse reactions to herbal products should be reported to the Food and Drug Administration, which has a monitoring program called Medwatch. Call the toll-free number, (800) FDA-1088, or contact the program online at www.fda.gov/medwatch.

Follow dosage recommendations on the label. More is not better; it may even be lethal. Do not take herbs for longer periods than experts recommend. And avoid mixtures of herbs; they generally have not been tested for safety or effectiveness.

Even if you have no known health problem and have experienced no known side effects, be sure to tell your doctor about any herbal products you use. When a routine blood test turns up an abnormal reading, you could end up having costly tests for a problem caused by an herb the doctor didn't know you were taking.

Never give herbs to babies or children except under medical supervision. Also, do not take herbal products if you are pregnant or trying to become pregnant or if you are breast-feeding; few if any of these products have been tested for safety during pregnancy and lactation.

Jane E. Brody, February 1999

PILLS AND POWDERS THAT PUT PATIENTS IN THE HOSPITAL

People trying to treat their own ailments with remedies from health food stores became severely ill from pills and powders sold as "dietary supplements," according to six reports in September 1998 in the *New England Journal of Medicine*.

Lead poisoning, impotence, lethargy, nausea, vomiting, diarrhea and abnormal heart rhythms were among the disorders described, resulting from powerful herbs, toxic contaminants or the presence of potent drugs or hormones in products that were supposed to be "all natural" and free of drugs. In addition, several children with cancer worsened when their parents rejected conventional therapy in favor of alternative methods.

The six reports—three articles and three letters to the editor—involved only about a dozen patients, but Dr. Marcia Angell, executive editor of the journal, said, "I think this is the tip of the iceberg." The six reports reached the journal over several months, Dr. Angell said, and were not solicited by the editors.

In a sharply worded editorial accompanying the reports, she and Dr.

Jerome P. Kassirer, the editor in chief of the journal, criticized supplement makers and practitioners of alternative medicine for advocating unproven and potentially harmful treatments. "Alternative treatments should be subjected to scientific testing no less rigorous than that required for conventional treatments," they wrote.

Taken together, the editorial and multiple cases from the medical establishment amount to throwing down the gauntlet before the booming supplement industry. The cases demonstrate that consumers can be harmed by seemingly innocuous herbs and nutritional supplements, authors of the reports say, and lend weight to the argument that the loosely regulated industry should be held more accountable.

Unlike drugs, dietary supplements do not have to be proved safe and effective before they are put on the market. Dr. Angell said that if supplements were held to the same standard as drugs, "the onus would be on the manufacturers to prove safety and efficacy, and I think most of them would shut down." She was especially critical of the Dietary Supplement Health and Education Act of 1994, which weakened the authority of the Food and Drug Administration to regulate vitamins, herbal remedies and other products classified as dietary supplements. The supplement industry boomed after the law was passed, to nearly $12 billion a year in 1997 from $8 billion in 1994.

Dr. Annette Dickinson, a spokeswoman for the Council for Responsible Nutrition, a trade association in Washington representing supplement makers, called the editorial an "unjustified broadside." Dr. Dickinson said that the law was adequate to safeguard the public, and that the industry had no more errors or mishaps than food or pharmaceutical producers.

Dr. William B. Schultz, deputy commissioner for policy at the FDA, said that before 1994, if the agency had concerns about a supplement it could order the substance off the market until the manufacturer proved it safe. "The biggest impact," Dr. Schultz said, "was that a lot of products probably never got to market." In 1994, he said, "Congress changed the rules." The law stipulated that to take a product off the market, the FDA would have to prove it unsafe. In practice, that means hazardous products may go undetected until someone is harmed by them, as in the cases reported in the journal.

In an especially impassioned letter, Dr. Max J. Coppes and his colleagues, pediatric cancer specialists at Alberta Children's Hospital in Calgary, described two cases in which parents of children with cancer decided to forgo chemotherapy and radiation in favor of alternative treatments.

One patient was a fifteen-year-old boy with Hodgkin's disease, a cancer of the lymphatic system that can be cured in more than 80 percent of patients if standard treatment is begun promptly. But the family rejected conventional therapy and instead used an herbal product. Within a few months, the boy had become sicker, and the family wanted to switch to conventional therapy. By then, the disease had progressed, requiring higher doses of chemotherapy that would pose more risk from side effects than the treatment that had been planned originally.

"Until now, neither I nor my three colleagues had encountered families choosing alternative treatments as the only therapy for children with cancer," Dr. Coppes said, adding that during the past year they have had four such cases.

Doctors also sounded a warning about herbal products from Asia. One of the journal letters reported that 83 of 260 samples tested by the California Department of Health Services contained poisonous heavy metals like lead, arsenic or mercury, or drugs not listed on the label.

The products have harmed people, said Dr. Richard Ko, a food and drug scientist with the health services department. In a telephone interview this week, Dr. Ko told of one patient who had taken an herbal preparation she got from an acupuncturist and developed a condition in which she essentially had no white blood cells.

The woman's doctor thought she had leukemia. But the acupuncturist alerted the health department about the herbal preparation, zhong gan ling. It turned out to contain a drug, dipyrone, not listed on the label, that has been kept off the market in the United States because it is known to wipe out white blood cells. The woman recovered, though she suffered a severe infection as a result of the lowered white cell count.

In another case reported in the journal, two women were hospitalized last year in the United States because of severe nausea and vomiting, and irregular heartbeats. Both had taken herbal mixtures that were marketed as a "program" to clean out the intestinal tract. Tests showed that one ingredient in the mixture, plantain (an herb, not the fruit of the same name), had been contaminated with digitalis, a powerful heart drug that can be deadly in overdose. In tracing the source of the contaminated plantain, FDA investigators led by Dr. Lori A. Love found it had been imported from Germany and shipped to more than 150 manufacturers, distributors and retailers. It was recalled, and later tests of other plantain supplies were negative for digitalis.

Dr. Dickinson, the spokeswoman for the supplement industry, said that the digitalis case actually showed that the law worked, because the FDA and industry worked together and quickly traced the contaminant and got products recalled.

Another letter to the journal describes an incident in which Scottsdale, Arizona, police officers stopped a driver who appeared drunk. He was lethargic, vomiting and sweating profusely, and was taken to an emergency room. But he had not been drinking. Rather, a half hour before being arrested he had taken two ounces of a liquid supplement called RenewTrient, marketed as a stimulator of growth hormone and an aid to body building.

Dr. Frank LoVecchio, an emergency-room doctor and toxicologist, and co-author of the letter about the case, said the supplement contained a chemical, gamma-butyrolactone, that is also used in paint remover. "There's no way it promotes muscle growth," Dr. LoVecchio said. The chemical depresses the central nervous system by acting on the same parts of the brain as alcohol and the drug Valium, he said.

The label on RenewTrient warns that one ounce will induce deep sleep for three to six hours, from which a person may be "unarousable." It also says that excessive doses will cause sweating, muscle spasms, vomiting, bed-wetting and diarrhea, and that the best treatment is to "sleep it off." A spokesman for RenewTrient's manufacturer responded to Dr. LoVecchio's report by saying that the patient had ignored the label and taken an overdose but recovered on his own within a few hours, and that the product is safe.

In another article, a team of doctors reported on a mixture of herbs called PC-SPES that many men are taking for prostate cancer. Dr. Robert DiPaola, an oncologist at the Cancer Institute of New Jersey in New Brunswick, said that some patients took the herbs on the assumption that they were a nonhormonal alternative to the female hormone estrogen, which has been used to slow the growth of prostate cancer.

But the researchers found that PC-SPES had "incredible estrogenic activity," Dr. DiPaola said. Like estrogen, the supplement did slow the progression of prostate tumors. But, also like estrogen, it caused marked adverse effects: sore, swollen breasts, loss of libido and, in one case, a blood clot in the foot. Dr. DiPaola said standard treatments like the drug Lupron were as powerful and less toxic than PC-SPES. Even so, he said, some patients chose to continue taking PC-SPES even after they learned the outcome of the study.

"This is an example of how patients can be taking herbal combinations and be unaware, and even the companies selling them can be unaware, of how they work and how potent and toxic they can potentially be," he said. "There is no such thing as a safe agent just because the word 'natural' is attached to it."

Denise Grady, September 1998

LOSE WEIGHT, RISK LIFE, WITH ONE CONVENIENT PRODUCT

In another round of its escalating battle with the dietary supplement industry, the Food and Drug Administration issued a health warning about a weight-loss product that is being marketed as a natural remedy but that the agency deems "an unapproved new drug."

The product, Triax Metabolic Accelerator, has been sold as a dietary supplement by Syntrax Innovations, Inc. of Cape Girardeau, Missouri. But FDA officials say Triax capsules can cause heart attack, stroke and other serious illness; they warn anyone who is taking them to stop immediately.

"This capsule contains an active ingredient that is the same as a minor metabolite of a thyroid hormone," said Dr. David Orloff, a medical officer at the agency. "The dose that they are recommending, which is two to four capsules a day, is the equivalent of as much as five to ten times a maintenance dose of thyroid hormone."

The owner of Syntrax said he had sold nearly one thousand bottles of Triax in its eight months on the market and insisted that it was safe. He vowed to continue selling it and threatened to sue the agency for what he called "irresponsible behavior."

"I have had many doctors who buy this product and give it to their patients with great results," declared the owner, Derek Cornelius, who said he founded Syntrax eighteen months ago. "We have had people lose one hundred to two hundred pounds on this."

The main ingredient in Triax is tiratricol, a derivative of a thyroid hormone. Dr. Orloff said a Los Angeles doctor had reported to the FDA that two of his patients, a husband and wife, had abnormal thyroid function tests while using the product. The woman, age thirty-eight, also suffered severe diarrhea, a symptom Dr. Orloff said was common in people with overactive thyroid glands.

If the issue does reach the courts, it will most likely intensify the five-year-old battle between the FDA and the dietary supplement industry. The dispute centers on a 1994 law, the Dietary Supplement Health and Education Act, which severely restricted the agency's ability to regulate vitamins, herbs and other dietary supplements. The law gave manufacturers the right to advertise the potential benefits of supplements, so long as they did not claim that the products could treat, cure or prevent disease. But in the view of critics, the statute muddled the line between what is and is not a drug.

Mr. Cornelius, the twenty-nine-year-old owner of Syntrax, described himself as a former military officer with an undergraduate degree in biochemistry. He maintains that because tiratricol occurs naturally in beef liver extract, it should be classified as a dietary supplement under the 1994 law.

Despite its warning, the FDA did not move to have Triax withdrawn from the market. The last time the agency tried to reclassify a dietary supplement as a drug, and so have the product removed, it lost in court. Legal experts say the law makes it difficult for the agency to win reclassification in such cases.

Instead, the agency has persuaded the contract laboratory that encapsulates Triax to stop manufacturing it for Syntrax. And Missouri officials have placed on the product an embargo that will prevent Syntrax from releasing for sale the supply it has on hand.

But Mr. Cornelius said he would continue selling Triax, although he would not explain how he intended to get around the embargo.

"There are other ways to distribute it," he said.

Sheryl Gay Stolberg, November 1999

HERBAL DIETERS LOSE MORE MONEY THAN WEIGHT

Two months after it forced the popular diet drug combination known as fen-phen off the market in 1997, the Food and Drug Administration issued a consumer warning about the possible dangers of herbal weight-loss cocktails, which are widely available in diet clinics and health food stores and over the Internet.

The FDA also threatened legal action against the manufacturer of Herbal Phen-Fen, the most popular of these alternatives. The agency accused the company of making false and illegal claims that its product promotes weight loss, and ordered it to stop using phen-fen in its name.

"It is not illegal for this company to sell this product," said Dr. Michael A. Friedman, the acting commissioner of food and drugs. "It is illegal for this company to call this product something that is exactly like a medication and to make medical claims that it will cause weight loss and treat obesity, like the prescription products do."

Herbal Phen-Fen—which contains neither phentermine nor fenfluramine, the two ingredients in the diet drug combination—was introduced by the Nutri/System weight-loss clinics, one industry analyst said. It gained such a big following that it was quickly marketed in health food stores. It is manufactured by HPF, LLC of Trevose, Pennsylvania, which would not disclose its relationship to Nutri/System except to say that they shared some of the same owners. Nutri/System is owned by Heico, Inc., of Chicago.

In an interview, the president of HPF, Brian Haveson, would not identify the company's owners but denied any wrongdoing. "We believe we are not violating any applicable laws," Mr. Haveson said. "We stand behind the product and the name. The product works."

Drug agency officials are precluded by federal law from regulating the diet supplement industry, and therefore they cannot take Herbal Phen-Fen off the market. But they can press for the product to change its name by asserting that the company is marketing it as a drug. The main ingredients in Herbal Phen-Fen are Saint John's-wort, a natural antidepressant, and ephedra, a natural stimulant that, Dr. Friedman said, has been linked to insomnia, headaches, palpitations, high blood pressure and heart attacks.

While fen-phen was removed from the shelves after reports it caused heart valve defects, Dr. Friedman said, "We have far less information, and far less good information, about these herbal products than we did with the medications."

Other experts are also concerned. "It's a marketing ploy; I'm very worried about it," said Dr. Richard A. Friedman, director of the psychopharmacology clinic at New York Hospital–Cornell Medical Center. "These natural biologics can be just as potent and dangerous as manufactured drugs."

Sheryl Gay Stolberg, November 1997

SURGERY AND HERBS DON'T MIX

Alarmed by what they see as the potential for mishaps with patients taking herbal remedies for everything from depression to memory loss, anesthesiologists have begun urging people to stop taking the herbs and supplements before having surgery.

Doctors say there is growing evidence that substances like Saint-John's-wort and ginkgo biloba may have dangerous interactions with the drugs used to anesthetize patients during surgery. Although hard scientific evidence of a problem is lacking, they say, anecdotal reports from hospitals suggest that herbal remedies may be putting some surgery patients at serious risk.

The American Society of Anesthesiologists and the New York State Society of Anesthesiologists both issued warnings to consumers using herbal medicines to stop taking them at least two to three weeks before any scheduled surgery. The New York group urged patients who could not go off the drugs in time to show the medication in its original container to the doctor.

Patients, however, are often reluctant to tell their doctors that they are using nontraditional approaches like herbal medications, said Dr. Carole W. Agin, director of the pain management clinic in Port Jefferson, New York. "I think patients fear that it will somehow drive a wedge between the patient-physician relationship," she said.

Americans spend about $5 billion a year on herbal products, which, unlike prescription drugs, are not fully regulated by the federal government. Often, little is known about the substances, their effects and their interactions with other drugs. And, in some cases, little is done to assure quality control. Only in rare cases, like the one involving the stimulant ephedra, when there are persistent reports of injury or death, does the government take action against an herbal product.

Anesthesiologists say they are taking no position on the use in general of herbal remedies, which are sometimes incorporated into the practice of traditional medicine.

Two of the most common herbals are Saint-John's-wort, which is said to help with mild depression, and ginkgo, which is taken to improve memory and blood circulation. Doctors also singled out two other popular remedies: feverfew, said to help ease migraine headaches, and ginseng, taken to improve vitality.

The possible interactions include an unintended deepening of the effects of some anesthetics and problems with blood pressure and bleeding. One situation that some doctors suspect might be happening in operating rooms involves ephedra, which, despite being banned by the federal Food and Drug Administration, is still being taken in other forms.

From time to time, said Dr. John B. Neeld Jr., president of the American Society of Anesthesiologists, patients in surgery suddenly show signs of a drop in blood pressure. The anesthesiologist will then administer a drug like ephedrine, to bring the pressure back up. In some cases, Dr. Neeld said, doctors have been surprised to see the blood pressure shoot back up to dangerous levels that could cause a stroke or heart attack. The patients later said they had been taking ephedra.

Doctors emphasize that much study needs to be done to establish whether there is a real risk for patients taking herbal remedies. "All of the concern may prove totally unwarranted down the line," Dr. Neeld said.

The growing herbal industry has raised no objection to the warning. Dr. Phillip W. Harvey, director of science and quality assurance at the National Nutritional Foods Association, whose four thousand members make and sell herbal remedies, called it common sense.

"I would wholeheartedly support that," Dr. Harvey said.

Eric Nagourney, July 1999

WHEN TO JUST SAY NO TO SAINT-JOHN'S-WORT

Saint-John's-wort, an herb commonly used by people to treat themselves for depression and anxiety, can interfere with a crucial drug used in AIDS cocktails as well as a drug used for transplant patients, researchers engaged in a pair of studies said today. Patients taking the AIDS drug, indinavir, sold by Merck & Company under the name Crixivan, were warned to be particularly careful about taking Saint-John's-wort.

Dr. Stephen Piscitelli of the National Institutes of Health, who led one of the studies, said, "When Saint-John's-wort and the protease inhibitor indinavir are taken together, the levels of indinavir in the blood drop dramatically." That could allow the AIDS virus to strengthen or, worse, start developing resistance.

"Patients and health care professionals need to be aware of this interaction," said Dr. Judith Falloon of the National Institute of Allergy and Infectious Diseases. "Most people taking medications to treat HIV infection should avoid using Saint-John's-wort."

It is well known that what patients eat and drink can affect the way drugs are absorbed and used by the body. For example, grapefruit juice is known to increase the effectiveness of some HIV drugs. Further, some of those drugs must be taken with food, while others must be taken on an empty stomach. Other research has shown that patients who take herbal or other alternative treatment often do not tell their doctors about it, in part for fear they will disapprove.

Dr. Piscitelli's study was published in the medical journal *Lancet*, which quoted him as saying: "There is a misconception that herbal products like Saint-John's-wort are safe, but this study demonstrates that there can be dangerous interactions when taken with other drugs prescribed to treat medical conditions. It is important for patients to tell their health care providers about their use of herbal products and complementary medicines."

Dr. Piscitelli had seen reports on how Saint-John's-wort affects the body, and feared that it might affect the protease inhibitor class of drugs used in treating HIV infection.

His team tested eight healthy volunteers, first giving them three daily doses of Crixivan alone on an empty stomach, testing levels of the drug in their blood and then adding capsules of Saint-John's-wort.

"The results were dramatically conclusive," Dr. Piscitelli said. "All the participants showed a marked drop in blood levels of indinavir after taking Saint-John's-wort. The drop ranged from forty-nine percent to ninety-nine percent."

Protease inhibitors are often crucial to making HIV drug cocktails work. They can keep the virus suppressed and keep patients healthy, but only if all the drugs are taken correctly. If drug levels fall—for instance, if something like Saint-John's-wort interferes or if the patient misses a few doses—the virus not only resurfaces with a vengeance but can mutate into forms that resist the drugs.

In the second report involving Saint-John's-wort, Frank Ruschitzka and colleagues at University Hospital in Zurich said it could also interfere with cyclosporine, a drug used to keep transplant patients from rejecting their new organs.

Reuters, February 2000

A CHEMICAL CONTAMINANT LURKING
IN A SUPPLEMENT

Researchers at the Mayo Clinic have found a potentially dangerous contaminant in the popular dietary supplement 5-hydroxy-L-tryptophan, or 5-HTP, which is sold in drug and health food stores as a remedy for insomnia, depression, anxiety, obesity, headaches, premenstrual syndrome and other ailments.

Although only six samples were tested and no recent cases of illness have been attributed to 5-HTP, the researchers said their finding still is cause for concern, because contaminated supplements have led to serious illnesses and deaths in the past. The suspected contaminant belongs to a class of compounds known as carboxylic acids.

In addition, they noted, in a letter in the journal *Nature Medicine*, self-help books recommend large doses of 5-HTP, which could expose users to large amounts of any impurity. Sales of 5-HTP reached $20 million in 1997, the *Nutrition Business Journal* reported.

The Food and Drug Administration, prompted by the scientists' warning, has begun testing samples of 5-HTP. The agency lacks authority to regulate the manufacture of vitamins, herbal products or other supplements, but it can take them off the market if they are found unsafe.

Dr. Randy Wykoff, associate commissioner for operations at the FDA, said, "We have issued a guidance to our offices to collect samples, and we have begun testing them." Dr. Wykoff could not predict when results would be available. In the meantime, he said, the agency does not have enough information to make recommendations to the public.

Products containing 5-HTP have come under scrutiny because the substance is a close chemical relative of another supplement, L-tryptophan, which was taken off the market in 1990, after 36 users died and an additional 1,500 became seriously ill with a disorder called eosinophilia-myalgia syndrome, or EMS. People with the syndrome developed extraordinarily high counts of white blood cells, known as eosinophils.

The outbreak was traced to a Japanese chemical company, Showa Denko, which has paid about $2 billion to EMS victims. But despite years of study, the exact cause of EMS was never identified. "There were sixty-three contaminants in L-tryptophan," said Dr. Roseanne Philon, chief of environmental hazards at the Centers for Disease Control and Prevention in Atlanta.

After L-tryptophan was banned, 5-HTP took its place. The substances are closely linked: chemically, they are similar, and in the body, L-tryptophan is converted to 5-HTP. L-tryptophan is an amino acid, which the body uses to build proteins.

The reason for so much interest in the two compounds is that in the brain, they are made into serotonin, a chemical believed to exert a powerful effect on mood. Low levels of it have been linked to depression and other problems. Popular books and manufacturers of supplements have cashed in on the serotonin connection by promoting 5-HTP as a nondrug means of boosting serotonin levels. That claim has not been proved.

Dr. John Hathcock, a spokesman for the Council for Responsible Nutrition, a Washington trade association for the supplement industry, said that the Mayo Clinic findings were cause for concern and that the industry needed to develop manufacturing and purity standards as well as careful dosage guidelines.

Denise Grady, September 1998

HERBAL REMEDIES NOT SAFE IN PREGNANCY

Many women trying to become pregnant are careful to avoid ingesting any substance that might impair their fertility or damage a developing embryo. According to a study published in 1999, several popular herbal remedies should be added to the list of substances that could have detrimental effects on men as well as women and could interfere with conception or a healthy pregnancy.

The herbal products include Saint-John's-wort, ginkgo biloba, echinacea and saw palmetto.

Despite the widespread belief, often fostered by advertising copy, that herbal preparations are "natural" and "drug-free," those that have druglike effects in the body do in fact contain potent chemicals that act like drugs. And, like many prescription and over-the-counter drugs that are known to be unsafe before or during pregnancy, some herbal remedies may also be expected to interfere with normal reproductive function. This expectation prompted researchers at Loma Linda University School of Medicine in Loma Linda, California, to explore the effects of four popular herbs on eggs and sperm. Their findings were published in March 1999, in *Fertility and Sterility*, the journal of the American Society for Reproductive Medicine.

Three of the herbs, Saint-John's-wort, echinacea and ginkgo biloba, had ill effects on either eggs or sperm or both. The damage, the researchers said, included a reduced ability of sperm to penetrate an egg, changes to the genetic material in sperm, poor sperm viability and, in the case of Saint-John's-wort, mutation of the tumor suppressor gene, BRCA1, a change that can increase the risk of breast and ovarian cancers in women who inherit the mutated gene.

Of the herbs tested, only saw palmetto, which is commonly taken by men to relieve the symptoms of an enlarged prostate, did not damage eggs or sperm in the doses tested. But even saw palmetto reduced the viability of sperm that were exposed to the herbal preparation for seven days.

The journal's editor, Dr. Alan H. DeCherney, said, "This is a very important study that could provide important information to patients suffering from infertility." He added, "The growing popularity of these herbal products means we must examine all their possible effects."

The researchers emphasized that their study, which was conducted in the laboratory on both human sperm and hamster eggs, indicated only a potential risk to those who take the herbs in question. They said it was possible that no untoward effects would occur in people who used the herbs in the usual recommended doses.

"To our knowledge, no data exist on concentrations of these herbs in semen or serum," the team, headed by Dr. Richard R. Ondrizek, noted. Thus, it is not possible to say whether the herbal doses tested represented an amount that may actually reach the eggs or sperm in people who use these preparations. Also, the remedies, which are sold over the counter as dietary supplements, are not required to undergo premarket tests for safety or accuracy of dosage.

In the studies, the researchers examined the effects of two concentrations of herbs, one high and one low, but in both cases the amounts that eggs and sperm were exposed to represented a tiny fraction of the recommended dosages on product labels. For echinacea, ginkgo and saw palmetto, the researchers examined amounts that represented one-thousandth and one-hundredth of the recommended daily doses. For Saint-John's-wort, they also looked at a concentration of one-millionth of the recommended dose.

Two types of studies were conducted. In one, hamster eggs that were prepared for fertilization were exposed to various concentrations of the herbs and then inseminated with sperm. Sperm were unable to penetrate the eggs exposed to higher doses of Saint-John's-wort and penetration was impaired by the higher doses of both echinacea and ginkgo. In the second study, human sperm were exposed for seven days to different herbal concentrations. This long-term exposure to Saint-John's-wort and echinacea resulted in significant changes to the sperm and reduced their viability.

In addition, the prolonged exposure to Saint-John's-wort caused some mutations.

Jane E. Brody, March 1999

A CHINESE HERB CAUSES KIDNEY FAILURE
AND MAYBE CANCER, TOO

In an example of the dangers of untested and unregulated herbal products, doctors have found that a Chinese herb, already linked to kidney failure, may cause cancer as well.

The herb, *Aristolochia fangchi*, was given to patients at a weight-loss clinic in Belgium from 1990 to 1992, according to a report published in June 2000 in the *New England Journal of Medicine*. By 1993 more than one hundred patients had kidney damage, and so far more than seventy of them have suffered kidney failure, requiring transplants or dialysis. Now, some of these patients are also developing cancers of the urinary tract. The report gave no indication how many patients might have taken the herb at the clinic.

Cases of kidney failure from the herb have also been reported in France, Britain, Spain, Japan and Taiwan. Dr. Christine Lewis, director of the office of nutritional products, labeling and dietary supplements at the Food and Drug Administration, said there had been no reports of Americans being harmed by aristolochia. But she also said the drug agency did not know how much of the herb might be on the market in this country.

In a check of fourteen stores in New York City yesterday, *Aristolochia fangchi* was available at two stores. At one, it was being sold under the name of Aristolochia sertentaria for $13.95 an once. The other store said that it had *Aristolochia fangchi* available under the name Senega snake root and that it was used to heal snake bites.

In May 2000, the FDA sent letters to doctors and to the supplement industry, with a six-page list of herbal remedies known to contain or suspected of containing aristolochia. The agency urged manufacturers to test their products for the presence of the herb. The FDA also prepared an "import alert" to ban importation of the herb, including every item on the six-page list, Dr. Lewis said.

Dr. John Cardellina, vice president for botanicals at the Council for Responsible Nutrition, a trade group for the supplement industry, said aristolochia had been found in some Chinese medicinal mixtures, but in few other products. Nonetheless, Dr. Cardellina said, because aristolochia is so dangerous, the supplement industry supports the drug agency's decision to list every item that might possibly contain the herb.

Herbs, amino acids, vitamins and other so-called dietary supplements are now a $15 billion industry, which is largely unregulated. Unlike drugs, supplements do not have to be proved safe and effective before they are marketed, and no outside agency even checks to make sure that the products actually contain the ingredients on the label. Regulation is lacking because in 1994, Congress passed the Dietary Supplement Health and Education Act, which cut back the authority of the Food and Drug Administration.

The report in the *New England Journal of Medicine* tells of thirty-nine patients who took the herb and, as a result, needed kidney transplants or dialysis at Erasme Hospital in Brussels, performed by a team led by Dr. Joelle L. Nortier. Eighteen of the thirty-nine also developed cancers of the urinary system. Nineteen others had abnormal cells in the urinary tract, possibly precancers.

In an editorial accompanying the article, Dr. David Kessler, former head of the Food and Drug Administration and now dean of the Yale School of Medicine, urged Congress to change the law to give the FDA more power over supplements.

Dr. Kessler said he had bought a bottle of aristolochia capsules, sold as "Virginia Snakeroot," from an American supplier via the Internet.

At the Belgian weight-loss clinic, aristolochia was given to patients by mistake; doctors had prescribed another herb, but the product that the patients were given was later found to contain aristolochia, possibly because of a manufacturing error or confusion over herbal ingredients with similar-sounding Chinese names. On average, the patients took the product for about a year. Aristolochia contains compounds called aristolochic acids, which are known to damage the kidneys and to cause cancer in rats in the laboratory. Symptoms of kidney failure in people can start within a few months of taking the drug, or even a few years after it is discontinued.

The FDA warning letter and a list of products that might contain aristolochia can be seen on the agency's Web site, www.fda.gov, by clicking on "what's new" and then on "dietary supplements."

Denise Grady, June 2000

Although the FDA had no reports of people in the United States being injured by aristolochia as of June 2000, a few months later American researchers did report a case, which they said was the first known case in the United States. In the October 2000 issue of Baylor University Medical Center Proceedings, *doctors from Oregon described the case of a forty-four-year-old woman whose kidneys deteriorated and failed completely over the course of eight months, necessitating a transplant. Her kidney problems began five months after she took Chinese herbs, which were later found to contain aristolochia.*

A BLACK CLOUD OVER BLUE COHOSH

Blue cohosh, an herbal dietary supplement that has long been used by midwives and American Indians to induce labor and is sold over the counter as a menstrual remedy, may be dangerous for women of child-bearing age, a new study suggests.

Dr. Edward J. Kennelly, an assistant professor of biological sciences at Lehman College of the City University of New York, studied the herb's effects in rat embryos while he was at the Food and Drug Administration from 1996 to 1998. The study, reported in October 1999 in an American Chemical Society publication, the *Journal of Natural Products*, found that blue cohosh produced significant birth defects in rats, resulting in nerve damage, twisted tails and poor or absent eye development.

"There's obviously evidence that people may want to be cautious with it," he said. "How it translates to humans is not known yet, but certainly this study has shown that there's a definite toxicity in the in vitro model. It will caution women of childbearing age who may become pregnant."

Dr. John Cardellina, a vice president of the Council for Responsible Nutrition, a trade association for the dietary supplement industry, says blue cohosh is not widely used in America and has never been highly recommended for menstrual use. He said many people may mistakenly associate it with black cohosh, an unrelated herb, which is widely used for menstrual and menopausal problems. A North American plant, blue cohosh is also known as blueberry root, papoose root and squawroot. It is sold in drug and health food stores and is not regulated by the Food and Drug Administration.

Dr. Victor Herbert, a professor of medicine at Mount Sinai and the Bronx Veterans Administration Medical Centers, said blue cohosh contains two powerful and potentially hazardous ingredients, N-methylcytisine and caulosaponin. "It's not surprising to me that it could produce birth defects," he said.

Nina Siegal, October 1999

VITAMIN O: SALT WATER CURE-ALL, FOR JUST $10 AN OUNCE

The Federal Trade Commission accused two companies of bottling salt water, labeling it "Vitamin O" and selling it as a dietary supplement for $10 an ounce, to treat cancer, high blood pressure, lung disease, headaches, infections, colds, flu and other ailments.

In advertisements in *USA Today* and other newspapers, and on the Internet, the companies—Rose Creek Health Products, Inc., and The Staff of Life, Inc., in Kettle Falls, Washington—asserted that their product "purifies your bloodstream, maximizes nutrients, eliminates poisons and toxins."

A testimonial on the companies' Web site, supposedly from someone with lung cancer, emphysema and heart disease, states: "Three days after starting the Vitamin O, I threw my cane away. In November, we went to Arizona and I bought myself a bicycle." Another testimonial, describing a man who had been suffering severe headaches for twenty years, says, "The day he began taking Vitamin O his headaches disappeared." The company also said that its product was used by American astronauts in space missions.

In a complaint filed on March 11, 1999, in Federal District Court in Spokane, Washington, the trade commission asserted that these claims were false and charged the two companies, both owned by Donald L. Smyth, with making false and unsubstantiated health claims. A spokesman for the companies' public relations office said Mr. Smyth was not available for comment.

Unlike drugs, products marketed as dietary supplements can be sold without the approval of the Food and Drug Administration. But the trade commission can move against companies that market these products, if it believes their advertising is misleading or deceptive. Joel Winston, assistant director of the division of advertising practices at the trade commission, said: "One of the things that makes this case of great significance to us is that they ran full and half-page ads in *USA Today*. This is not the back pages of some alternative medicine journal or late-night cable TV. Ads like this should not be running in mainstream publications like this."

Bruce Dewar, director of advertising operations for *USA Today*, said, "We screen our ads, as any newspaper does."

The O stands for oxygen, which the product purports to deliver to cells and tissues. But Mr. Winston said the product had been analyzed by the FDA and found to contain nothing but salt water. "The company claims it's salt water into which they have introduced something they call stabilized oxygen," Mr. Winston said, but he noted that scientists who searched the scientific literature to find out about stabilized oxygen could not find a single reference to it.

Even if the product did contain high levels of dissolved oxygen, a notion that chemists dismiss, it would be of no medicinal use. Mr. Winston said medical experts had said people could not absorb oxygen by drinking water containing it. Only animals with gills can do that.

Mr. Winston said officials at the National Aeronautics and Space Administration said Vitamin O had never been given to astronauts.

Denise Grady, March 1999

CULT OF THE COLON: FROM LITTLE LIVER PILLS TO BIG OBSESSIONS

In a grand leap of logic about one hundred years ago, doctors declared that they had pinpointed the cause of violent crime, suicide, headaches, bad skin, baldness, cancer, spinsterhood and a host of other maladies and misfortunes. The culprit was intestinal stasis, which led to an even more horrible condition, autointoxication. It was, please pardon the term, constipation.

And it was universal. Astute doctors could spot victims everywhere, even on city streets, by their telltale greasy skins and "septic open mouths." Autointoxication meant that toxins from backed-up, rotting wastes were seeping into their bloodstreams, poisoning their bodies and minds. They needed help, in the form of laxatives, roughage, special exercises, trusses, gut-pounding massages, abdominal vibrating machines and a menacing array of equipment to administer "internal baths" and restore muscle tone to their flaccid innards. Sometimes, they needed drastic surgery to rearrange their insides.

This obsession with the bowels was more than a mad moment in the history of medicine. It went on for a century or more, and it is not over yet, according to a book published in March 2000, *Inner Hygiene* (Oxford

University Press), by Dr. James C. Whorton of the University of Washington in Seattle. The book is exhaustive and scholarly, but, thank goodness, it is also a wry chronicle.

To anyone who grew up puzzling over delicately worded radio ads for peculiar products like Serutan ("'natures' spelled backwards"), Sal Hepatica and Carter's Little Liver Pills, or wondering how Grandma could have become addicted to Feen-A-Mint laxative chewing gum, Dr. Whorton's book will explain it all.

There is no denying that constipation causes a great deal of suffering and can be serious, especially in elderly or chronically ill people. But the notion that it is the root of every illness is, well, more than a bit far-fetched. The idea, however, had been around for centuries, and it was truly embraced by doctors and the public in the United States and Europe in the 1800s. It kept its hold on medicine until well into the twentieth century.

By Dr. Whorton's account, a giant in the fight against constipation was the London surgeon Dr. William Arbuthnot Lane, who had his heyday during the first decade or so of the twentieth century. He convinced people that virtually everyone was chronically constipated, and he made up a theory to explain it: the human digestive system had evolved in four-footed ancestors, and when people stood up on two legs, gravity was too much for their intestines, which drooped, kinked and got clogged. Dr. Lane was a great believer in mineral oil, and he gulped it down several times a day himself and also dosed everyone around him with it, including his family, his servants and his parrot.

But advanced cases were too far gone for mineral oil, and Dr. Lane, who was said to be a brilliant surgeon, devised ever-bolder and more useless operations, taking out more and more of people's intestines to relieve them of kinks and blockages. Most of his patients were women, some of whom married after the surgery, for which Dr. Lane took credit, claiming that no one would have married them before he straightened out their knotted bowels, improving both their looks and their dispositions.

By the 1920s Dr. Lane's theories and operations had been discredited and even ridiculed by his colleagues, one of whom pointed out that by his gravitational theory, penguins, gorillas and especially bats, since they hang upside down, should suffer terribly from constipation. But the cult of the colon still ruled, and gave rise during the 1920s to a laxative industry and volumes like *Intestinal Management for Longer, Happier Life*. No matter that doctors said anything from three times a day to once every three days was normal, there was money to be made by convincing people of the great peril of "irregularity."

An American ad during that era warned that poisonous gases would spread through the body unless "bowel bloat" was cleaned out gently but thoroughly with Cascarets Candy Cathartic. Other ads claimed that laxatives were a marvelous way to lose weight, and Ex-Lax called itself "the secret of natural beauty." Food crazes for bran, yeast, yogurt and sour milk to prevent constipation also sprang up during the 1920s, and Battle Creek, Michigan, home of Kellogg's All-Bran and Post Grape-Nuts, became the cereal capital of the world, marketing products to promote regularity.

All this might seem like a quaint and amusing chapter in the history of weird medical beliefs. But is it history? Given Americans' current preoccupation with high-fiber diets, and their endless parental fussing over the contents of children's diapers, one could easily argue that old fears of autointoxication must still be with us. As late as 1986, the National Institutes of Health was still writing pamphlets to reassure the public that the human body did not absorb poisons from retained feces.

Today, herbal and alternative medicine magazines carry ads for "cleansing programs" that promise to rid the body of toxins that linger in the intestines in a slimy layer of something called "mucoid plaque." And Americans still spend $847 million a year on laxatives.

Denise Grady, May 2000

THE HERBAL POTIONS THAT MAKE SCIENCE SICK

In San Diego on a Tuesday in November 1998, two major drug companies rolled out studies showing the safety and effectiveness of a new class of prescription pain relievers; they had been duly tested on thousands of patients, some for up to a year. Such testing was a minimum requirement before the drugs could be prescribed to millions of Americans.

On the same day, the prestigious *Journal of the American Medical Association* held a news conference in Washington to hail the publication of six papers "evaluating" studies of alternative medical treatments.

But these treatments were already on the market. The studies came after the fact. The testing involved only dozens of patients and only weeks of trials. Yet these studies, which any large drug company would have considered tentative and inconclusive, were presented as resolving questions of safety and efficacy.

An accompanying editorial, titled "Alternative Medicine Meets Science," used decisive words like *found*, as in the study "found" that moxibustion—the burning of herbs to stimulate acupuncture points—is helpful for breach pregnancy; that a particular treatment "is helpful" for a medical condition; that researchers were able to "document" that a mixture of Chinese herbs "improves symptoms of irritable-bowel syndrome."

Is there a double standard? One thing is sure: the issue has stirred up supporters and skeptics. Dr. Phil B. Fontanarosa, an editor of the *Journal of the American Medical Association* who helped write its editorial, said that "the trials were all well done and the usual caveats were in place." The resulting news coverage was exuberant. But Dr. Fontanarosa said that was the result of interest in the topic.

Exactly, said some critics of alternative medicine, who were stung by what they saw as an exaggeration of the importance of such modest studies.

Double standard? "Absolutely," said Dr. Richard A. Friedman, director of the psychopharmacology clinic at Cornell Hospital–New York Medical Center. With all the hoopla, the message that alternative treatments were still a scientific terra incognita got lost. "The public will be sold" on the notion that such treatments have passed muster, Dr. Friedman said.

Dr. John Hathcock, the director of nutritional and regulatory science for the Council for Responsible Nutrition, argued that the double standard works the other way by hurting the vitamin and mineral industry. His group represents the dietary supplement industry. Dr. Hathcock said that an epidemiological study came out about a month ago linking folic acid in the diet with protection from colon cancer.

"I was talking with a high official at the National Cancer Institute, and he said, 'That's very intriguing, we're very interested, but it needs to be confirmed with a clinical trial,'" Dr. Hathcock said. "I said, 'Give me a break. There is no risk, and the effective period is fifteen years.'" A study is likely to take that long to assess the effects of folic acid on colon cancer rates.

If a treatment has a low risk, the consumer does not have to be as certain of the benefit in order to use it, said Dr. Stephen DeFelice, chairman of the Foundation for Innovation in Medicine in Cranford, New Jersey. With actual pharmaceuticals, "we require more evidence because it is an unknown entity, an artificial molecule," he said. Drugs "are not nature's way of handling disease," Dr. DeFelice added.

Alternative medicine is different, he said. "These things are not nearly as toxic as drugs," said Dr. DeFelice, adding that "when we go for benefits, we accept less evidence."

But that is not to say that most Americans are indifferent about evidence on whether alternative treatments work, said Lisa Meyer, a spokeswoman for the Council for Responsible Nutrition. "People are hungry for additional information," she said.

Critics of America's acceptance of alternative medicine trace it to the Dietary Supplement Health and Education Act of 1994, which enabled makers of supplements containing herbs, amino acids, botanical extracts, vitamins and minerals to sell them without the approval of the Food and Drug Administration. These companies also can claim benefits for their products—without any supporting scientific studies. But unlike manufacturers of pharmaceuticals and devices, they are not required to report adverse effects to the agency.

With no regulations forcing them to test for product safety, no protocol for tracking bad side effects and no requirement that products demonstrate effectiveness, the alternative medicine industry has been able to sidestep the rules of drug development. Critics like Dr. Allen Roses, a vice president at the drug company Glaxo Wellcome, Inc., say that is inherently dangerous.

If an alternative medicine company is selling its product as a substitute for a drug, it should show that it works and that its benefits outweigh its risks, said Dr. Roses, who questioned studies like those in the medical journal. One of those studies involved 116 patients divided into three groups and studied for fourteen weeks. Such a study, he said, cannot detect deleterious side effects that, as so often happens with drugs, occur only in a small percentage of people or only after people take the drug for a long time.

"If you are going to take anything, it should be based on efficacy and not on hope," Dr. Roses said. "You are crushing people's hope by giving them a treatment that is not efficacious and implying it will be."

The result has been a clash of two cultures, said Dr. William M. Wardell, the executive director of the Covance Institute for Drug Development Studies in Princeton, New Jersey. "The culture for conventional medicine comes out of a history of fraud and disaster," he said. "The presumption is that drugs are ineffective and unsafe unless they are proven to be effective and safe."

Alternative medicine's philosophy has been the presumption that treatments are safe and effective unless proven otherwise. Now, Dr. Wardell said, "There is a confusion of gullibility with credibility. If sales go up from $2 million to $67 million, people say, 'This proves it works.' If you can put yourself in the mind of a marketer, it's true. It works."

Gina Kolata, November 1998

CASTING A COLD EYE ON ALTERNATIVE MEDICINE

With Americans spending billions of dollars a year on alternative medicine, the time would seem right for a scientific journal dedicated to examining unorthodox treatments like acupuncture, homeopathy and shark cartilage.

Such a journal, the *Scientific Review of Alternative Medicine*, began publication in October 1997, with the stated purpose of applying "rational analysis" to alternative treatments. The founder and editor of the journal, Dr. Wallace Sampson, a clinical professor of medicine at Stanford University, said the journal was needed because the few devoted to alternative medicine did not take a sufficiently rigorous approach.

Dr. Sampson, a practicing doctor, is a longtime skeptic of any treatment that has not been subjected to stringent scientific testing. At times, he said, he has been exasperated to hear of people spending time and money on unproved therapies promoted by practitioners who appeared to be either misguided, or, in some cases, charlatans. As an oncologist, he was especially disturbed to see cancer patients during the 1970s being taken in by claims for laetrile, an extract of apricot pits that was ultimately proved useless as a cancer treatment.

To start the new journal, Dr. Sampson teamed up with Paul Kurtz, who is the publisher, another confirmed skeptic and debunker and chairman of the Committee for the Scientific Investigation of Claims of the Paranormal. That group publishes its own journal, the *Skeptical Inquirer*, which regularly dissects faith healers, psychics and UFO sightings.

The new journal carries an endorsement from a group calling itself the Council for Scientific Medicine. The council consists mostly of doctors and scientists, including other renowned scourges of health and nutrition fads, like Dr. Victor Herbert of Mount Sinai Medical Center in New York, and the author Martin Gardner. Five Nobel Prize winners (two of them in physics) are also prominently featured.

Decrying the lack of reliable information about the efficacy of alternative treatments, the council's statement said the potential harm from such treatments was incalculable, and described some promoters as "naive, greedy, or unscrupulous." Readers looking for the pros and cons of alternative therapies will find that the first issue comes down heavily on the con side, with detailed articles that skewer homeopathy, therapeutic touch and the popular self-help writer Dr. Andrew Weil.

The hard-nosed approach does not surprise people familiar with those who have shaped the new journal. "Their history is very serious, hardworking, determined opposition to unconventional ideas," said Dr. David Hufford, a behavioral scientist at Pennsylvania State College of Medicine in Hershey, who has studied the alternative medicine movement in the United States since the 1970s.

Dr. Sampson described the intended audience for the journal as "physicians and scientists and interested and educated adults." Just six hundred copies of the first issue were mailed out. He said he did not expect to change the minds of believers in alternative therapies, noting that many have little interest in science.

Dr. Daniel Callahan, a biomedical ethicist at the Hastings Institute in Briarcliff, New York, noted that the first issue of the new journal was for the most part negative. "Will they publish things that are favorable?" Dr. Callahan asked. "Something or other is going to work. Are they prepared to say some good things?"

Dr. Sampson said the journal would include any properly done studies or reasoned analyses. "We'll publish anything logical," he said.

Denise Grady, December 1997

[1 0]

Ginkgo Candy Bars and Ketchup for What Ails You

Food as Medicine

Chicken soup for a cold. Tea with honey for a sore throat. Ginger ale for a queasy stomach. The urge to find cure as well as comfort in food and drink dates back to the ancients. In its modern incarnation it has taken on high-tech trappings: our grandmothers took ginger ale at face value, but consumers today are more impressed by a list of active ingredients, like gingerols, terpenoids and shogaols.

The idea of food having medicinal properties is seductive: so many tempting things are bad for you that it is sheer relief to hear about anything that might be good.

Research during the past decade has provided new evidence about the benefits of eating tomatoes and tomato products, tea, fruits, vegetables, whole grains and moderate amounts of soy. But consumers are advised to resist the temptation to overdose on particular foods; boring as it may be, the old advice to eat a little bit of everything may still be the wisest course. And "a little bit" may prove to be the most important advice of all: studies in animals, including monkeys, show that the only diet that appears to slow down the aging process and prolong life is one in which the daily intake of calories is cut back sharply, by 20 to 40 percent.

328

Food manufacturers, of course, are all too happy to sing the praises of their own products. A tub of "buttery spread" promises to "help balance fats in the diet." A can of soup boasts, "good source of fiber." The label on soy milk says it "may reduce heart disease." Green tea brags about antioxidants that "neutralize harmful molecules in your body known as free radicals." Breakfast cereal announces that it contains soluble fiber, which, "in a diet low in saturated fat and cholesterol, may reduce the risk of heart disease." So what if you have to eat three cups of oats a day? You'll be as healthy as a horse.

If food by itself can be good for you, why not take it one step further? Manufacturers have done so. It is now possible to buy chicken broth spiked with echinacea, pea soup with Saint-John's-wort and ice tea and soft drinks with ginseng. The products, called nutraceuticals or functional foods, are a fast-growing industry, with yearly sales of more than $17 billion. Major producers have either entered the market or expressed interest in it, including Nabisco, Coca-Cola, Quaker Oats, General Mills and Lipton.

But are these products foods, drugs, or dietary supplements? Manufacturers that want to make health claims, saying, for instance, that a product lowers cholesterol, have to go through a complex approval process that the Food and Drug Administration requires for drugs or food additives. If, on the other hand, the manufacturers are content with vague pleasantries like "defender of your health," they are free to lace their candy bars with ginkgo and the FDA cannot touch them.

Will Americans live longer, healthier lives thanks to herbally fortified ice tea? Probably not, but the companies that make the tea just might.

AMERICANS NEED A BETTER DIET: THIS IS NEWS?

Americans are eating better than they were in the 1980s, but the diets of nine out of ten still need improvement, federal officials reported in May 2000. People should reduce their intake of saturated fats, seek a healthy body weight, reduce sodium in their diet and choose foods and drinks that "moderate" their sugar consumption, the government said.

Those recommendations are contained in the government's dietary guidelines, which are updated every five years, and determine, among other things, the nutritional content of lunches served to 26 million schoolchildren every day.

President Clinton devoted his weekly radio address today to the guidelines, choosing a holiday weekend to address "our family and friends at picnics and backyard barbecues." Despite progress in eating less fat and more vegetables, "the vast majority of Americans still don't have healthy diets," Mr. Clinton said. He faulted lifestyle changes for aggravating the problem. "We're eating more fast food because of our hectic schedules, and we're less physically active because of our growing reliance on modern conveniences, from cars to computers to remote controls," he said. As a result, Mr. Clinton said, more Americans are obese—including one in ten children—placing them at greater risk for heart disease, stroke, cancer and diabetes.

Mr. Clinton, who is 6-feet-2-inches tall and has a reputation for a hearty appetite and a fondness for fast food, lost about twenty pounds in the year before his 1997 physical examination. He later regained it all, and last November his doctors reported that he weighed 218 pounds. As a result, the White House said at the time, his doctors "recommended that the president focus again on a low-calorie diet and focus more attention also on his exercise regimen."

The guidelines, which are drafted by a joint advisory committee of the Agriculture Department and the Department of Health and Human Services, may seem tame, but twice a decade virtually every phrase is cause for battle between public-interest advocates and food producers. This year, sugar growers and soft drink manufacturers scored a victory by persuading the administration to alter a draft recommendation from "go easy on beverages and foods high in added sugars" to "choose beverages and foods to moderate your intake of sugars."

"It's unfortunate the government caved in to pressure from junk food makers," said Margo G. Wootan, the director of nutrition policy at the Center for Science in the Public Interest, a nonprofit consumer advocacy group. "The sugar industry was out in full force." Ms. Wootan, who has a doctorate in nutrition, nevertheless praised the administration for ignoring pressure from salt producers and issuing an explicit message on sodium, "Eat less."

Among the key recommendations:

- Choose a diet that is low in saturated fat and cholesterol. Limit fatty meats and high-fat dairy products like cheese; opt for fish and lean poultry, use vegetable oils rather than solid fats.
- Aim for a healthy weight. One in three adults is overweight, up from one in four just a decade ago. Choose sensible portions at mealtime and get regular physical activity to reduce the risk of heart disease and other maladies.
- Cut your salt intake. Substitute spices and herbs to flavor food; go easy on soy sauce, ketchup, mustard, pickles and olives; choose plain foods like grilled or roasted entrees when dining out.
- Moderate your intake of sugars. The number-one source of added sugars is in nondiet soft drinks. Other sources include cakes and cookies, fruit drinks and candy. Do not let such foods ruin your appetite for healthful items like low-fat milk.
- Drink alcohol in moderation. That means no more than one drink per day for women—a 12-ounce beer or a 5-ounce glass of wine—and no more than two drinks a day for men.

The government offered guidance on exercise and handling and storing food safely. Americans can improve their health by exercising moderately every day, the guidelines said. Exercise that speeds up the heart rate and breathing and that builds strength and flexibility is particularly beneficial.

"Just a brisk thirty-minute walk five times a week, for instance, can cut the chance of developing or dying from heart disease in half," Mr. Clinton said.

People can avoid food-borne illnesses by being careful with perishable items like eggs, meats, fish, fresh fruits and milk products. The government urged Americans not to drink unpasteurized juices, raw sprouts and raw or undercooked meat, eggs, fish or shellfish.

Cooks should wash their hands, utensils and surfaces after handling raw meat, poultry or fish and store those foods, if necessary, apart from other foods.

Christopher Marquis, May 2000

"FUNCTIONAL FOODS": EATING YOUR WAY TO WISDOM AND HARMONY

Et tu, Ben and Jerry?

The men who brought us the alternative ice cream are once again adding odd ingredients to cream, sugar and egg yolks. Only now it is gingseng, echinacea and chamomile that they have put in their latest smoothies.

This time, however, the ice cream guys are not setting the trend but following it, as they join the food manufacturers who are making so-called functional foods. These foods have been pumped up with enough herbs, vitamins, minerals and other supplements to qualify as medicines. At least, that is what their advertising leads you to think.

Functional foods fall into two categories: those that are based on science and those that are based on wishful thinking. Products like Benecol and Take Control salad dressings have the scientific evidence to back up claims: each contains substances that can lower cholesterol. But most companies "are adding whatever the herb of the moment is without any proof that they work," said Phil Lempert, editor of the *Lempert Report Newsletter*, which tracks marketing trends in the food industry.

"We are going to see more and more products coming up with herbs as ingredients, whether they do any good or not," he said. "It's the same thing that happened in the late 1960s, when everyone was using the term *natural*, whether it was or not, and for years people were fooled."

According to the Grocery Manufacturers Association, a trade group, sales of functional foods reached $14.7 billion in 1997 and are projected to reach $17 billion by 2001. Many of these products suggest that they can bring well-being, relaxation, wisdom and harmony into your life. The label on Knudsen's Simply Nutritious peach berry Saint-John's-wort beverage states that Saint-John's-wort "has been widely used to reduce anxiety and exhaustion," while the SoBe Energy drink maintains that it has "health benefits enhanced by addition of herbs, nutrients and other natural supplements."

Hansen's Anti-OX drink suggests in its name what it provides, antioxidants, and the package for Think!, a candy bar with ginkgo and choline, calls it an "interactive bar" for "concentration, calmness and stamina." Whatever that means.

Some of these products taste as if they want you to remember that they aspire to some medicinal purpose. Aqualibra, whose copy is about its alkalizing effect, has such an unpleasant odor that you know it must be good for you. Simply Nutritious Mega Green looks like old mown grass, which is also what it tastes like. Think! tastes like all those other sports bars, sort of sweet, sort of crunchy and sort of inedible. Benecol tastes like any soft margarine. In other words, no one would ever confuse it with butter.

The trend goes beyond herbs. Fresh Samantha Desperately Seeking C juice contains 100 percent of the federally suggested daily requirement of vitamin A, ten times that for vitamin C and 100 percent of that for vitamin E. But it's an antioxidant pill in drink form. It is not a good idea to get ten times the suggested daily requirement of vitamin C in this form, because it just might cause diarrhea.

Campbell's Soup is introducing Campbell's Plus, four soups fortified with the B vitamins, as well as A, C, E and calcium. Kraft's new Taste of Life salad dressings "celebrate a life of wellness," or so their labels say, because they have been fortified with vitamins A, C and E.

But before you run out to buy Knudsen's Lemon Ginger drink with echinacea or SoBe Wisdom, which contains ginkgo biloba, Saint-John's-wort and gotu kola, consider this: there is no point in drinking echinacea to prevent colds because evidence shows that it doesn't. Proof that echinacea shortens the length of a cold and reduces symptoms is still inconclusive, and no one knows what the proper dose should be, or which of the three kinds of echinacea plants works best. And experts warn against using echinacea for more than eight weeks at a time.

While research has shown that Saint-John's-wort is useful for mild to moderate clinical depression, it must be taken for at least four weeks to be effective. At what dosage, no one is certain.

Some drinks like Odwalla Serious Energy contain ginseng. But David Schardt, the associate nutritionist at the Center for Science in the Public Interest, a nutrition advocacy group, said, "All the best research in the United States and Canada shows that ginseng has no effect on energy whatsoever."

All the research that has been done on ginkgo biloba, Mr. Schardt said, "is almost entirely with those who have dementia, particularly Alzheimer's."

Effectively marketing the functional foods that have some valid scientific evidence to back them has not been easy. Some, like Hain's Herbal Kitchen Prescription soups, have already come and gone. Kellogg's had very little success selling its line of Ensemble foods, which contain psyllium, a fiber that helps reduce cholesterol.

Now, Benecol, made by McNeil Consumer Healthcare, comes in a margarine product, in salad dressing and in candy bars. Eating a certain amount of Benecol a day will reduce cholesterol levels by 10 percent, because the product contains stanol esters. Take Control, which comes in salad dressing and margarine, makes similar claims.

But to be effective, Benecol should be used in a low-fat, low-saturated-fat diet with five servings of fruits and vegetables a day, said Dr. Tu Nguyen, director of the lipid clinic at the Mayo Clinic.

"You don't want to go to McDonald's and think by taking Benecol you are still doing a good thing for yourself," he said.

Whatever happened to real food and a healthy diet?

Marian Burros, November 1999

AND NOW FOR A PRESUMPTUOUS LITTLE DRINK

Soft drinks used to have modest goals. Basically, they slaked thirst while delivering a mild sugar-caffeine rush, plus a few intangibles dreamed up by the advertising agencies, like instant membership in the Pepsi Generation.

That was then. Fast-forward, please, and reach for a bottle of Wisdom, a new orange-mango herbal drink from a New Age beverage company in Norwalk, Connecticut, called SoBe. Read the fine print. Be amazed. Wisdom is more than a soft drink—it's an invitation to a new way of life. The drink contains Saint-John's-wort, an herbal antidepressant some-times referred to as nature's Prozac. It also has ginkgo, an extract from the leaves of the ginkgo biloba tree, "to sharpen the mind," and gotu kola, a kind of cola nut, to help "rejuvenate the brain." Working together, this herbal troika promotes "calm and focused thought." The pitch is irre-sistible, the psychic equivalent of a grand-prize mailing from Publishers Clearing House.

Could one soft drink really do all this? To answer the question, I entered a well-stocked health food store and purchased several weeks' supply of Wisdom, planning to drink one 20-ounce bottle a day and take note of any mental and emotional changes that took place along the way.

One bottle a day seemed about right. Too much intelligence added too quickly might have undesirable consequences, like the jealousy of fel-low workers or a heightened output of brilliant work that my employers would start demanding as a matter of course. Better to take it slow—or is that "slowly"? I gulped my first bottle.

In doing so, I joined the swelling ranks of consumers who want more, much more, than a caffeine jolt or fresh-fruit flavor when they put a bot-tle to their lips. The young, health-oriented market tapped by companies like Snapple, Mistic and Arizona now wants ginseng, guarana, schizan-dra, echinacea and yohimbe in its teas and fruit drinks. Let us not forget kava, a rising herbal superstar from the South Pacific, reputed to ease stress and anxiety. The magic herbs, it is said, can do everything from preventing the common cold to relieving the symptoms of premenstrual tension.

The new glamour herbs, along with the occasional berry, almost invariably come from the mysterious East or the deepest recesses of the Amazonian rain forest, their secret properties long treasured by ancient peoples but only now coming to the attention of dim Westerners.

Tribal Tonics—"One Tribe! One Vibe!"—captures the ethos perfectly with its new lineup of herbally enhanced green teas, made by Apple and Eve, a juice company in Roslyn, New York. Relaxation Cocktail, for example, harnesses the power of kava, supplemented by extracts of hawthorn berry and chamomile, to soothe nerves jangled by our senseless postindustrial way of life.

Pepsi, taking note of the trend, is gradually rolling out Josta, a carbonated drink flavored with guarana. Guarana, the bottle text proclaims, grows "deep within the jungle" where ancient tribes used it to release "raw, primal power." Guarana also finds its way into a new Venezuelan rum, Ocumare, whose promotional copy describes the berries as "mystical, sensual and exotic."

"This is a small niche, but it's the area of the beverage industry where there's been the most innovation," said Gary Hemphill, a vice president of the Beverage Marketing Corporation. The new-wave sodas, sometimes called functional or nutriceutical drinks, are so new that precise statistics on their growth or present market size have not been compiled. Beverage Marketing lumps functional drinks in the New Age category, a loosely defined market worth $7 billion in wholesale sales annually, encompassing everything that is not a carbonated, flavored soft drink. Mr. Hemphill estimated the herbally enhanced beverage niche at about $100 million.

The first bottle of Wisdom, fruity and sweet, went down easily. The lush mango flavor comes through strongly, its cloying qualities held in check by the acidity of the orange juice.

It was far too early to do a self-check for feelings of well-being. Saint-John's-wort takes about two weeks to kick in and four weeks to achieve maximum effect when prescribed to depressed patients. It is usually administered in daily doses of 300 milligrams, which means that I would have to drink fifteen bottles of Wisdom a day for a proper comparison, a daunting task, considering that each bottle contains 275 calories. On the other hand I was not actually depressed, so the math might work out fine. Perhaps the depression would come with calm and focused thinking, since seeing the world clearly invites dark thoughts. At that point the Saint-John's-wort would begin to earn its keep. On the ginkgo front, my mental processes seemed fine, but I sensed no unusual brain-wave activity after the first Wisdom treatment. The gotu kola did not seem to be rejuvenating my brain yet, but then again, that was a big job.

The weeks passed. The bottles of Wisdom, glowing radioactively in my refrigerator, began to disappear as I drank deeply at the well of ancient knowledge. From time to time, I noticed changes in my mood and outlook. A large Visa bill arrived, casting a pall over my personal universe. Calm and focused thought led me to an insight: deep debt is natural, the white-collar equivalent of the farmer's drought or crop failure. The wise man does not seek to change the course of the planets, nor to turn the tides. Is this not so? My depression lifted. A victory for Saint-John's-wort?

Meanwhile, in a mysterious development, I began cashing tickets at Oaklawn Park, a racetrack that has perplexed me for years. In race after race, I was betting against the crowd, and winning. The fools. My mind, sharpened to a fine edge by daily infusions of ginkgo, was making mincemeat of the opposition. I want to retake my SAT. On the other hand, I spent an entire hour transfixed by a behind-the-scenes documentary on the making of the *Jerry Springer Show*.

The brain-rejuvenation project may take some time.

William Grimes, April 1998

LYCOPENE: TOMATOES AND THEIR COLLEAGUES IN DIETARY FIGHT AGAINST CANCER

The buzzword of a few years ago was beta-carotene, a substance found in fruits and vegetables that was supposed to protect against cancer. Then scientific studies showed no particular benefit from taking beta-carotene in pill form. In fact, questions were raised about potential harm, especially to smokers. Now it seems another substance in fruits and vegetables may account for the health protection long associated with eating carotene-rich foods.

It is called lycopene (pronounced LIKE-o-peen), and it is what makes tomatoes red. It had previously been strongly linked to a reduced risk of developing various deadly cancers, including those of the prostate, colon and rectum.

A large study of 1,379 European men has indicated that those who consumed the most lycopene from foods were half as likely to suffer a heart attack as those who consumed the least lycopene. The study is especially valuable because it assessed lycopene consumption and absorption by measuring its presence in body fat rather than by using a less reliable method of asking men how much lycopene-rich food they regularly consumed.

Like beta-carotene, lycopene is fat soluble. Dietary fat is needed for it to be absorbed through the intestines, and the amount stored in body fat is considered a reliable reflection of how much people absorb from their diets. Lycopene's protective role, however, stems not from fat stores but from its ability as a potent antioxidant, which means it can prevent free radical damage to cells, molecules and genes as it circulates in the blood. Free radicals are highly reactive molecules that can combine with other substances and change them in a harmful way.

Such damage can, for example, transform freely circulating cholesterol into a form that sticks to arteries and clogs them, setting the stage for a heart attack. It can cause genetic changes that may in time result in cancer. Free radical damage is also involved in cataracts caused by exposure to sunlight and lung disease caused by inhaling pollutants like ozone. Lycopene was recently shown to become depleted in skin that is exposed to ultraviolet light, suggesting that the nutrient's antioxidant role is called into play to protect the skin from sun damage.

Findings from the new study indicate that lycopene is most likely the substance responsible for the protection against heart disease and cancer that had long been thought to result from consuming beta-carotene. When the research team, headed by Dr. Lenore Kohlmeier, simultaneously examined levels in body fat of lycopene, alpha- and beta-carotene and lutein, another carotenoid, lycopene alone seemed to account for the reduced risk of heart disease.

Dr. Kohlmeier, a professor of epidemiology and nutrition at the University of North Carolina at Chapel Hill, and her colleagues at ten European medical centers published the findings in October 1997 in the *American Journal of Epidemiology.*

In an interview, Dr. Kohlmeier cautioned against assuming, first, that the protection the researchers observed resulted directly from lycopene and not some other as-yet-unknown nutrient that "travels with lycopene" and, second, that if lycopene is in fact protective, the same benefit can be gained from taking it in pill or powder form, instead of getting it from food.

"We made that mistake with beta-carotene," Dr. Kohlmeier said. "We should not repeat it." She was referring primarily to two large costly studies that sought to determine whether supplements of beta-carotene could reduce the risk of cancer. Instead, the studies showed that those who took beta-carotene supplements had higher cancer rates than those given a dummy pill.

Just as beta-carotene turned out to be a red herring, "it is possible that lycopene is a marker for something else not yet identified," Dr. Kohlmeier explained. She also cited a study, however, by chemists at Jefferson Medical College in Philadelphia that revealed lycopene to be a much more potent antioxidant than alpha-carotene, beta-carotene and vitamin E.

Lycopene is most prominent in tomatoes. But it is not well absorbed into the body unless the tomatoes are cooked. Thus, the best sources are concentrated processed tomato products like tomato paste, ketchup and tomato sauce. Tomato juice is a reasonably good source if it has been heated, as would occur when it is canned or bottled. In addition, tomatoes ripened on the vine have more lycopene than those that ripen after they are picked. Other sources of lycopene include watermelon, red grapefruit and, to a lesser extent, shellfish like lobster and crab meat.

Dr. Kohlmeier explained that cooking tomatoes releases the lycopene and makes it available for absorption. Heat breaks down cell walls and frees the lycopene from a matrix of proteins and fiber that keep it locked in the raw food.

"Once again we have to revise an old recommendation—to eat fresh fruits and vegetables," Dr. Kohlmeier remarked. "You get five times more lycopene from tomato sauce as you would get from the equivalent amount of fresh tomatoes." Furthermore, she said, when tomatoes are consumed as part of a processed food, that food is likely to contain some fat that makes it possible for the lycopene to be absorbed.

Participants in the new study were middle-aged men, 662 of whom had suffered heart attacks. Lycopene was most strongly associated with protection against heart disease among men with the highest levels of polyunsaturated fatty acids in their body fat. Since these acids are highly susceptible to oxidation, this finding, too, suggests that lycopene's role as an antioxidant accounts for the benefits, Dr. Kohlmeier said.

She added that a second study is under way to determine whether a diet rich in processed tomato products can protect people's lungs against oxidative damage caused by ozone. Preliminary results indicate that lycopene from foods does indeed find its way to lung cells, although beta-carotene does not. The researcher said that participants would be examined for genetic damage to their lung cells after exposure to ozone and their lung capacity would be measured to determine whether lycopene was protective.

Jane E. Brody, October 1997

GREEN TEA WITHOUT THE TASTE OF OLD SOCKS

In recent years, several studies have pointed to the health benefits of green tea. Regular drinkers have less lung, stomach and esophageal cancer, lower rates of cardiovascular disease and fewer strokes.

But for some, the pungent drink is, at best, an acquired taste, the cod liver oil of the '90s. So green tea pills have begun to appear on the market, promising all the benefits of the drink without the bouquet of old gym socks. A pill or capsule that contains the essential chemicals found in the liquid from of green tea should provide the same benefits. The key ingredients seem to be an assortment of polyphenols, a broad class of antioxidants found in plants. Antioxidants prevent or delay cell damage that may cause cancer, heart disease and other ailments. A cup of green tea contains about 60 milligrams of polyphenols. One commonly sold capsule contains 242 milligrams, but the amounts vary by manufacturer.

With little clinical research to guide them, experts caution that something essential may be lost in the process of extracting chemicals from tea. Still, the leap from liquid tea to its essential elements is logical, so studies are under way.

At the M. D. Anderson Cancer Center in Houston, researchers have completed the first phase of a study of green tea extracts. The most important finding is that the human limit for green tea seems to be about forty cups per day, said Dr. Waun Ki Hong, the chairman of the Department of Thoracic, Head and Neck Oncology at the center. Higher doses caused tremors, nervousness, nausea and vomiting.

Having established the maximum tolerable dose, the researchers will try to determine whether the extract has any effect on the cancers. The subjects are mostly lung cancer patients whose tumors have recurred, Dr. Hong said. Others have recurring head, neck, ovarian or colon cancer, or lymphoma. All are undergoing conventional treatments while they participate in the study.

Another study is under way at the Memorial Sloan-Kettering Cancer Center in New York. Researchers there are also trying to establish a tolerance level and may eventually focus on establishing optimum levels of green tea for regular use as a dietary supplement, said Dr. Vincent A. Miller, the principal investigator. Dr. Miller said he and his team hoped to look at whether green tea supplements could prevent cancer.

It is not known, Dr. Miller said, whether extracts will prove as effective as liquid tea seems to be. His patients are up to the equivalent of twenty to thirty cups of tea a day, he said, and are beginning to complain of nausea and shaking. But at least, Dr. Miller added, no one has complained about the taste.

Jane Fritsch, October 1998

FOR SOY, THE TIME MAY HAVE FINALLY COME . . .

It has taken thirty years for soy to lose its hippie image. There has been no mainstream movement to replace hamburgers with soy burgers or pork with tofu. But thanks to a number of studies suggesting that foods made from soybeans may have impressive health benefits, soy is finally getting some respect.

The Food and Drug Administration has proposed adding soy to its list of foods whose labels can make health claims, in this case that soy can reduce the risk of heart disease. The agency says it takes 25 grams of soy protein a day to lower cholesterol, as long as the soy is part of a diet low in cholesterol and saturated fat.

Consuming that amount is getting easier. At a health food supermarket in suburban Washington, I found forty varieties of soy substitutes for cow's milk, nine soy substitutes for yogurt and twenty-two for hamburger. I found a soy margarine, three soy ice creams, three soy versions of mayonnaise; textured soy protein to replace ground beef, soy flour and, of course, tofu. The varieties of tofu or bean curd alone numbered twenty-six: flavored tofu, soft tofu, firm tofu, very firm tofu, low-fat tofu. Someone must be eating this stuff, and don't be surprised if it's one of your closest friends.

Studies have suggested that soy products also offer protection against breast and prostate cancer and may ease menopausal symptoms. Soy contains phyto-estrogens called isoflavones that do have a weak estrogenic effect. But as with green tea, oat bran and ever so many other silver bullets, evidence about soy's benefits is still not proven except for the cholesterol-lowering effect. No long-term human clinical trials have been conducted. Studies have found a lower incidence of breast cancer in Chinese and Japanese women who eat a lot of soy, but the lower rate could be due to other cultural differences.

Studies in monkeys and a few small studies in women have shown a decrease in LDL cholesterol (the bad cholesterol) and a reduced risk of clogged arteries from eating soy. Rat studies indicate that one isoflavone found in soy can block the growth-stimulating effects of estrogen in the breast. Data on bone loss are conflicting. And one study has shown that 8 ounces of a soy beverage daily reduced the number and severity of hot flashes.

Taking phyto-estrogen supplements is not a good idea: no one knows the effects of concentrated phyto-estrogens. But adding actual soy to the diet may be beneficial. It's a good low-fat source of protein. But soybeans, like other beans, may produce gas, so introduce them slowly. If that fails, Beano usually works.

If you are using tofu as a source of soy, check the label to get the maximum grams of soy protein, which can vary from 5 to 13 grams per 4 ounces. The average I found was about 12.

Do not buy the loose tofu that is sold in stores in containers of water. In a survey the *New York Times* conducted in 1995, extremely high levels of bacteria were found in the eight containers that were analyzed. Four contained *E. coli* bacteria. Not all *E. coli* is deadly, but it is indicative of fecal contamination. So stick with packaged tofu.

About 55 percent of the soybeans grown in this country are genetically engineered. If you are concerned about the impact of bioengineered foods on the environment, or about the lack of long-term studies on their impact on health, buy organic soy. Health food stores carry a considerable amount of it.

Here are two recipes using tofu. The chocolate mousse does not taste like one made with eggs, sugar and cream, but when I served it without revealing what it was beforehand, it was lapped up. The main dish uses the tofu as a substitute for ground pork and is good hot or cold.

Marian Burros, August 1999

Chocolate Amaretto Tofu Mousse with Raspberry Sauce

Adapted from *The Strang Cookbook for Cancer Prevention*, by Laura Pensiero and Susan Oliveria, with Dr. Michael Osborne and Jacques Pepin (Dutton, 1998)

Time: 10 minutes

For the mousse:

20 ounces silken firm or extra-firm organic tofu

¼ cup maple syrup

¼ cup dark brown sugar

3 tablespoons amaretto

6 tablespoons good-quality unsweetened cocoa like Valrhona

2 teaspoons coffee flavoring or 2 teaspoons instant espresso

For the raspberry sauce:

12 ounces raspberries

⅓ cup orange juice

Juice of ½ lemon

2 tablespoons granulated sugar

1. Place all the ingredients for the mousse in a food processor, and blend completely, about 2 minutes, scraping down the sides once or twice. Place in bowl, cover and chill while making the sauce.

2. Wash raspberries; measure out 1 cup, and set aside. Place remaining berries, orange juice, lemon juice and sugar in food processor, and blend until smooth.

3. Stir in the whole berries. Into each of four parfait glasses or small glass bowls, spoon about an inch of the mousse. Top with a couple of spoonfuls of raspberry sauce; repeat until the rim is reached, topping with raspberry sauce.

Yield: 4 servings

Note: Each serving contains 15 grams of soy protein.

Hot Gingered Broccoli with Tofu

Time: 20 minutes

12 ounces firm or extra-firm regular or low-fat organic tofu

1 tablespoon toasted sesame oil

2 large cloves garlic, minced

1 tablespoon coarsely shredded ginger

1 to 2 teaspoons hot chili-garlic paste

2 tablespoons Asian sesame paste

2 pounds broccoli, tough stems trimmed and heads cut into bite-size florets

2 tablespoons rice wine or dry sherry

    1 tablespoon reduced-sodium soy sauce

    ⅔ cup chicken stock or broth, no salt added

    12 ounces fresh thin noodles, Chinese or American

    2 green onions, washed, trimmed and chopped

1. Bring a pot of water to a boil. Drain tofu, and press between paper towels to remove moisture. Cut into ¼-inch cubes.
2. Heat oil in a wok or large skillet over very high heat. Add garlic, ginger, chili paste and sesame paste, and stir. When mixture begins to color, reduce heat, add tofu, and cook over low heat for 2 minutes. Add broccoli, rice wine, soy sauce and stock; cover, and simmer until broccoli is tender but still firm, 3 to 5 minutes.
3. Meanwhile, cook noodles in boiling water according to package directions. When noodles are done, drain and stir into broccoli mixture. Sprinkle with green onions, and serve.

Yield: 4 servings

Note: Each serving contains 9 grams of soy protein.

BUT NEW DOUBTS CLOUD ROSY NEWS ON SOY . . .

Over the last several years, millions of Americans who had turned a deaf ear to the virtues of soy have had a change of heart. Sales of the lowly bean, which has been a staple of the Asian diet for millennia, have been skyrocketing because preliminary research suggested that soy has many life-enhancing benefits, from preventing bone density loss to easing some symptoms of menopause.

In October 1999, the federal government put its imprimatur on soy when it allowed food companies to make the claim that soy protein reduces cholesterol and the risk of heart disease. The other claims are still unproved, even though soy in all its forms, from tofu and veggie burgers to shakes and supplements, is being heavily promoted by its sellers as a panacea. The news media, too, have been almost unanimous in praising its safety and efficacy.

Against the backdrop of widespread praise, however, there is growing suspicion that soy—despite its undisputed benefits—may pose some health hazards. The scientific world is divided over many of the claims for efficacy and over some safety issues, but there are two points on which there is agreement. Soy is useful for reducing cholesterol. And there may be an increased risk of cancer associated with consuming the components of soy called isoflavones in supplement form, particularly for post-menopausal women; and for these women, there may also be hazards in adding soy foods to their diets.

Isoflavones, particularly genistein and daidzein, are phyto-estrogens. These plant chemicals, which have estrogenlike hormonal effects on the body, occur naturally in soybeans and foods made from them. Compared with chemical estrogens, the kind taken by women to reduce the symptoms of menopause, phyto-estrogens are weak, but they act the same way: they can both inhibit and stimulate the growth of certain types of cells.

Not one of the eighteen scientists interviewed for this column was willing to say that taking isoflavones was risk-free. Some particularly cautioned against it. Dr. Margo Woods, an associate professor of medicine at Tufts University School of Medicine, who specializes in nutrition and breast cancer, said: "As a food, soy does a lot of great things, but once you start looking at different components like phyto-estrogens, you are talking about pharmacological things. It's wiser to talk about soy and soy foods. A whole food behaves very differently in the body than when you take one compound. We are looking into the components, but we haven't been studying in the area long enough. I would not recommend to anyone that they take isoflavones."

Even before the Food and Drug Administration approved the cholesterol-lowering health claim for soy, sales were booming. In 1998, 770,000 metric tons of soybeans were sold in this country to be turned into food products; in 1999 the figure rose to 1.007 million metric tons. Total sales of soy foods in supermarket chains during the twelve months ending in October 1999 were almost $420 million, up 45 percent from the previous year's, according to Spins, a natural products market research company in San Francisco. In natural food stores, sales in the six months ending in October were up 37 percent from the previous six-month period. Many large companies like Kellogg's, General Mills,

Campbell's Soup and ConAgra are developing new soy products in response to the demand.

The biggest jump has been in soy supplements, the isoflavone pills, whose sales were up 246 percent in the twelve months ending in October. But the carefully worded health claim the Food and Drug Administration permits for cholesterol reduction is for soy protein, not for isoflavones. To have that health claim on its label, a food must be low in fat, saturated fat and cholesterol and contain 6.5 grams of soy protein per serving. For the cholesterol-lowering effect, 25 grams of soy protein must be added daily to a diet low in saturated fat and cholesterol.

The scientists are worried that the public is interpreting the approval of soy protein as a recommendation to take soy supplements, which generally have higher levels of isoflavones than occur naturally in food. The highest levels of naturally occurring isoflavones are found in soy beverages, cooked soybeans and tempeh, and the range is wide. Some processed products, like sports bars, have added isoflavones. Supplements can contain more than 85 milligrams of isoflavones in a single pill, and some manufacturers advise taking two pills a day. There are soy protein concentrate powders with as much as 160 milligrams of isoflavones in a single serving.

"People don't distinguish isoflavones from soy protein," said Dr. Daniel Sheehan, a research biologist at the FDA's National Center for Toxicological Research in Jefferson, Arkansas. He also directs a program that studies endocrine disrupters, which are chemicals like isoflavones with hormonal activity that disrupts the endocrine system. "The approval of soy protein for cardiovascular disease is going to lead to tremendous increase in the use of isoflavones, and this rachets up concern levels," he added. For that reason, Dr. Sheehan opposed the Food and Drug Administration's health claim label.

Dr. Gregory Burke, chairman of the public health sciences department at Wake Forest University School of Medicine in Winston-Salem, North Carolina, worries that Americans will overdose on these supplements. "To Americans, more is better," he said. "Adding soy to a healthy diet makes a lot of sense. If you have to take soy through food, you are not going to overdose on isoflavones, but if you take it through pills you could take doses up to ten times what folks consume in Japan"—where soy is a staple of the diet. "I don't know what the risk-benefit is on those high doses," Dr. Burke said.

No one is really willing to put a number on the maximum safe level of isoflavones, because human studies have not been done, said Dr. Daniel Doerge, a research chemist in biochemical toxicology at the National Center for Toxicological Research. "Nobody knows what high levels are," he added.

Dr. William Helferich, an associate professor of nutrition at the University of Illinois, who specializes in diet and breast cancer, pointed out that regulators, food companies and some scientists are willing to make the assumption that 50 milligrams of isoflavones a day are safe. One gram of soybeans contains about 1 milligram of isoflavones. "That amount may be perfectly safe and beneficial for the vast majority of the population," he said. "However, the potential for some individuals to be harmed, such as postmenopausal women with estrogen-dependent breast cancer, still remains unclear. Because it is a natural food component, there is no requirement to put any indication or contraindication on the products. I don't know how anyone can commit to any number, because data are not there for all populations." The typical daily consumption in Japan, for example, is 25 to 50 milligrams of isoflavones.

Whether soy or its isoflavones reduce the risk of breast cancer or increase it has not been sorted out. Data on estrogens are mixed so far, said Dr. Helferich. "Estrogens are a mixed bag," he said. "Given early they will prevent, given late they will likely promote. Taking natural estrogens late in life to prevent symptoms of menopause may be a real problem."

Epidemiological studies suggest that soy may reduce the risk of breast cancer, but there are animal and even human studies that suggest that soy may increase the risk. Dr. Stephen Barnes, a professor of pharmacology and toxicity at the University of Alabama, said that in countries like Japan, where there is a lot of soy in the diet, women have lower rates of breast cancer than American women. But American-born daughters of Japanese immigrants have higher levels of breast cancer than their Japanese-born mothers. This statistic is often cited as proof that soy reduces the risk of breast cancer. Dr. Barnes said that consumption of soy early in life may make the difference. "But," he added, "I don't know what happens if you are fifty years old and go on soy."

Dr. Sheehan said it was a mistake to compare Asian and Western populations. "You are making an assumption they are biologically identical, but there are significant differences in the way humans handle chemicals, depending on their ethnic background," he said.

Yet another study, reported in the *American Journal of Clinical Nutrition* in December 1998, showed that there was increased breast cell proliferation in women given soy. The greater the cell proliferation, the greater the chance for cancer cells to develop.

A number of studies that may answer these questions are being underwritten by the National Cancer Institute, but Dr. Peter Greenwald, the director of the institute's division of cancer prevention, said: "The results are mixed and far from definitive. I don't think we are in a position to give advice for or against."

The public looks for black-and-white answers, said Dr. Sheehan, adding: "We don't have enough information to be able to give the public good advice, and that's why we need to do the studies. Not only can there be some outcomes that are beneficial and some adverse in the same individual; there are also going to be different degrees of susceptibility in different organs, depending on age. This sort of confusion and attempting to sort through the confusion is characteristic of science, but people don't understand it."

For adults, Dr. Barnes offers this advice: "Examine your family history. If there is premature cardiac death, it may be worthwhile to eat soy. If you've got breast cancer in the family, I wouldn't advise it, because we don't know. There is enough evidence out there to raise concerns."

Marian Burros, January 2000

AND SOY MAY NOT EVEN BE BEST FOR BABIES

Sales of infant formula based on soy protein rather than cows' milk have risen in recent years, driven in part by the vegetarian allure. But some parents are worried that the estrogenlike substances found in soy, a popular alternative to pharmaceutical hormone replacements among menopausal women, may not be good for a baby.

In recent years the debate has focused on those substances known as phyto-estrogens. In 1997, a study published in *Lancet* found that phyto-estrogen levels in babies fed soy formula were several thousand times higher than in babies who drank breast or cows' milk. This finding led to concerns among parents that puberty could be delayed in boys and accelerated in girls. A New Zealand group led an effort to ban soy formula; the effort failed, but sales there fell more than one-third.

In August 1999, one of the researchers involved in the *Lancet* study suggested at a Stanford University conference that new studies should take the opposite approach, and look at what he said were the likely health benefits of greater exposure to phyto-estrogens. The researcher, Dr. Kenneth Setchell of the University of Cincinnati College of Medicine, said he had long been interested because in countries where soy was consumed in large quantities, like Japan, "the incidence of hormone-dependent diseases like breast cancer and prostate cancer are very low."

"We know that what you eat early in life has a big effect on later health," Dr. Setchell said. "We know that in animal studies phyto-estrogens have had a protective effect. And we know that in the adult model they clearly have anticancer effects."

So what is a parent to believe?

Dr. Susan Baker, the chairwoman of the nutrition committee of the American Academy of Pediatrics, said the realistic if uninspiring answer was that nobody knew, but it seemed unlikely that after thirty years of widespread use there were either hidden dangers or hidden benefits to be found for soy milk.

In 1998, the academy adopted a policy that essentially ranked soy as a third choice behind breast milk and cows' milk formula. Dr. Baker, a professor of pediatrics at the Medical University of South Carolina in Charleston, said the academy "takes a very strong stand that mothers' milk is the most important nutrient and should be the sole food for the first four to six months of life."

Iron-fortified cows' milk formula is ranked ahead of soy because the protein quality seems higher, and premature or low-weight babies do not create bone mass as quickly on soy milk, she said. Soy is the right choice for children whose mothers cannot breast-feed, who choose not to and who are lactose intolerant—that is, have an allergic reaction to cows' milk. But true lactose intolerance, as opposed to temporary reactions caused by gastrointestinal infections, is far rarer than is commonly thought, Dr. Baker said.

"Throughout the American population, people attribute all sorts of difficulties to lactose intolerance" that are in fact due to something else, she said.

While Dr. Baker says she is befuddled by the appeal of soy formula, which accounts for 25 percent of formula sales in some parts of the country, she does not believe it is a bad thing, either. "We do know that babies fed on soy demonstrate normal growth and development; so far we have not identified any long-term health problems."

Dr. Setchell says he, too, is a strong believer that "breast is best" but adds that doctors must "face the reality that many women are unable or choose not to." Because so many babies drink formula, it would be worthwhile to investigate what extra benefits different types of formulas might have, as well as setting to rest parental concerns about possible hazards, he said.

John O'Neil, August 1999

DIET CHANGES MAY CALM THE HYPER,
AVERTING THE NEED FOR RITALIN

My sister-in-law, Cindy Brody, thought that large amounts of sugary foods turned Sam, her otherwise normally active son, wildly aggressive. But well-designed studies have failed repeatedly to find a relationship between sugar per se and hyperactivity.

Then, through careful observation, Cindy realized that sugar itself was not the culprit; rather, she concluded, it was chocolate that typically made Sam hard to control.

For a quarter of a century now, parents of hyperactive children have been besieged with claims that various common foods, food additives and preservatives were the cause of the syndrome that is now called attention-deficit/hyperactivity disorder, or ADHD. And over and over again, many leading health organizations, bolstered by a collection of mostly small and often poorly done studies, have disputed such claims.

Children with the disorder are hard to manage, disruptive at home and in the classroom, and they often fail in school. The main symptoms are difficulty concentrating, short attention spans, easy distractibility, excessive activity and impulsiveness. The vast majority of children with diagnoses of the disorder are given Ritalin (methylphenidate), a stimulant that has the paradoxical effect of calming them down and helping them to get a better focus on the task at hand. The use of Ritalin in children has skyrocketed in the last decade, increasing two and a half times in the first five years of the 1990s.

While Ritalin is highly effective—it helps 70 percent to 90 percent of children with the disorder, often significantly—there is growing concern about its extensive use and occasional abuse, its common side effects and its possible and still unknown long-term effects on children who take it for many years.

Various estimates hold that 3 to 5 percent of schoolchildren have the disorder, which affects twice as many boys as girls. But in some schools as many as 20 percent of boys in the upper elementary grades are being given Ritalin. Critics say that many boys exhibiting normal (testosterone-induced?) activity and aggressiveness are being improperly labeled hyperactive and treated with a drug that may ultimately do them more harm than good.

Prompted by these concerns and nagging questions about the effects of diet on behavior, the Center for Science in the Public Interest, a nutrition advocacy group, has taken a new hard look at the studies that explored various dietary factors in ADHD and the pronouncements by health authorities that there is little or no evidence to support such a relationship.

A new report reviews twenty-three of the best studies conducted since the mid-1970s and public statements from the Food and Drug Administration, the American Academy of Pediatrics, the International Food Information Council and the American Council on Science and Health, among others. It concludes that the evidence strongly indicates that for some children, behavioral disorders are caused or aggravated by certain food additives, artificial food colors, the foods themselves or a combination.

In seventeen of the twenty-three studies, behavioral improvements were noted when the children's diets were modified. Eleven other studies, ones that were not as well designed, showed even greater improvements on restricted diets.

The center and a group of physicians and scientists who share this conclusion have urged the Department of Health and Human Services to advise parents and health professionals to try changing the diets of children with ADHD before placing them on stimulant drugs (Ritalin or amphetamines) that may suppress their appetites and cause weight loss, insomnia, stomachaches and, in rare cases, tics. The petitioners also expressed concern about a laboratory study that found an increase in liver tumors in mice (but not rats) given doses of Ritalin not much greater than what children receive.

The center has also asked the Health and Human Services Department to commission new and better studies on the relationship between diet and behavior in children, and the Food and Drug Administration to require behavioral tests for certain food additives.

In 1998, a consensus conference convened by the National Institutes of Health noted in its final report that "some of the dietary elimination strategies showed intriguing results suggesting future research" but then failed to include diet in its research recommendations. Meanwhile, the report suggested that the food industry refrain from using suspect additives and that the government "consider banning synthetic dyes in foods and other products widely consumed by children," including cupcakes, candies, sugary breakfast cereals, vitamin pills, drugs and toothpaste.

Although only a small percentage of children with the disorder are expected to benefit significantly from changes in their diets, the new report urges parents to try the changes before resorting to drugs. Children who suffer from asthma, eczema or hives are especially likely to benefit, some research has indicated.

Controlling behavior through diet requires first identifying and then removing from the child's diet those foods or chemicals that seem to cause the unwanted behaviors. The task is not easy, but it has been done successfully for many children with food allergies.

There are several ways to approach the problem. One is to start with a very basic diet of foods that are beyond suspicion and one at a time add back possible culprits for a few days and carefully monitor the results. Another is to eliminate one suspect food or substance at a time from the child's usual diet and see if there is an improvement.

The substances that have most often been linked to worsening ADHD symptoms include artificial colors and flavors; foods that naturally contain salicylates, like apricots, berries and tomatoes; and foods that sometimes cause allergic reactions, like milk, wheat and corn. Some children may also react to chocolate.

Parents, and children when they are old enough, will have to become compulsive label readers to avoid the offending foods. And of course, keeping a child away from problem foods can be a daunting task, especially when the child eats lunch in school, goes out to eat or eats in other people's homes. Some children may be teased about their dietary restrictions; others may rebel at being deprived of foods and treats they love. On the other hand, as one eleven-year-old from Waldorf, Maryland, put it, "I would rather be different because of what I eat than because of how I behave."

Jane E. Brody, November 1999

BLUEBERRIES, THE NEW FOUNTAIN OF YOUTH

An antidote to aging may be as close as a nearby farm or the supermarket shelves: blueberries.

Elderly rats fed the human equivalent of at least half a cup of blueberries a day improved in balance, coordination and short-term memory, according to a study published in September 1999 in the *Journal of Neuroscience*. A cup of blueberries is a normal serving. Like other fruits and vegetables, blueberries contain chemicals that act as antioxidants. Scientists think antioxidants protect the body against "oxidative stress," one of several biological processes that cause aging.

Barbara Shukitt-Hale, a co-author of the study at the Agriculture Department's Human Nutrition Research Center on Aging at Tufts University in Boston, says people "are told that once you're old, there's nothing you can do." But, she said, "That might not be true."

Blueberries, strawberries and spinach all test high in their ability to subdue molecules called oxygen free radicals, which are created when cells convert oxygen into energy. In normal amounts, free radicals help rid the body of toxins, but they can also harm cell membranes and DNA, which results in cell death. The Tufts study said strawberry and spinach extracts produced some improvement in memory, but only blueberry extract had a significant impact on balance and coordination. (Other fruits and vegetables high in antioxidants include alfalfa sprouts, beets, broccoli, brussels sprouts, garlic, grapes and kale.)

Other studies have suggested that antioxidants in fruits and vegetables could prevent cancer and heart disease. Previous research by the Tufts scientists indicated that antioxidants slowed the aging process in rats that started taking the dietary supplement at six months of age. Their latest study was the first to show that antioxidants could actually reverse age-related declines, they said. But the researchers do not know why blueberries were more effective than strawberries and spinach or exactly how the chemicals work in the laboratory animals.

"Fruits and vegetables in general are very good for you; that's without question," said Marcelle Morrison-Bogorad, who directs the neuroscience and neuropsychology program at the National Institute of Aging. "It's another thing to know why."

Clinical trials are needed to see whether humans could benefit, she said. The institute, which helped finance the Tufts research, is already sponsoring studies to test the effects of vitamin E, another antioxidant, as well as aspirin and B vitamins, on the mental processes of older women.

The rats used in the Tufts study were nineteen months old, the equivalent of sixty-five to seventy years in humans. They begin losing motor skills at twelve months. By nineteen months, the time it takes a rat to walk a narrow rod before losing its balance drops from thirteen seconds to five seconds. After eating daily doses of blueberry extract for eight weeks, the rats could stay on the rod for an average of eleven seconds. They also performed better in negotiating mazes, which signals improved short-term memory. The rats fed strawberry and spinach extracts did well on those tests, too, but they were no better at staying on the rod than rats who got no fruit extract. The scientists think that antioxidants improve cell membranes so important nutrients and chemicals can flow through more easily.

James Joseph, one of the Tufts scientists, starts his day by mixing a handful of berries in a protein drink. "Motor behavior is one of the first things to go as you age," he said.

Associated Press, September 1999

EATING TO REACH YOUR LIFE SPAN. OR, TO EXTEND IT

Is there anything you can eat that might make you live a lot longer? The answer is yes, but it's not entirely pleasant.

Researchers at Tufts University reported in September 1999 that elderly rats fed servings of blueberries performed much better in everyday lab rat tasks like walking along a narrow rod. One of the scientists was so impressed with his rodents' regained skills that he has started eating berries every day.

Nutritionists, an often fractious crowd, agree that fruit and vegetables are good for you. But there's a difference between eating for good health—which may improve the chances of attaining one's maximum life span—and eating to extend that natural maximum.

To improve the odds that no disease gets you before old age does, the greengrocer is your friend. Even blueberries may help, if you don't mind flashing blue smiles and scrubbing crimson stains from your shirt. But it's unlikely that any one food is the true ambrosia. The real hope lies in genetics, where scientists are beginning to make real progress. But until they hit the fountain of youth, there's only one diet that has been proved to extend life. If it works as well in people as it does in rodents, it will lengthen your life by twenty-five years. Guaranteed.

So why isn't it touted in all those $30 health books that promise longevity if one bets on the author's prescribed diet? Doubtless because it can be described in eight words, not a book: reduce your intake of calories by 40 percent.

Rats and mice fed on this diet—which means 40 percent less than they will eat when allowed as much food as they want—live a third longer. Note that this isn't a malnutrition diet: the animals are given all the vitamins and minerals they need. It's just that their calories are cut way down.

The upside: you can eat whatever you like. It doesn't seem to matter whether the calories are in the form of fat or protein or carbohydrate.

Would a calorically restricted diet work in people as well as it does in laboratory rodents, which live only a couple of years? Because people are generally more like monkeys than mice, two monkey-feeding trials are under way. But since rhesus monkeys can live forty years and the trials started only in the late 1980s, no simian Methuselahs have had time to emerge.

A possible shortcut to finding if caloric restriction helps people was reported in August 1999 by Richard Weindruch, a leader in animal aging studies, and his colleague, Tomas A. Prolla, both of the University of Wisconsin. They used a new biological tool called an Affymetrix chip to measure aging at the cellular level. The chip can tell what cells are doing by monitoring which genes are switched on or off.

The chip supported a longstanding theory of aging: that cells get damaged by oxygen-derived chemicals known as free radicals, which are created as a by-product of energy production. Cells from old mice had switched on the genes that deal with free radical damage, the chip found, whereas in calorically restricted mice of the same age the damage control genes were quiescent.

Fewer calories, less energy production, less damage to the cell's mitochondria, as its miniature batteries are called. If the chip provides a true measure of cellular aging, then it may be possible to tell whether the monkeys are aging more slowly on their calorically restricted diet as soon as an appropriate chip can be developed.

Dr. Weindruch says that until he conducted the chip experiment he had not tried to restrict the calories in his own diet. Like a true scientist, he wasn't going to assume the truth of the hypothesis he was testing. But he changed his mind after seeing the effects of dietary intervention. "Although I have studied caloric restriction for twenty-five years, the power of the intervention was such that it changed my behavior and I'm eating less food," he says.

The study of why organisms age has long been a hopeless backwater of science. The secrets were locked deep in the cell beyond researchers' reach. In the past few years, much has changed. Biologists have begun contemplating ways to reverse aging. In 1998 researchers supported by the Geron Corporation made two spectacular advances—they learned how to "immortalize" ordinary cells of the human body, and how to isolate a naturally immortal class of cells known as human embryonic stem cells.

Immortal, in biologists' parlance, refers to the ability of cells grown in glassware to grow and divide indefinitely without becoming cancerous—an ability in marked contrast to that of normal body cells, which can divide only fifty or so times before hitting senescence.

Immortality of the cell is not the same as immortality of the entire organism, but the two are not necessarily unrelated. The very existence of a perpetually enduring cell is proof that biological systems don't have to rust and decay as man-made machines do. They can renew themselves indefinitely, suggesting that there is no biological limit on longevity. The bristlecone pine, for example, lives five thousand years.

That evolution does not design mice or people to live so long is not because it could not, many biologists believe, but because there would be no advantage in terms of natural selection. In a world full of predators, it's better to design organisms that breed prolifically and die young than ones that can live forever but are bound to get zapped by saber-toothed tigers at an early age.

But if that's the case, perhaps just a few patches in evolution's genetic programming might confer immortality. Biologists have already learned how to make the roundworm, a standard laboratory organism, live four to six times its normal life span by changing certain of its genes.

Genetically contrived life extension for people may come one day, but it's not around the corner. For those who wish to do something now, caloric restriction seems to be the best—in fact, the only—bet, even though not yet proved in primates. And Dr. Weindruch, working with mice, has already worked out the answers to many obvious questions: Don't begin young—undernutrition stunts growth. You can start later in life and still get a substantial benefit.

It's also not necessary to cut calories the full 40 percent: mice live longer even with a 10 percent calorie reduction, though the effect is not as pronounced. In a recent article in *Scientific American*, Dr. Weindruch figured that people would do best "by consuming an amount that enabled them to weigh 10 to 25 percent less than their personal set point," which (though often hard for a person to define) is the weight the body naturally tries to keep itself at.

So eat what you like—blueberries, chocolate liqueurs, ice cream. But *mal appétit!*

Nicholas Wade, September 1999

UPS AND DOWNS FOR DIET GUINEA PIGS

Like many people discussing the rigors of being on a diet, Jeffrey A. Behrendt, a lawyer in Ottawa, sounds both plaintive and hopeful.

"I still eat chocolate!" Mr. Behrendt wrote in a note, starting with the good news. "Just a lot less than before."

Then came the downside. There is the problem of buying a suit when one's jacket size is 36 tall and one's waist is 28. ("This is not easy to find in stores!") There is the problem of sitting down. ("If the chair is not well padded, I find it uncomfortable.") And then there is the problem of how people react to Mr. Behrendt's new look. ("Very negative! People started thinking I was very ill and I got comments that I looked like a concentration camp survivor.")

This is not your ordinary diet.

Mr. Behrendt is among a small group of people who have put themselves on what they call a calorie-restricted diet. They consume 20 percent to 40 percent fewer calories than what would be considered normal, with a single goal: prolonging their lives to age 100, 120, even 140.

The technique has appeared promising in tests on mice, and current experiments on monkeys also suggest that their aging has been slowed. In September 2000, Dr. Leonard Guarente of the Massachusetts Institute of Technology published a paper in *Science* that explains just how calorie restriction prolongs life span in yeast. But no one knows whether calorie reduction works in humans.

Undeterred, Mr. Behrendt follows the regimen, along with hundreds of others he communicates with through a computer newsgroup. They, and possibly many others, are a bold band of experimenters, one part guinea pig, one part scientist. Still, some freely own up to being a tad grumpy. Maybe it is the cold hands and feet that many of them experience. Maybe it is the decline in sexual interest many report. Maybe it is the social isolation some say such a radical diet imposes on them. Or maybe it is just that much of the time, they are just a little bit hungry.

Many followers of the CR (for calorie-restricted) diet, as the practice is known, were inspired by the writings of Dr. Roy Walford, a pathologist at the University of California at Los Angeles. For many of them, there are no forbidden foods: the only thing that matters is controlling the total calories taken in and ensuring that nutritional needs are met. As a practical matter, most eat vast quantities of vegetables.

Michael A. Sherman, a software company owner in Mountain View, California, said a friend gave him one of Dr. Walford's books about three years ago, when he turned forty.

"It sort of hit me pretty suddenly; everything's fine, but you're just moving in the wrong direction," he recalled. "It just suddenly struck me that I was going to die."

Mr. Sherman went from consuming about 3,200 calories a day to taking in 1,725. At 5 feet 5, he weighs 122 pounds, down from about 145. And he says he has seen tangible improvements in health indicators like his cholesterol levels and heart rate. He says that he is rarely hungry, that his mental energy is good and that he is able to work out and run several times a week.

But Mr. Sherman, who is married and has two children, says he has seen a decline in sexual interest, which he is combating by trying different preparations of testosterone. He has no qualms about whether he is following a "natural" approach.

"I know what nature's plan is for me," Mr. Sherman said. "It wants me to decay and die pretty soon. So I don't really put a lot of stock in sort of trying to be natural. So far, there's been about fifty billion humans—and they all died, except for the last six billion. So that's what you get if you do things the natural way."

Mr. Sherman has other plans. He wants to see the twenty-second century, and to do so, he needs to live to age 143. Still, he said that, unlike some CR followers, he is not fixated on his diet. He goes out to restaurants often, ordering carefully.

T. Francesca Skelton, a sixty-year-old Washington woman who has been on the diet for about four months, said that it seemed to attract some fanatics. "They really wouldn't eat a bread crumb if it wasn't on the diet," she said.

And that, said Dr. Gail C. Frank, a nutrition professor at California State University at Long Beach, is the big drawback. While she admires the intent behind the diet, Dr. Frank said the approach was too extreme.

"What good is the aging if there can't be the pleasure to go with it?" she asked.

For Mr. Behrendt, thirty, it has not been easy. He has lost 20 pounds and now weighs 120. He is 6 feet tall. In a telephone interview, he said that he felt better on the whole. But on just 1,800 calories day, he can no longer do the long-distance running he once enjoyed because it burns too many calories. He feels more prone to irritability and depression.

And he has had trouble getting others to accept his choice, especially his family.

"A lot of families, mine included, show their love by cooking a big meal for you," Mr. Behrendt said. "They're really insulted. You go there and you hardly eat anything."

Eric Nagourney, September 2000

HEALTH FOOD HOMILIES

My husband and I recently moved to a new apartment with an excellent health food market nearby. The convenience has improved our eating habits (more soy milk, less Coca-Cola), as well as the way we keep house (recycled-plastic garbage bags and 80 percent post-consumer-waste paper towels).

But now when I open a cupboard or the refrigerator, on every package I find snippets of philosophy, aphorisms and quotations attributed to people who lived long before the advent of Tofutti.

For instance, a box of echinacea tea bags offers this thought from Elizabeth Cady Stanton: "Nature never repeats herself, and the possibilities of one human soul will never be found in another."

Our trash bags come in boxes carrying the following message: "In our every deliberation, we must consider the impact of our decisions on the next seven generations—From the Great Law of the Iroquois Confederacy."

One side of a chocolate soy milk carton has this slightly mangled quotation from Harry Truman: "I've found that the best way to give advice to my children is to find out what they want to do and then advise them to do it."

Another panel on the same carton features a seven-paragraph screed imploring soy milk drinkers to help save not the harp seal or the rain forest, but, of all things, the caboose: "The caboose has been replaced by little metal shoe boxes stuck to the butt-end of every train." Running vertically up the same panel in tiny type is this claim: "Remember the

Monkees? Stephen Stills, Paul Williams, Harry Nilsson and Charles Manson all auditioned and were turned down."

Finally, under the nutrition facts box is the image of an AIDS ribbon with this appeal: "Please Be Safe." Safe soy. Safe sex. It's a logical continuum, I guess. Nice of them to care.

And that's what all this is: an effort, either sincere or calculated, to show that these companies care about me. It's a harsh world out there, they seem to say, full of pesticides and virgin plastic and bovine growth hormone. But we, your groceries, will take care of you! Buy us and we will comfort you with quotations from early feminists when you're getting a cold. (Really? No soul like mine? They must be missing me at the office today!) And ex-presidents will help you raise your children.

When I think about it I do feel better buying recycled products and more healthful foods. But as for their recycled wisdom, the sagest words in my kitchen are to be found on a container of plain old (nonorganic) cottage cheese: "Discard after date on bottom."

Allison Adato, October 1999

MEDICARE WILL TEST AN EXTREME DIET IN CRITICALLY ILL HEART PATIENTS

Eva Hebenstreit remembers a trip to Israel in January 1986, when her seventy-one-year-old husband, Werner, could not get across the street before the light changed.

"He was a cripple," said Mrs. Hebenstreit. "A permanent coronary cripple."

At his doctor's recommendation, Mr. Hebenstreit, who had had two heart attacks, joined a program run by Dr. Dean Ornish, who for more than twenty years has studied whether changes in diet and daily activities can reverse coronary heart disease. It was a radical program combining an extremely low-fat, vegetarian diet with exercise, meditation and smoking cessation.

Within four months, Mr. Hebenstreit said, he felt a difference.

Fourteen years later, he has a very different life. Now eighty-five, he starts the morning with twenty-five push-ups, does yoga stretches and walks a half hour a day. He takes no heart medication, unless you count a baby aspirin every other day.

"At seventy-one, I was convinced I would die very soon," said Mr. Hebenstreit, who lives in San Francisco. "I feel healthier now than when I was forty years younger."

Now, in a first-ever experiment on critically ill elderly people, Medicare will examine whether what worked for Mr. Hebenstreit will work on a large scale and bring down medical costs. Enrollment of volunteers started in April 2000. The nutrition and exercise experiment is designed to determine whether drastic changes in lifestyle and eating habits can prevent the need for angioplasty and heart bypass surgery.

"The challenge for us is how to modernize Medicare from a medical, acute-care model to a comprehensive health-care model emphasizing successful and healthy aging through health promotion and risk-factor reduction," said Jeffrey Kang, chief clinical officer with the Health Care Financing Administration, which oversees Medicare.

Officials with the Health Care Financing Administration defended the choice of Dr. Ornish's program, saying that studies had been sufficient to warrant a pilot project. The program has been criticized by some health experts as too restrictive, and, they say, the studies that point to the program's success have been too small to draw such conclusions.

Dr. Michael Hash, deputy administrator of the Health Care Financing Administration, said the Ornish program was selected after Dr. Ornish made a proposal to the agency, which wanted to see if the results could be replicated. The agency is advertising for another similar program to test.

Over the next three years, about 1,800 elderly heart patients, at a cost of $7,200 each, will each spend a year on the program, which will be run out of at least fifteen centers whose staffs are trained by Dr. Ornish. While the demonstration project, financed by Medicare, tests a form of treatment, it exemplifies a broad shift toward preventive medicine being examined by Medicare. In 1997, Medicare took major steps in this direction when coverage was expanded to include colorectal cancer screening, bone mass measurement for osteoporosis and expanded benefits for screenings like mammograms and pelvic exams.

In December 1999, a panel of experts from the Institute of Medicine, part of the National Academy of Sciences, recommended that Medicare pay for outpatient nutrition counseling. According to the report, 86 percent of the estimated 34 million Americans over sixty-five have at least one chronic condition like high blood pressure or diabetes that might be helped by nutrition counseling.

Many see the moves as long overdue. While Medicare has traditionally covered nutrition therapy for hospitalized patients, some health experts said that with the current emphasis on cost cutting, such services were often lost and in any case had rarely been offered to outpatients.

"Hospital stays are shorter and shorter, so work that used to be done in the hospital isn't being done very much," said Dr. Virginia A. Stallings, chairwoman of the institute's panel of experts and the chief of the nutrition section at Children's Hospital of Philadelphia. At the same time, she said, growing evidence indicates that nutrition therapy can be a cost-effective way to deal with outpatients with chronic disease. "The science supports nutrition in the management of a number of important diseases," Dr. Stallings said. "There really is a place for this."

Some critics, however, while praising the concept, questioned whether large numbers of people would be able to stick to the highly regimented Ornish program. For instance, Dr. Ornish recommends that fat intake be no more than 10 percent daily, while the United States Department of Agriculture's guidelines allow 30 percent.

Officials from the American Heart Association said many of the studies showing results with the Ornish program had been small and that more information was needed on which parts of the program had the most effect. They also said that such a restrictive program might have negative effects on the day-to-day quality of life of patients and their families.

"We don't feel the situation is at all clear as to whether this approach is going to be applicable to the general population," said Dr. Ronald M. Krauss, past chairman of the nutrition committee of the heart association. "They should have looked into potentially less expensive ways of doing that."

But Dr. Hash said: "We wouldn't be proceeding to demonstrate this with the Medicare population if we didn't have confidence that it had produced evidence of effectiveness in reducing heart disease. We have determined it is promising as a possible alternative to bypass surgery." Coronary heart disease, he added, is the leading cause of death among people receiving Medicare.

Medicare's test of the Ornish program is not a clinical trial, but will instead follow the progress of volunteers who enroll at the centers. Rather than testing the effectiveness of the program as a health measure per se, the Medicare experiment is intended to show whether people who stick with it end up costing the program less. It is the first time Medicare has run a payment demonstration on a lifestyle-modification program.

Johanna Dwyer, director of the nutrition clinic at New England Medical Center Hospital, said that many elderly patients did not get nutrition counseling and that such steps could help. She recalled the case of an elderly woman with emphysema who was taking a large amount of medicine that affected her appetite. Nutrition counselors were able to find foods she could eat and get her back on track. "Nutrition isn't a cure-all, but it's part of the solution," Ms. Dwyer said.

Dr. Ornish said he began looking for a new approach to heart surgery twenty-three years ago when he was a medical student learning to do bypass surgery. Patients would come in for surgery, go home to the same food and stresses and soon be back for another bypass.

The Ornish diet is vegetarian, relying on combinations of complex carbohydrates to replace proteins found in meat, fish and poultry. The only animal products allowed on the diet are egg whites and nonfat dairy products. No oils can be added to food, but moderate amounts of sugar, alcohol and salt (unless otherwise restricted for health reasons) can be used. No caffeine is allowed. The bulk of the diet is made up of a large variety of whole grains, vegetables, fruits and legumes.

Mr. Hebenstreit, while no longer part of an official Ornish program, still maintains the strict regimen. The Hebenstreits start each day with whole-grain cereal, sweetened only with fruit juice. They each eat a whole orange as opposed to drinking orange juice, which is more concentrated and has a higher sugar content. Mr. Hebenstreit also has a piece of toast, spread with ripe banana and orange marmalade. Rather than coffee, the Hebenstreits have a substitute made from grain.

Lunch is typically a sandwich on whole grain bread with soy cheese, bean paste, tomato, onion and some type of green like spinach or baby lettuce, followed by fruit. Or they make soup with a variety of beans and grains. For dinner, they have pasta or polenta with steamed vegetables and grapefruit or fat-free fig bars.

Don Vaupel, sixty-one, a retired professor from Oakland, California, and an Ornish patient of eleven years, said he decided to try the program as an alternative to bypass surgery. Looking back to his early days on the diet, he said, "all I can remember is that lots of things were dark green and brown and not very tasty." In the early days, he said lunch might have been a sweet potato and salad with nothing on it. Dinner consisted of steamed vegetables and steamed rice. Now, with all the new low-fat foods, things have gotten more interesting.

As he arrived home from the store recently, Mr. Vaupel was carrying the ingredients for a frittata he would make with an egg substitute for dinner: portobello mushrooms, fat-free Parmesan and ricotta and spinach.

He generally starts his day with green tea and a soy-powder protein shake, which he pours over a whole-grain cereal like Grape-Nuts. For lunch he might have a grilled low-fat cheese sandwich on whole-wheat bread.

"I just walked three miles," he said. "I don't mean walk like, oh look at the pretty flower. I walk, break a sweat, and then slow down."

He meditates for an hour each morning and night although he prefers to call it "my appointment with me." He lost 110 pounds in the first nine months of the program, 85 of which have stayed off permanently, and there has been reversal in the blockages of his heart, his doctors tell him. For all his accomplishments, though, he said he still needed nutritional counseling. Three years ago he received a diagnosis of adult diabetes, which he also works to control through diet.

"I didn't go on a diet," Mr. Vaupel said. "This was a lifestyle change. I had to change everything."

Barbara Whitaker, April 2000

TEA: THE LATEST HEALTH FOOD (BUT HOLD THE CLOTTED CREAM)

Coffee lovers, take heed. For the sake of your health, you might consider switching at least some of those daily cups of java for tea. Not herbal tea but "real" tea—green tea, black tea, Chinese tea, fruit-flavored tea, with or without caffeine, lemon, milk or sugar.

As long as the leaves come from the plant *Camellia sinensis,* tea will contain potent antioxidant chemicals that have been linked to protection against major diseases like cancer and heart disease. Even the caffeine in tea may be somewhat beneficial, emerging evidence suggests. The popularity of tea in Japan and China may partly explain why heart disease rates are so much lower in the Far East than in Western countries.

There are three types of real tea: green, black and oolong. Green tea, which is most popular in Japan and China, has in recent years found a small but growing following here as word about its potential health benefits has leaked out. It is the least processed of all the teas, made by quickly steaming or heating the leaves of *Camellia sinensis.*

Black tea, by far the most popular in Western countries and India, is prepared by exposing tea leaves to air. That exposure causes oxidation, which turns them a deep brown and intensifies their flavor. The leaves are then crushed. According to Dr. Gary Beecher, food chemist with the United States Department of Agriculture, black tea contains as much of the protective chemicals as green tea, though the form may differ.

Oolong is between the two: more processed than green tea but less so than black tea. It is exposed to heat, light and crushing for less time than black tea.

Herbal teas, on the other hand, come from a wide variety of plants other than the tea plant and may include roots and flowers as well as leaves. Most herbal teas do not possess the antioxidant properties of real tea, although they may contain certain other biologically active compounds. A few also contain caffeine.

Contrary to common belief, green tea has as much caffeine as black tea, though all teas have less caffeine than drip-brewed coffee. A typical eight-ounce cup of tea prepared from one tea bag brewed for three to five minutes contains 40 milligrams of caffeine, compared with 100 milligrams in a cup of brewed coffee.

The caffeine content of tea can range from 20 to 90 milligrams a cup, depending on the blend of tea leaves, method of preparation and length of brewing time, whereas a cup of coffee may contain from 60 to 180 milligrams of caffeine. Decaffeinated tea, like decaffeinated coffee, has about 4 milligrams of caffeine per cup. Instant teas and prepared ice teas, which can be purchased with or without caffeine, may be too highly processed to contain much of the protective chemicals.

Throughout the 1990s researchers exploring the health effects of tea have gradually accumulated highly suggestive, though not definitive, evidence for tea's ability to prevent or ameliorate several common serious diseases. Most of the presumed health effects are related to polyphenols, chemicals that act as antioxidants, preventing cell damage caused by highly reactive molecules called free radicals. The polyphenols in tea, especially green tea, are more potent antioxidants than well-known antioxidants like vitamins C and E, experts say.

The bulk of evidence for tea's health benefits comes from studies in animals that were treated with amounts of tea polyphenols equivalent to what might be consumed by a regular tea drinker. For example, in a study published in April, a research team from Case Western Reserve University School of Medicine added green tea polyphenols to the drinking water of eighteen mice and none to the water of eighteen other mice. All the animals were then injected with a substance that causes a condition like rheumatoid arthritis in people. Of the group that got the polyphenols, only eight developed arthritis; in the group that got plain water, all but one developed arthritis.

With regard to cancer, several dozen animal studies indicate that the polyphenols and related compounds in tea are protective, especially against cancers of the oral cavity and digestive tract. Tea chemicals are believed to act by preventing damage to DNA that could result in a loss of control over cell growth.

According to cancer researchers at Rutgers University College of Pharmacy, "Tea is one of the few agents that can inhibit carcinogenesis at the initiation, promotion and progression stages." However, they added, it is not yet known how effective tea can be in preventing human cancer, what dose is most effective or what is the best way to administer the active compounds.

Studies in people have yielded inconsistent results, in part because in some studies other factors may have entered into the picture to distort the findings, like the heat of the tea and the use of tobacco or alcohol. In one well-designed study conducted in Beijing, China, among fifty-nine patients with precancerous mouth lesions, those treated for six months with capsules of oxidized green tea polyphenols experienced a decrease in the size of the lesions; in the untreated group, the lesions got larger.

A study of more than 35,000 postmenopausal women in Iowa suggested that women who drank two or more cups of tea daily were less likely to develop cancers of the digestive tract and urinary tract. However, no protection was found against other cancers.

Likewise, a study in the Netherlands among 58,000 men and 62,000 women found no link between tea drinking and a reduced risk of cancers of the lung, breast or colon. However, in a study in laboratory mice and rats, Dr. Fung-Lung Chung of the American Health Foundation found that both green and black tea and caffeine given in drinking water protected the animals against lung cancer caused by a major carcinogen in tobacco.

Another study in mice showed that both green and black tea inhibited the growth of both malignant and nonmalignant skin tumors. And a study in rats conducted by Dr. Roderick H. Dashwood of Oregon State University showed that both green and black tea inhibited the formation of precancerous lesions in the colon.

With regard to heart disease and stroke, a study of 1,330 Chinese men found a significantly lower level of serum cholesterol and triglycerides among those who drank more than ten cups of green tea a day.

Some studies in Western countries have indicated that tea drinkers may be less likely to develop heart disease and stroke. A Harvard study by Dr. Howard Sesso indicated that people who drank one or more cups of black tea a day were half as likely to suffer a heart attack as those who did not drink tea, regardless of other risk factors for heart disease.

However, much more research is needed to sort out the effects of tea on blood vessel diseases as well as cancer. For example, in a study of 880 Japanese men, researchers found that heavy tea drinkers were also likely to eat more fruits and vegetables, which may account for or contribute to their lower risk of heart disease and cancer.

Still, the evidence to date is sufficiently suggestive to prompt the National Cancer Institute to conduct studies of the capacity of the biologically active chemicals in green and black tea to curb the development of cancer in people at high risk for developing cancers of the colon, lung, esophagus and skin.

And Japanese researchers have suggested that the ability of green tea and its chemicals to inhibit a substance called tumor necrosis factor-alpha may make it useful in treating a wide range of health problems that include Crohn's disease, multiple sclerosis, malaria and sepsis as well as rheumatoid arthritis.

Jane E. Brody, September 1999

INDEX

About the Authors

Jane E. Brody is the Personal Health columnist for the *New York Times*, and the author of several best-selling books, including *Jane Brody's Good Food Book* and *Jane Brody's Nutrition Book*. She lives in New York City.

Denise Grady is a health and science reporter for the *New York Times*. She lives in New York.